Psychotherapeutic Drug Identification Guide

This guide contains color reproductions of some commonly prescribed major psychotherapeutic drugs. This guide mainly illustrates tablets and capsules. A † symbol preceding the name of the drug indicates that other doses are available. Check directly with the manufacturer. *(Although the photos are intended as accurate reproductions of the drug, this guide should be used only as a quick identification aid.)*

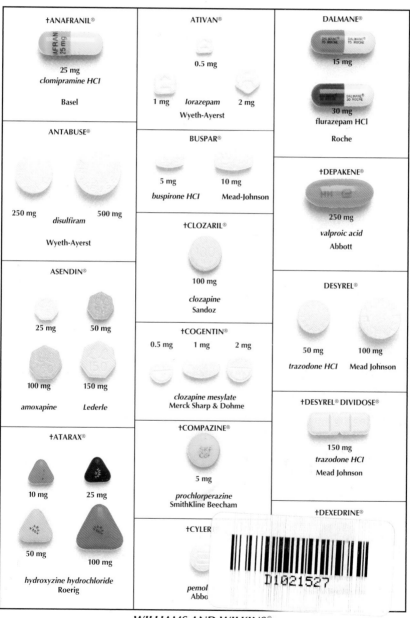

†ANAFRANIL®

25 mg

clomipramine HCl

Basel

ANTABUSE®

250 mg   500 mg

disulfiram

Wyeth-Ayerst

ASENDIN®

25 mg   50 mg

100 mg   150 mg

amoxapine   Lederle

†ATARAX®

10 mg   25 mg

50 mg   100 mg

hydroxyzine hydrochloride
Roerig

ATIVAN®

0.5 mg

1 mg   *lorazepam*   2 mg

Wyeth-Ayerst

BUSPAR®

5 mg   10 mg

buspirone HCl   Mead-Johnson

†CLOZARIL®

100 mg

clozapine
Sandoz

†COGENTIN®

0.5 mg   1 mg   2 mg

clozapine mesylate
Merck Sharp & Dohme

†COMPAZINE®

5 mg

prochlorperazine
SmithKline Beecham

†CYLER

pemol
Abbo

DALMANE®

15 mg

30 mg
flurazepam HCl

Roche

†DEPAKENE®

250 mg

valproic acid
Abbott

DESYREL®

50 mg   100 mg

trazodone HCl   Mead Johnson

†DESYREL® DIVIDOSE®

150 mg

trazodone HCl
Mead Johnson

†DEXEDRINE®

WILLIAMS AND WILKINS©

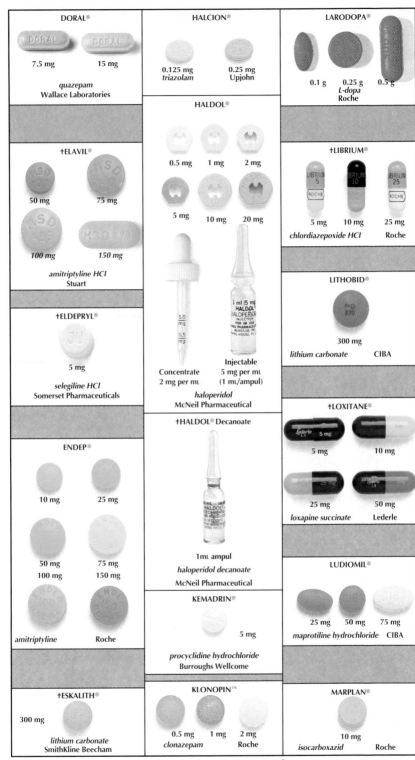

DORAL®

7.5 mg   15 mg

quazepam
Wallace Laboratories

HALCION®

0.125 mg   0.25 mg
triazolam   Upjohn

LARODOPA®

0.1 g   0.25 g   0.5 g
L-dopa
Roche

†ELAVIL®

50 mg   75 mg
100 mg   *150 mg*

amitriptyline HCl
Stuart

HALDOL®

0.5 mg   1 mg   2 mg

5 mg   10 mg   20 mg

1.0 mg
0.5 mg

Concentrate
2 mg per mL

1 mL (5 mg)
HALDOL
HALOPERIDOL
INJECTION
FOR IM USE

Injectable
5 mg per mL
(1 mL/ampul)

haloperidol
McNeil Pharmaceutical

†LIBRIUM®

LIBRIUM 5   BRIUM 10   LIBRIUM 25
ROCHE   ROCHE

5 mg   10 mg   25 mg
chlordiazepoxide HCl   Roche

LITHOBID®

PD
270

300 mg
lithium carbonate   CIBA

†ELDEPRYL®

5 mg

selegiline HCl
Somerset Pharmaceuticals

†HALDOL® Decanoate

1 mL
HALDOL
DECANOATE

1 mL ampul
haloperidol decanoate
McNeil Pharmaceutical

†LOXITANE®

Lederle
LT 5 mg   10 mg

25 mg   50 mg
loxapine succinate   Lederle

ENDEP®

10 mg   25 mg

50 mg   75 mg
100 mg   150 mg

amitriptyline   Roche

KEMADRIN®

5 mg

procyclidine hydrochloride
Burroughs Wellcome

LUDIOMIL®

25 mg   50 mg   75 mg
maprotiline hydrochloride   CIBA

†ESKALITH®

300 mg

lithium carbonate
SmithKline Beecham

KLONOPIN™

0.5 mg   1 mg   2 mg
clonazepam   Roche

MARPLAN®

10 mg
isocarboxazid   Roche

WILLIAMS AND WILKINS©

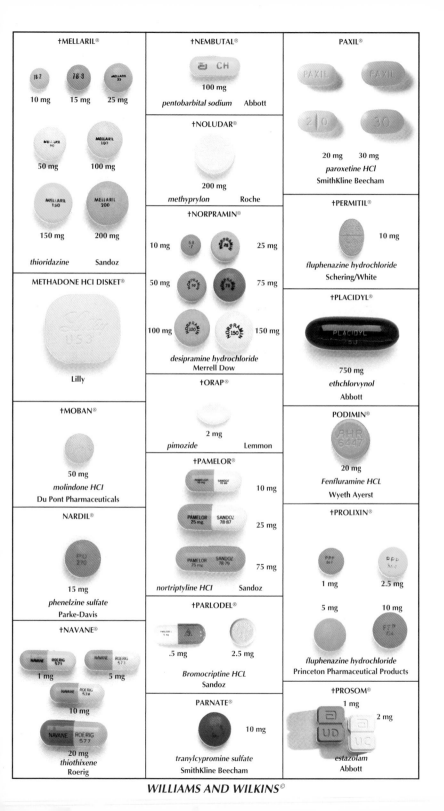

†MELLARIL®

10 mg   15 mg   25 mg

50 mg   100 mg

150 mg   200 mg

thioridazine   Sandoz

METHADONE HCl DISKET®

Lilly

†MOBAN®

50 mg

molindone HCl
Du Pont Pharmaceuticals

NARDIL®

15 mg

phenelzine sulfate
Parke-Davis

†NAVANE®

1 mg   5 mg

10 mg

20 mg
thiothixene
Roerig

†NEMBUTAL®

100 mg

pentobarbital sodium   Abbott

†NOLUDAR®

200 mg

methyprylon   Roche

†NORPRAMIN®

10 mg   25 mg

50 mg   75 mg

100 mg   150 mg

desipramine hydrochloride
Merrell Dow

†ORAP®

2 mg

pimozide   Lemmon

†PAMELOR®

10 mg

25 mg

75 mg

nortriptyline HCl   Sandoz

†PARLODEL®

.5 mg   2.5 mg

Bromocriptine HCL
Sandoz

PARNATE®

10 mg

tranylcypromine sulfate
SmithKline Beecham

PAXIL®

20 mg   30 mg

paroxetine HCl
SmithKline Beecham

†PERMITIL®

10 mg

fluphenazine hydrochloride
Schering/White

†PLACIDYL®

750 mg

ethchlorvynol
Abbott

PODIMIN®

20 mg

Fenfluramine HCL
Wyeth Ayerst

†PROLIXIN®

1 mg   2.5 mg

5 mg   10 mg

fluphenazine hydrochloride
Princeton Pharmaceutical Products

†PROSOM®

1 mg

2 mg

estazolam
Abbott

WILLIAMS AND WILKINS©

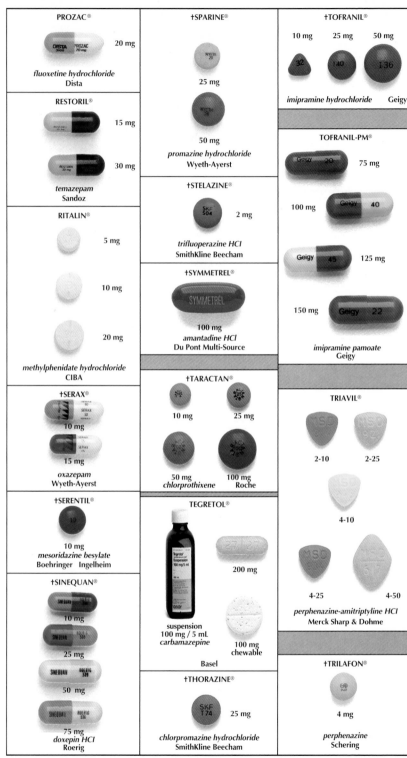

PROZAC®

20 mg

fluoxetine hydrochloride
Dista

RESTORIL®

15 mg

30 mg

temazepam
Sandoz

RITALIN®

5 mg

10 mg

20 mg

methylphenidate hydrochloride
CIBA

†SERAX®

10 mg

15 mg

oxazepam
Wyeth-Ayerst

†SERENTIL®

10 mg
mesoridazine besylate
Boehringer Ingelheim

†SINEQUAN®

10 mg

25 mg

50 mg

75 mg
doxepin HCl
Roerig

†SPARINE®

25 mg

50 mg

promazine hydrochloride
Wyeth-Ayerst

†STELAZINE®

2 mg

trifluoperazine HCl
SmithKline Beecham

†SYMMETREL®

100 mg
amantadine HCl
Du Pont Multi-Source

†TARACTAN®

10 mg   25 mg

50 mg   100 mg
chlorprothixene   Roche

TEGRETOL®

200 mg

suspension
100 mg / 5 mL
carbamazepine   100 mg
chewable

Basel

†THORAZINE®

25 mg

chlorpromazine hydrochloride
SmithKline Beecham

†TOFRANIL®

10 mg   25 mg   50 mg

imipramine hydrochloride   Geigy

TOFRANIL-PM®

75 mg

100 mg

125 mg

150 mg

imipramine pamoate
Geigy

TRIAVIL®

2-10   2-25

4-10

4-25   4-50

perphenazine-amitriptyline HCl
Merck Sharp & Dohme

†TRILAFON®

4 mg

perphenazine
Schering

WILLIAMS AND WILKINS©

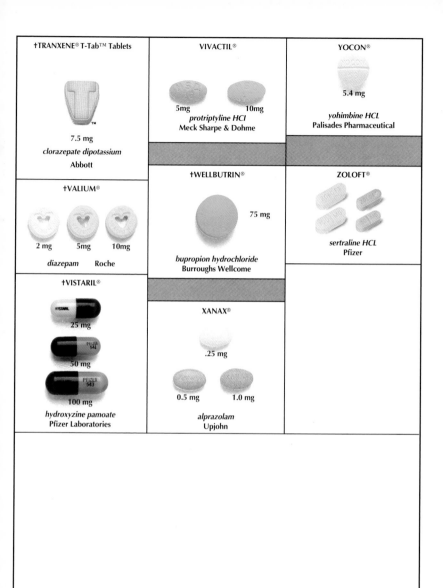

†TRANXENE® T-Tab™ Tablets

7.5 mg

clorazepate dipotassium
Abbott

†VALIUM®

2 mg   5mg   10mg

diazepam   Roche

†VISTARIL®

25 mg

50 mg

100 mg

hydroxyzine pamoate
Pfizer Laboratories

VIVACTIL®

5mg   10mg

protriptyline HCl
Meck Sharpe & Dohme

†WELLBUTRIN®

75 mg

bupropion hydrochloride
Burroughs Wellcome

XANAX®

.25 mg

0.5 mg   1.0 mg

alprazolam
Upjohn

YOCON®

5.4 mg

yohimbine HCL
Palisades Pharmaceutical

ZOLOFT®

sertraline HCL
Pfizer

POCKET
HANDBOOK
OF
EMERGENCY
PSYCHIATRIC
MEDICINE

SENIOR CONTRIBUTING EDITOR

Robert Cancro, M.D., MED.D.Sc.

Professor and Chairman, Department of Psychiatry,
New York University School of Medicine;
Director, Department of Psychiatry, Tisch Hospital
of the New York University
Medical Center, New York, New York;
Director, Nathan S. Kline Institute for
Psychiatric Research, Orangeburg, New York

CONTRIBUTING EDITOR

James C.-Y. Chou, M.D.

Assistant Professor of Psychiatry,
New York University School of Medicine,
New York, New York;
Research Psychiatrist, Nathan S. Kline Institute
for Psychiatric Research, Orangeburg, New York;
Attending Psychiatrist,
Bellevue Hospital, New York, New York;
Attending Psychiatrist,
Westchester County Medical Center, Valhalla, New York;
Attending Psychiatrist,
Phelps Memorial Hospital, Tarrytown, New York

POCKET HANDBOOK OF EMERGENCY PSYCHIATRIC MEDICINE

Harold I. Kaplan, M.D.

Professor of Psychiatry, New York University School of Medicine;
Attending Psychiatrist, Tisch Hospital
of the New York University Medical Center;
Attending Psychiatrist, Bellevue Hospital,
New York, New York

Benjamin J. Sadock, M.D.

Professor and Vice Chairman,
Department of Psychiatry,
New York University School of Medicine;
Attending Psychiatrist, Tisch Hospital of the
New York University Medical Center;
Attending Psychiatrist, Bellevue Hospital,
New York, New York

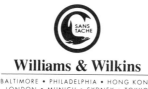

Williams & Wilkins

BALTIMORE • PHILADELPHIA • HONG KONG
LONDON • MUNICH • SYDNEY • TOKYO

A WAVERLY COMPANY

Editor: David C. Retford
Associate Editor: Molly Mullen
Copy Editor: Joan Welsh
Designer: Norman W. Och
Illustration Planner: Wayne Hubbel
Production Coordinator: Barbara J. Felton
Project Editor: Lynda Abrams Zittell, M.A., N.Y.U. School of Medicine

Copyright © 1993
Williams & Wilkins
428 East Preston Street
Baltimore, Maryland 21202, USA

Accurate indications, adverse reactions, and dosage schedules for drugs are provided in this book, but it is possible that they may change. The reader is urged to review the package information data of the manufacturers of the medications mentioned.

Printed in the United States of America

Library of Congress Cataloging-in-Publication Data

Kaplan, Harold I., 1927-
   Pocket handbook of emergency psychiatric medicine / Harold
I. Kaplan, Benjamin J. Sadock.
      p.   cm.
   Includes index.
   ISBN 0-683-04539-3
   1. Psychiatric emergencies—Handbooks, manuals, etc.   I. Sadock,
Benjamin J., 1933-   .   II. Title.
   [DNLM: 1. Psychiatry—handbooks.   2. Emergencies—handbooks.
3. Mental Disorders—diagnosis—handbooks.   4. Mental Disorders—
therapy—handbooks.   WM 39 K17pa 1993]
   RC480.6.K36   1993
616.89'02'5—dc20
DNLM/DLC
for Library of Congress   93-18379
                                                               CIP

93 94 95 96 97
1 2 3 4 5 6 7 8 9 10

*Dedicated
to our wives,
Nancy Barrett Kaplan
and
Virginia Alcott Sadock,
without whose help and sacrifice
this book would not have been possible*

Preface

Emergency medicine is one of the most rapidly expanding medical specialties, and psychiatric emergencies make up a large part of the conditions that emergency room physicians treat. Most psychiatric emergencies are first seen by nonpsychiatrists in the medical emergency room, at the hospital bedside, or in the office setting. *Pocket Handbook of Emergency Psychiatric Medicine* is geared not only to the needs of those physicians but also to the needs of practicing psychiatrists, psychiatric residents, medical students, psychiatric social workers, nurses, and other mental health professionals who work in busy hospital emergency rooms. This book meets the needs of all those clinicians who deal with psychiatric crises. As in all our books, the humanistic aspects of medical care are emphasized. The qualities of compassion, empathy, and understanding are as important in emergency medicine and emergency psychiatry as they are in any other field.

ORGANIZATION

This book is divided into two major areas. *Area A* consists of a series of succinctly written chapters that cover the field of emergencies in psychiatry. They include (1) an introduction to emergency psychiatry, covering treatment settings, staffing, the integration of psychiatry into emergency medical services, and models of emergency care; (2) the evaluation of the psychiatric patient, including the psychiatric history and the mental status examination; (3) an overview of medical and surgical problems that are accompanied by or that cause emergency psychiatric signs and symptoms; (4) a section on telephone emergencies and the use of hotlines in the prevention, the diagnosis, and the treatment of emergency disorders; (5) a section on legal issues, dealing with involuntary hospitalization, the rights of mental patients to refuse and to receive treatment, and the responsibilities of the psychiatrist to protect patients from doing harm to themselves or others; and (6) an overview of psychiatric emergencies in children, with special emphasis on child abuse, which has become a national crisis of almost epidemic proportions during the past few years.

Area B contains discussions of 145 disorders that may be encountered in the emergency room or your office. Such conditions may present as a sign or a symptom of a major mental disorder, such as delusions in schizophrenia, or as the early manisfestation of a potentially fatal illness, such as dementia in acquired immune deficiency syndrome (AIDS).

Content

The decision to include a particular psychiatric emergency condition in this book was based on many factors: frequency of presentation, incidence, prevalence, severity, type of symptoms, potential lethality, and risk of danger to self or others. Reports from emergency room physicians around the country were reviewed, and conditions drawn from those experiences were included. In addition, the psychiatric emergency room at Bellevue Hospital, which is renowned as a receiving center, provided additional examples of psychiatric emergencies. Bellevue draws patients from the entire New York metropolitan area and also cares for visitors from around the world who become impaired psychiatrically. Almost all the emergency conditions discussed in this book have been treated at Bellevue Hospital at one time or another during its long history.

Alphabetized Emergency Listing

The 145 emergency conditions are listed alphabetically for easy and rapid access and sufficient data to diagnose and treat the specific disorders are provided. The data frequently include (1) a definition of the emergency; (2) the criteria used to diagnose the disorder, including, when necessary, the differential diagnosis; (3) interviewing guidelines to use with the patient and with friends or relatives who are in attendance; (4) practical guidelines about treatment and proper disposition; and (5) a special section on drug treatment, including the specific drugs and dosages used to manage the emergency situation.

Teaching System

Pocket Handbook of Emergency Psychiatric Medicine is one in a series of concise practical guides that deal with specific issues in the treatment of psychiatric disorders. Other books in this series include *Pocket Handbook of Clinical Psychiatry* and *Pocket Handbook of Psychiatric Drug Treatment.* The handbooks form one part of a comprehensive system we developed to facilitate the teaching of psychiatry and the behavioral sciences. The handbooks are compactly designed and concisely written books to be carried in the pocket by the clinical clerk or practicing physician to provide a ready reference.

The keystone of the system is *Comprehensive Textbook of Psychiatry,* now in its fifth (1989) edition; that textbook is global in its depth and scope and encyclopedic in its breadth of information. *Synopsis of Psychiatry,* another part of the system, is now in its sixth (1991) edition; it is designed for practicing psychiatrists, psychiatric residents, and medical students. Another part of the system, *Study Guide and Self-Examination Review for Synopsis of Psychiatry and Comprehensive Textbook of Psychiatry,* is now in its fourth (1991) edition; it contains multiple-choice questions keyed to those books. Finally, the system includes *Comprehensive Glossary of Psychiatry and Psycholoy* (1991), which provides simply written definitions of terms of interest for psychiatrists and other physicians, psychologists, students, other mental health professionals, and the general public.

The teaching system is unique in that it provides a comprehensive library of psychiatry that can fulfill all the educational needs of the student and the practitioner.

SPECIAL SECTIONS

Specific Poisons and Toxic Substances

A section on the symptoms and the treatment of specific poisons and toxic substances is included in the appendix. Almost all such substances can cause mental changes, such as confusion, depression, and emotional lability.

Illustrated Drug Identification Guide

A unique aspect of this book is the inclusion of colored plates of all the major drugs used in psychiatry. Both the forms in which they are commercially available and their doses are indicated to help the physician recognize and prescribe the medications. The plates are completely up-to-date. Many emergencies are due to the misuse, abuse, or intentional overdose of drugs that can be identified by using the colored plates.

Indications

In the appendix, a chart of the drugs and the classes of drugs used in the treatment of major psychiatric disorders is found. This chart indicates the various medications that are used to treat a particular disorder and is completely up-to-date.

References

We have not included specific references at the end of each section; however, a reference list of papers that represent the most up-to-date information available about emergency psychiatry is included in an appendix. For further information, the reader is referred to the fifth (1989) edition of our standard work, *Comprehensive Textbook of Psychiatry*, or the sixth (1991) edition of *Synopsis of Psychiatry*, in which each of the topics included in this book is discussed in depth.

ACKNOWLEDGMENTS

We thank James C.-Y. Chou, M.D., Assistant Professor of Psychiatry at New York University Medical Center, who served as contributing editor. We also thank our collaborating authors for their participation and help in this project.

Lynda Abrams Zittell, M.A., served as project editor, as she has for many of our other publications and for which we are deeply appreciative. She carries out her complex tasks with skill and alacrity. Laura Marino processed the manuscript, and we thank her for her extraordinary efforts. We especially thank Joan Welsh, who is an outstanding, highly skilled editor and a much-valued friend.

Virginia Sadock, M.D., Clinical Professor of Psychiatry and Director of Graduate Education in Human Sexuality at New York University Medical Center, deserves special mention and thanks for her help in every aspect of this book.

Finally, we thank Robert Cancro, M.D., Professor and Chairman of the Department of Psychiatry at New York University Medical Center, who served as senior contributing editor. We are deeply grateful for the inspiration and support he offers in all our academic endeavors.

Harold I. Kaplan, M.D.
Benjamin J. Sadock, M.D.

June 1993
New York University Medical Center
New York, New York

In Collaboration With

Michael Allen, M.D.
Clinical Assistant Professor of Psychiatry, New York University School of Medicine; Director of Psychiatric Emergency Services, Bellevue Hospital, New York, New York

Laura Bernay, M.D.
Clinical Instructor of Psychiatry, New York University School of Medicine; New York, New York

Rebecca M. Jones, M.D.
Assistant Professor of Psychiatry and Behavioral Sciences, University of Washington School of Medicine, Seattle, Washington

Caroly Pataki, M.D.
Clinical Assistant Professor of Psychiatry, New York University School of Medicine, New York, New York

Eugene Rubin, M.D.
Clinical Instructor of Psychiatry, New York University School of Medicine, New York, New York

Howard Silbert, M.D.
Clinical Assistant Professor of Psychiatry, New York University School of Medicine, New York, New York

Contents

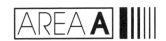

Overview of Emergency
Psychiatric Medicine

1 / Emergency Psychiatric Medicine: An Introduction

A psychiatric emergency is any disturbance in thoughts, feelings, or actions for which immediate therapeutic intervention is necessary. For a variety of reasons—such as the growing incidence of violence, the increased appreciation of the role of organic disease in altered mental status, and the epidemic of alcoholism and other substance use disorders—the number of emergency patients is on the rise. Physicians are performing an expanded role as the primary clinician or consultant as part of integrated emergency medicine services. The widening scope of emergency psychiatry goes beyond general psychiatric practice to include such specialized problems as the abuse of substances, children, and spouses; violence in the form of suicide, homicide, and rape; and such social issues as homelessness, aging, competence, and acquired immune deficiency syndrome (AIDS). The emergency psychiatrist must be up-to-date on medicolegal issues and managed care.

TREATMENT SETTING

Most emergency psychiatric evaluations are done by nonpsychiatrists in a general medical emergency room setting, but specialized psychiatric emergency rooms, sometimes offering comprehensive psychiatric services, are increasingly favored. Regardless of the type of setting, an atmosphere of safety and security must prevail. An adequate number of staff members—including psychiatrists, nurses, aides, and social workers—must be present at all times. Additional personnel to help out in times of overcrowding should be available. Specific responsibilities, such as the use of restraints, should be clearly defined and practiced by the entire emergency team. Clear communication and lines of authority are essential. The organization of the staff into multidisciplinary teams is desirable.

Children and young adolescents are best served in a pediatric setting. Unless there is a risk of behavioral problems or of their leaving the hospital against advice, they need not be sent to the adult psychiatric emergency service.

Immediate access to the medical emergency room and to appropriate diagnostic services is necessary because many (5 to 30 percent) medical conditions present with psychiatric manifestations. The full spectrum of psychopharmacological options should be available to the psychiatrist.

Violence in the emergency service cannot be condoned or tolerated. The code of conduct expected of staff members and patients must be posted and understood from the time of the patient's arrival in the emergency room. Security is best managed as a clinical issue by the clinical staff, not by law enforcement personnel. Whenever possible, agitated and threatening

3

patients should be sequestered from the nonagitated. Seclusion and restraint rooms should be located close to the nursing station for close observation.

The entire staff must understand that patients in physical and emotional distress are fragile and that various expectations and fantasies, often unrealistic, influence their responses to treatment. For example, a man suffering from impaired reality testing who is brought in by the police against his will may not understand that the clinician is interested in helping him. Other patients, influenced by previous unsatisfactory treatment experiences, may be hostile. A high percentage of patients believe that psychiatrists can read minds or are only interested in admitting patients to lock them away. Such people see little point in openly discussing their problems. Many people have an inaccurate understanding of their rights as patients. All clinical interventions must take those expectations and attitudes into account to minimize the possibility of misunderstanding and consequent problems.

EVALUATION

The primary goal of an emergency psychiatric evaluation is the timely assessment of the patient in crisis. To that end, the physician must make an initial diagnosis, identify the precipitating factors and immediate needs, and begin treatment or refer the patient to the most appropriate treatment setting. In view of the unpredictable nature of emergency room work, with many patients presenting both physical and emotional complaints, and in view of the limited space and the competition for ancillary services, a pragmatic approach to the patient is required. Sometimes moving the patient out of the emergency room into the most appropriate diagnostic or treatment setting is best for the patient. Medical emergencies, interpersonal conflicts, and support services are generally better managed elsewhere in the system. Keeping the number of emergency patients in one place to a minimum reduces the chance of agitation and violence.

The standard psychiatric interview—consisting of a history, a mental status examination, and, when appropriate and depending on the rules of the emergency room, a full physical examination and ancillary tests—is the cornerstone of the emergency room evaluation. However, the emergency room psychiatrist must be ready to introduce modifications as needed. For example, the emergency psychiatrist may have to structure the interview with a rambling manic patient, medicate or restrain an agitated patient, or forgo the usual rules of confidentiality to assess an adolescent's risk of suicide. In general, any strategy introduced in the emergency room to accomplish the goal of assessing the patient is considered consistent with good clinical practice as long as the rationale for the strategy is documented in the medical record.

What constitutes a psychiatric emergency is highly subjective. The emergency room has increasingly come to serve as an admitting area, a holding room, a detoxification center, and a private office. Such medical conditions as head traumas, acute intoxications, withdrawal states, and AIDS encephalopathies may present with acute psychiatric manifestations. The emergency psychiatrist must rapidly assess and distinguish the truly emergency psychiatric patients from those who are less acutely ill and from nonpsychiatric emergencies. A triage system using psychiatrists, nurses, and psychiatric social workers is an efficient and effective way to identify emergency, urgent, and nonurgent patients, who can then be prioritized for care (Figure A.1-1).

In one model, every patient who comes to the emergency room is assessed by a triage nurse on arrival to ascertain the patient's chief complaint, clinical condition, and vital signs. The psychiatrist then briefly meets with the patient and other significant people involved in the case—family members, emergency medical service technicians, and police—to assign the patient to one of the three categories—emergency, urgent, and nonurgent—or to refer the patient to an appropriate treatment setting, like the medical emergency room. Having a senior clinician perform that task ensures a rapid identification of the most urgent and troublesome cases, an appropriate allocation of resources, and an answer to the most common question heard in the emergency room: "When am I going to see a doctor?"

The psychiatrist then assigns clinical responsibility for each patient to the appropriate personnel. As the evaluation often stretches over more than one shift, a careful procedure to transfer responsibility and to pass along information from tour to tour must be built into the system by using visual, oral, and written communications. A request for old records should be made automatically for every patient who is assigned to the emergency room. Each emergency should be judged on its own merits, but information from previous records and from workers in the field and family members can be of crucial importance in assessing patients, especially patients who are psychotic, frightened, or otherwise unable or unwilling to cooperate in giving a good history.

A multilingual staff and a hospital language bank that lists bilingual staff members and other translation services should be readily available to the psychiatrist. The use of the patient's friends or family members as translators is not desirable because of the possibility of unconscious or deliberate denial or distortion of the clinical picture stemming from their involvement with the patient.

An initial assessment of the patient's total biopsychosocial needs is optimal, but the patient's emergency status, other patients waiting to be seen, and the constraints of the emergency room setting often make such a full assessment a moot point. At a minimum, the emergency evaluation should address the following five questions before any disposition is decided on: (1) Is it safe for the patient to be in the emergency room? (2) Is the problem organic or functional or a combination? (3) Is the patient psychotic? (4) Is the patient suicidal or homicidal? (5) To what degree is the patient capable of self-care?

Patient Safety

Physicians should consider the question of the patient's safety before evaluating every patient. The answer must address the issues of the emergency room's physical layout, staffing patterns and communication, and

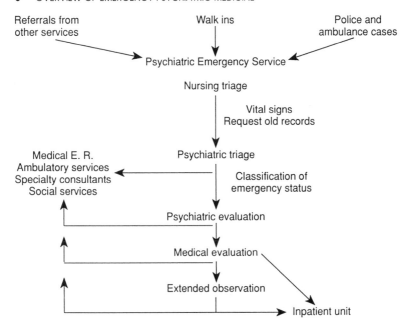

Figure A.1–1. Evaluation and treatment of psychiatric emergencies.

patient population. Psychiatrists must then take stock of themselves: Are they in the proper frame of mind to conduct an evaluation? Do any issues in the case spark countertransference reactions? The self-assessment should go on throughout the evaluation. The physical and emotional safety of the patient takes priority over all other considerations. If verbal interventions fail or are contraindicated, the use of medication or restraints must be considered and, if necessary, ordered. Careful attention to the possible outbreak of agitation or disruptive behavior beyond acceptable limits is often the best insurance against untoward occurrences.

Organic or Functional (Psychological)

The most important question for the emergency psychiatrist to address is whether the problem is organic or functional or both. Organic conditions—such as diabetes mellitus, thyroid disease, acute intoxications, withdrawal states, AIDS, and head traumas—can present with prominent mental status changes that mimic common psychiatric illnesses. Such conditions may be life-threatening if not treated promptly. Generally, the treatment of a medical illness is more definitive and the prognosis is better than for a functional psychiatric disorder. The psychiatrist must consider all causal possibilities.

Unfortunately, once patients are labeled psychiatric, their complaints may not be taken seriously by nonmental health professionals, and the patients' conditions may deteriorate, especially if the patients suffer from major Axis I syndromes. Because of such factors as deinstitutionalization, homelessness, and chronic alcoholism, the mentally ill are at great risk of tuberculosis, vitamin deficiencies, and other easily overlooked but easily treated conditions. Symptoms such as paranoia, internal preoccupation, and acute psychosis can make a routine medical diagnosis exceedingly difficult. Each patient must be assessed for the possibility that an organic illness is combined with an underlying psychiatric illness. A young man who comes to the emergency room intoxicated or in alcohol withdrawal two or three times a month may come one day with a subdural hematoma suffered in a fall.

The psychiatrist who is functioning as a consultant to other branches of the emergency service must also answer the question of whether the patient's condition is organic or functional or both, even if the patient has been declared medically cleared.

Psychosis

Whether the patient is psychotic refers not so much to the patient's diagnosis as to the severity of the patient's symptoms and the degree of life disruption. The patient's degree of withdrawal from objective reality, level of affectivity, intellectual functioning, and degree of regression are other important parameters. Impairment in any of those areas may lead to difficulties in conducting an evaluation. Agitated, assaultive behavior or failure to comply with treatment recommendations may also result. A paranoid, hypervigilent patient may misperceive a staff member's offer of help as an attack and may lash out in self-defense. Command auditory hallucinations may cause a patient to deny symptoms and to throw prescriptions in the garbage immediately after leaving the emergency room. The psychiatrist should be alert to the complications that may arise with patients whose reality testing is impaired and should modify the approach accordingly.

All communication with patients must be straightforward. All clinical interventions should be briefly explained in language they can understand. Psychiatrists should not assume that the patient trusts or believes them or even wants their help. Clinicians must be prepared to structure or to terminate an interview to limit the potential for agitation and regression.

Suicidal or Homicidal

By definition, suicidal and homicidal patients are dangerous to themselves and to others. Suicidal ideation is the most common chief complaint in the psychiatric emergency service. All suicidal threats, gestures, and thoughts must be taken seriously until proved otherwise. Suicidal patients must be observed closely. Outside the safe confines of the hospital, violent impulses are much more difficult to control. Violence toward others in an emergency room setting is most often the result of the patient's misperceptions or a reaction to intrusive, insensitive, or indifferent staff members. The patient must always be asked about suicidal or violent feelings.

Self-Care

Whether the patient is capable of self-care is important beyond the immediate concerns in the emergency service. It must also be considered in admission criteria and initial inpatient orders. Self-neglect is now considered an adequate reason for involuntary psychiatric hospitalization in some states. The psychiatrist must make the assessment before releasing the patient from the emergency room. The physician's responsibility for a patient's well-being after release from the hospital has come under increased scrutiny in recent years. It is not sufficient to decide that a patient does not warrant inpatient care. The psychiatrist must judge the patient's ability to follow through with the outpatient recommendations and capacity to adjust to problems in case of any delays in effecting the treatment plan. A case manager or a social worker can offer the patient assistance and support in the treatment process. At a minimum, the patient should have adequate food and shelter. Patients should always be reminded of their option to call or to return to the hospital if any difficulty arises.

DIAGNOSTIC AND TREATMENT CONSIDERATIONS
Diagnosis

The emergency assessment is not expected to be complete, but it must address certain important questions. Toxicology screening, chest X-rays, an electrocardiogram (ECG), and other relevant laboratory tests, such as serum lithium (Eskalith) and phenytoin (Dilantin) levels, should be done as soon as possible for the most accurate information. Initial medical clearance and specialty consultations should be done in the emergency room whenever feasible. If available, old records should be reviewed, and all information from outside sources, such as family members and the police, should be gathered before making a disposition. Although safety is always the highest priority, it should not unduly delay the completion of the diagnostic evaluation.

Treatment

When medications or other restraints are indicated, they should be ordered according to the principle of maximum tranquilization with minimum sedation. The goal is to help the patient regain control, to ease the pain, and to allow the evaluation to proceed to its conclusion. A patient who is asleep cannot hurt anyone but cannot give a history or undergo a mental status examination. Low-dose high-potency antipsychotics are fast-acting and have a wide margin of safety. Intramuscular (IM) benzodiazepines have short half-lives. Sometimes they are very effective when used in combination. Intravenous (IV) administration is risky because of the danger of working with agitated patients. Universal precautions should be observed with all patients because of the risk of human immunodeficiency virus (HIV) and other infections.

The most common medication errors made by doctors are (1) overmedication (using too powerful a preparation or too high a dose, resulting in delayed evaluation or disposition), (2) undermedication (using an inadequate preparation or too small a dose, again resulting in delay because of the patient's continued agitation or other disruption), and (3) premature switching of the medication—for example, giving a patient haloperidol (Haldol), chlorpromazine (Thorazine), and lorazapam (Ativan)—all within one hour.

Patients who require restraints or seclusion place a burden on the staff members who must monitor vital signs, hydration, and range of motion. Patients must be evaluated frequently for continued need of control.

Disposition

In some cases the usual option to admit or to discharge the patient is not felt to be optimal. Suspected toxic psychoses, brief decompensations in a patient with a personality disorder, and adjustment reactions to traumatic events, for example, may be best managed in an extended-observation setting. Allowing the patient additional time in a secure environment can result in sufficient improvement or clarification of the issues to make traditional inpatient treatment unnecessary. Also, doing so can spare the patient the trauma and the stigma of a psychiatric admission and can free up bed space for more needy patients. Crisis intervention for victims of rape and other traumas can also be done in an extended-observation setting.

When the decision is to admit the patient to the hospital, it is preferable to do so on a voluntary status. Allowing patients that option gives them a sense of control over their lives and of participation in the treatment decisions. Patients who clearly meet involuntary admission criteria on the basis of dangerousness to themselves or to others cannot leave the hospital without further review and can always be converted to involuntary status if warranted.

Because the initial evaluation is often inconclusive, definitive treatment is best deferred until the patient can be further assessed on the inpatient unit or in the outpatient department. However, when the diagnosis is clear and the patient's response to previous treatment is known, nothing is gained by delay. For example, a patient suffering from chronic schizophrenia who has decompensated after discontinuing the usual regimen of antipsychotic medication is best served by the prompt resumption of treatment.

Even if patients feel comfortable coming to the emergency room in times of need, the emergency psychiatrist should always direct or redirect them to the most appropriate treatment setting. Patients in the psychopharmacology clinic who have missed their regular appointments should be given only enough medication to sustain them until they can be seen in the clinic. Feedback to their other treaters should be a matter of course.

The emergency room is often the gateway to the department of psychiatry or the general hospital. First impressions carry a great deal of weight. The kind of attention and concern shown to patients on arrival in the emergency room has important implications for how they will respond to staff members and treatment recommendations and even in their treatment compliance long after they have left the emergency room.

Documentation

In the interests of good quality care, respect for patients' rights, cost control, and medicolegal concerns, documentation has become a central focus for the emergency physician. The medical record should convey a concise picture of the patient, highlighting all pertinent positive and negative findings. Gaps in information and the reasons why the information could not be obtained should be mentioned. The names and the telephone numbers of interested parties should be noted. A provisional diagnosis or differential diagnosis must be made. An initial treatment plan or recommendations should clearly follow from the findings of the patient's history, mental status examination, and other diagnostic tests and the medical evaluation. The writing must be legible. The emergency physician has unusual latitude under the law to perform an adequate initial assessment; however, all interventions and decisions must be thought out, discussed, and documented in the patient's record.

2 / Evaluation of the Patient as a Psychiatric Emergency

In a psychiatric emergency the person poses a significant risk to self or others. Common examples include violence, suicide, self-mutilation, markedly impaired judgment, and severe self-neglect. Often, an emergency evaluation of a psychiatric patient involves determining how much of a risk the patient poses to self or others and to what degree the patient requires immediate hospitalization versus outpatient treatment. The patient may come voluntarily to the emergency room or be brought involuntarily by family members, teachers, or the police.

The primary tools for evaluating a psychiatric emergency include a physical examination, a psychiatric interview, a mental status examination, and relevant laboratory tests.

PHYSICAL EXAMINATION

Initially, all psychiatric patients must have their vital signs assessed. Blood pressure, temperature, and pulse readings are easy, straightforward measurements that can reveal significant information quickly. For instance, an agitated and hallucinating patient who is febrile with an elevated blood pressure (BP) and a pulse of 120 may be suffering from delirium tremens (DTs), rather than from some clear-cut psychiatric disorder. Whatever the patient's actual illness, the vital signs can help direct the clinician down the correct diagnostic path.

Common medical findings that are significant in psychiatric emergency room patients are listed in Table A.2-1. Many of the findings reflect the severe level of self-neglect found in many psychiatric emergency patients. The findings are also indicative of the often severely impaired judgment found in many of those patients that prevents them from seeking needed and timely medical care. The findings listed in Table A.2-1 are not meant to be all-inclusive. A psychiatric emergency patient may present with virtually any medical disorder or finding not listed in that table.

Table A.2–1
Common Medical Findings in Psychiatric Emergency Patients

Signs and Symptoms	Common Associated Findings
Lice infestation	Anemia Secondarily infected skin excoriations
Emaciation Dehydration	Fever Anemia Electrolyte disturbances Positive: HIV Positive: VDRL Positive: CXR, PPD
Cellulitis Stasis ulcers Gangrene Maggots	Fever Sepsis Elevated WBC Abnormal blood glucose Abnormal LFT Positive: CXR, PPD
Cough Shortness of breath	Fever Positive: CXR, PPD Positive: HIV
Alcohol on breath Distended abdomen Spider angioma Visual and tactile hallucinations	Abnormal LFT Ascites Elevated BP and pulse Fever Elevated blood alcohol
Drug intoxication	
Pupillary changes Somnolence or agitation Disorientation Lability of mood and affect Visual and tactile hallucinations	Positive: urine toxicology screen Labile BP, pulse, and temperature
Anticholinergic Intoxication	
Sweating Dilated pupils Flushed, red skin Dry mouth Disorientation and agitation Visual and auditory hallucinations	Elevated, labile BP and pulse Fever Absent bowel sounds
Dementia	Positive: HIV Positive: VDRL Abnormal LFT Abnormal TFT Abnormal CT scan Abnormal LP Abnormal B_{12}/folate Abnormal urobilinogens
Disorientation	Positive: urine toxicology screen Positive: HIV Abnormal TFT Abnormal LFT Abnormal blood glucose Toxic lithium level Electrolyte disturbances Elevated BP and pulse Fever CBC disturbances

Table A.2–1—*continued*

Signs and Symptoms	Common Associated Findings
Somnolence, stupor, and coma	Rapid response to naloxone Rapid response to glucose infusion Abnormal blood glucose Positive: drug toxicology screen Abnormal CT scan Abnormal LP Toxic lithium levels Toxic antidepressant levels Electrolyte disturbances Abnormal LFT Elevated CPK
Seizures	Toxic lithium levels Toxic antidepressant levels Elevated antipsychotic doses Positive: urine toxicology screen Positive: HIV Abnormal blood glucose Abnormal CT Abnormal LP Fever
Dystonic reactions Akathisia Pseudoparkinsonism	Recent initiation or increase in antipsychotic medication
Neuroleptic Malignant Syndrome	
Severe muscle rigidity Palpitations Diaphoresis Agitation Possible disorientation Possible respiratory failure Stupor and coma	Labile hypertension Fever Elevated pulse Elevated CPK Myoglobinuria Renal failure Pulmonary embolism
Lithium Toxicity	
Tremor Ataxia Vomiting Severe diarrhea Seizure Disorientation Hyperreflexia Dysarthria Coma	Abnormal UA, BUN, and CR Electrolyte disturbances Leukocytosis Abnormal TFT Abnormal ECG
Dizziness	Orthostatic hypertension Elevated antidepressant levels Elevated thorazine levels Elevated lithium levels Anemia Electrolyte disturbances

BP: blood pressure
BUN: blood urea nitrogen
CBC: complete blood count
CPK: creatine phosphokinase
CR: creatinine
CT: computed tomography
CXR: chest X-ray
ECG: electrocardiogram
HIV: human immunodeficiency virus

LFT: liver function test
LP: lumbar puncture
PPD: purified protein derivative of
  tuberculin
TFT: thyroid function test
UA: urinalysis
VDRL: Venereal Disease Research
  Laboratory
WBC: white blood count

When a medical problem is discovered and assessed as severe, the patient may need to be admitted first to a medical ward for the problem to be managed aggressively and effectively. Once the medical problem is addressed, the patient may be transferred to a psychiatric ward.

EMERGENCY PSYCHIATRIC INTERVIEW

The emergency interview is similar to the standard psychiatric interview except for the time limitation imposed by the other patients waiting to be seen and by the potential sense of urgency in assessing the risk to the patient or others. In general, the physician focuses on the presenting complaint and the reasons that the patient has come to the emergency room at that time. The time constraint requires that the clinician structure the interview, particularly with patients who may respond with long, rambling accounts of their illness. If friends, relatives, or the police accompany the patient, a supplemental history should be obtained from them, especially if the patient is mute, negativistic, uncooperative, or otherwise unable to give a coherent history.

Patients may be highly motivated to reveal themselves to gain relief from suffering, but they may also be both consciously and unconsciously motivated to conceal innermost feelings that they perceive to be shameful or threatening. If the patient has been brought to the hospital involuntarily, willingness or ability to cooperate may be impaired for that reason. The psychiatrist's relationship with the patient strongly influences what the patient does and does not say, even within the context of a first interview in an emergency room; therefore, a large portion of the psychiatric emergency interview involves the specific and sophisticated techniques of listening, observation, and interpretation that provide the foundation of psychiatric training in general. Being straightforward, honest, calm, and nonthreatening is of utmost importance, as is the ability to convey to patients the idea that the clinician is in control and will act decisively to protect them from hurting themselves or others.

Table A.2–2 summarizes a number of necessary initial factors in the evaluation of a psychiatric emergency.

Sometimes the contact with the emergency room is by telephone. In such cases the psychiatrist should obtain the number from which the call is made and the exact address. Those items are important in case the call is interrupted; they allow the psychiatrist to direct help to the patient. If the patient is alone and the psychiatrist ascertains that the patient is in danger, the police should be alerted. If possible, an assistant should call the police on another line while the psychiatrist keeps the patient engaged until help arrives. The patient should not be told to drive alone to the hospital. Rather, an emergency medical team should be dispatched to bring the patient to the hospital.

The emergency psychiatrist must consider a wide range of conditions that may account for the presenting signs or symptoms. The most common complaints fall within the large general categories of anxiety, depression,

Table A.2–2
General Strategy in Evaluating the Patient

I. Self-protection

A. Know as much as possible about the patients before meeting them.

B. Leave physical restraint procedures to those who are trained.

C. Be alert to risks of impending violence.

D. Attend to the safety of the physical surroundings (e.g., door access, room objects).

E. Have others present during the assessment if needed.

F. Have others in the vicinity.

G. Attend to developing an alliance with the patient (e.g., do not confront or threaten patients with paranoid psychoses).

II. Prevent harm

A. Prevent self-injury and suicide. Use whatever methods are necessary to prevent patients from hurting themselves during the evaluation.

B. Prevent violence toward others. During the evaluation, briefly assess the patient for the risk of violence. If the risk is deemed significant, consider the following options:
   1. Inform the patient that violence is not acceptable.
   2. Approach the patient in a nonthreatening manner.
   3. Reassure, calm, or assist the patient's reality testing.
   4. Offer medication.
   5. Inform the patient that restraint or seclusion will be used if necessary.
   6. Have teams ready to restrain the patient.
   7. When patients are restrained, always closely observe them, and frequently check their vital signs. Isolate restrained patients from surrounding agitating stimuli. Immediately plan a further approach—medication, reassurance, medical evaluation.

III. Rule out organic mental disorders.

IV. Rule out impending psychosis.

---

mania, and thought disorders. Those conditions may overlap and have multiple causes, from psychiatric to overtly medical.

The greatest potential error in emergency room psychiatry is overlooking a physical illness as the cause of the emotional illness. Head traumas, medical illnesses, drug abuse (including alcohol), cerebrovascular diseases, metabolic abnormalities, and medications may all cause abnormal behavior, and the psychiatrist should take a concise medical history that concentrates on those areas. Table A.2–3 lists those factors that require a high index of suspicion for underlying organic disorders.

Specific Interview Situations

Depressed and potentially suicidal patients. The clinician should always ask about suicidal ideas as part of every mental status examination, especially if the patient is depressed. The patient may not realize that such symptoms as waking during the night and increased somatic complaints are related to depressive disorders. The patient should be asked directly, "Are you or have you ever been suicidal?" "Do you want to die?" "Do you feel so bad that you might hurt yourself?" Eight out of 10 persons who eventually kill themselves give warnings of their intent. If the patient admits

Table A.2–3
Features Requiring a High Index of Suspicion for Organicity

1. Acute onset (within hours or minutes, with prevailing symptoms)
2. First episode
3. Geriatric age
4. Current medical illness or injury
5. Significant substance abuse
6. Nonauditory disturbances of perception
7. Neurological symptoms—loss of consciousness, seizures, head injury, change in headache pattern, change in vision
8. Classic mental status signs—diminished alertness, disorientation, memory impairment, impairment in concentration and attention, dyscalculia, concreteness
9. Other mental status signs—speech, movement, or gait disorders
10. Constructional apraxia—difficulties in drawing a clock, a cube, intersecting pentagons, Bender-Gestalt design
11. Catatonic features—nudity, negativism, combativeness, rigidity, posturing, waxy flexibility, echopraxia, echolalia, grimacing, mutism

to a plan of action, that is a particularly dangerous sign. If a patient who has been threatening suicide becomes quiet and less agitated than before, that may be an ominous sign. The clinician should be especially concerned with the factors listed in Table A.2–4.

A suicide note, a family history of suicide, or previous suicidal behavior on the part of the patient increases the risk for suicide. Evidence of impulsivity or of pervasive pessimism about the future also places the patient at risk. If the physician decides that the patient is in imminent risk for suicidal behavior, the patient must be hospitalized or otherwise protected. A difficult situation arises when the risk does not seem to be immediate but the potential for suicide is present as long as the patient remains depressed. If the psychiatrist decides not to hospitalize the patient immediately, the doctor should insist that the patient promise to call whenever the suicidal pressure mounts.

Violent patients.   Patients may be violent for many reasons, and the interview with a violent patient must attempt to ascertain the underlying cause of the violent behavior, since cause determines intervention.

The differential diagnosis of violent behavior includes psychoactive substance-induced organic mental disorder, antisocial personality disorder, catatonic schizophrenia, medical infections, cerebral neoplasms, decompensating obsessive-compulsive personality disorder, dissociative disorders, impulse control disorders, sexual disorders, alcohol idiosyncratic intoxication, delusional disorder, paranoid personality disorder, schizophrenia, temporal lobe epilepsy, bipolar disorder, and uncontrollable violence secondary to interpersonal stress.

The psychiatric interview must include questions that attempt to sort out the differential for violent behavior and questions directed toward the prediction of violence.

The best predictors of violent behavior are (1) excessive alcohol intake; (2) a history of violent acts, with arrests or criminal activity; and (3) a history of childhood abuse. Table A.2–5 lists some of the most significant factors in assessing and predicting violence.

Table A.2–4
History, Signs, and Symptoms of Suicidal Risk

1. Previous attempt or fantasized suicide
2. Anxiety, depression, exhaustion
3. Availability of means of suicide
4. Concern for effect of suicide on family members
5. Verbalized suicidal ideation
6. Preparation of a will, resignation after agitated depression
7. Proximal life crisis, such as mourning or impending surgery
8. Family history of suicide
9. Pervasive pessimism or hopelessness

Table A.2–5
Assessing and Predicting Violent Behavior

1. Signs of impending violence
   a. Very recent acts of violence, including property violence
   b. Verbal or physical threats (menacing)
   c. Carrying weapons or other objects that may be used as weapons (e.g., forks, ashtrays)
   d. Progressive psychomotor agitation
   e. Alcohol or drug intoxication
   f. Paranoid features in a psychotic patient
   g. Command violent auditory hallucinations—some but not all patients are at high risk
   h. Organic mental disorders, global or with frontal lobe findings; less commonly with temporal lobe findings (controversial)
   i. Patients with catatonic excitement
   j. Certain patients with mania
   k. Certain patients with agitated depression
   l. Personality disorder patients prone to rage, violence, or impulse dyscontrol

2. Assess the risk of violence
   a. Consider violent ideation, wish, intention, plan, availability of means, implementation of plan, wish for help.
   b. Consider demographics—sex (male), age (15–24), socioeconomic status (low), social supports (few).
   c. Consider past history: violence, nonviolent antisocial acts, impulse dyscontrol (e.g., gambling, substance abuse, suicide or self-injury, psychosis).
   d. Consider overt stressors (e.g., marital conflict, real or symbolic loss).

PSYCHIATRIC HISTORY

The psychiatric history is the record of the patient's life that allows the physician to understand who the patient is, where the patient has come from, and where the patient is likely to go in the future. In the emergency setting, there is usually an increased sense of urgency because of the acute nature of the situation, and often the psychiatrist must take a directive approach in calming the patient and eliciting information. It may be necessary, for instance, to medicate or to restrain the patient before the psychiatrist is able to speak with the patient. Many times the history also includes information about the patient obtained from other sources, such as a parent, a spouse, or a police officer. Obtaining a comprehensive history from the patient and, if necessary, from informed sources is essential to making a correct diagnosis and formulating a specific and effective treatment plan. It may be impossible in an emergency setting to fully determine a diagnosis, but as much information as possible needs to be obtained to begin to make a reasonable, if tentative, diagnosis.

Many patients in a psychiatric emergency setting are unable to give any history at all, thus making witnesses and other informed sources extremely important. The mental status examination also becomes correspondingly more important as the history becomes more difficult or impossible to obtain.

Identifying Data

The identifying data provide a succinct demographic summary of the patient by name, age, marital status, sex, occupation, language if other than English, ethnic background and religion insofar as they are pertinent, and current circumstances of living. The information can also include the place or the situation where the interview took place, the sources of the information, and whether the emergency is the first episode of that type for the patient. The identifying data are meant to provide a thumbnail sketch of potentially important patient characteristics that may affect the diagnosis, the prognosis, the treatment, and patient compliance.

An example of the identifying data part of the interview is as follows:

Jane Jones is a 45-year-old white single Catholic woman, currently unemployed and homeless, living in public shelters and on the street. The current interview occurred in the emergency room (ER) with the patient in four-point restraints in the presence of four clinical staff members and two police officers. It was approximately the fifth such visit to the ER for Ms. Jones in the past year. The source of information on Ms. Jones was the police officer who brought the patient to the ER. Ms. Jones herself remained mute throughout the interview.

Chief Complaint

The chief complaint, in the patient's own words, states why he or she has come or been brought in for help. The complaint should be recorded even if the patient is unable to speak, and a description of the person who provided the information should be included. The patient's explanation, regardless of how bizarre or irrelevant it is, should be recorded verbatim in the section on the chief complaint. The other sources of information can then give their versions of the presenting events in the section on the history of the present illness. Example:

Although the patient remained mute, police officers reported that she had been standing naked in Grand Central Terminal, stating, "Take me to God."

History of Present Illness

This part of the psychiatric history provides a comprehensive and chronological picture of the events leading up to the current moment in the patient's life. An understanding of the history of the present illness helps answer the question "Why now?" Why did the patient come or why was the patient brought to the emergency room at this time? What immediate precipitating events triggered the current episode? What were the patient's life circumstances at the onset of the symptoms or the behavioral changes, and how did they affect the patient, so that the presenting episode became manifest? Knowing what the personality was of the previously well patient also helps give perspective on the currently ill patient.

Previous Illnesses

Past episodes of both psychiatric and medical illnesses are described. The patient's symptoms, the extent of the incapacity, the type of treatment received, the names of the hospitals entered, the length of each illness, the effects of the prior treatments, and the degree of compliance should all be explored and recorded chronologically if possible. Particular attention should be paid to the first episode that signaled the onset of illness, as first episodes can often provide crucial data about precipitating events, diagnostic possibilities, and coping capabilities. Each patient should also be specifically asked about past suicidal and homicidal ideas and acts.

The physician should obtain a medical review of past medical symptoms and note any major medical or surgical illnesses and major traumas, particularly those requiring hospitalization, that the patient experienced. Episodes of craniocerebral traumas, neurological illnesses, tumors, and seizure disorders are especially relevant to psychiatric histories and so is a history of having tested positive for the human immunodeficiency virus (HIV) or of having acquired immune deficiency syndrome (AIDS). Specific questions need to be asked about the presence of a seizure disorder, episodes of loss of consciousness, changes in usual headache patterns, changes in vision, and episodes of confusion and disorientation. A history of infection with syphilis is critical and relevant. All patients must be asked about alcohol and drug abuse, including details about the quality and the frequency of use.

Past Personal History (Anamnesis)

In addition to studying the patient's present illness and current life situation, the physician needs a thorough understanding of the patient's past life and its relation to the present emotional problem. However, a detailed developmental history is generally not indicated or possible in an emergency situation. A brief history, if possible, may be helpful in placing the present episode in some perspective. For instance, knowing the patient's highest level of functioning before the current emergency is essential, and knowing the patient's highest level of education, work history, history of legal troubles, and social relationships can be helpful.

Family history.　A brief statement about any psychiatric illnesses, hospitalizations, and treatments in the patient's immediate family members should be placed in this part of the report and can be helpful in constructing an emergency differential diagnosis. Is there a family history of alcohol and drug abuse or of antisocial behavior? Is there a history of schizophrenia, mood disorders, suicide, or violence? Can some family members be contacted for information or assistance?

MENTAL STATUS EXAMINATION

The mental status examination is the essential part of the emergency clinic assessment. It describes the sum total of the examiner's observations and impressions of the psychiatric patient at the time of the interview. Whereas the emergency patient's history remains stable, the patient's mental status can change from hour to hour, even minute to minute. Even when a patient is mute or incoherent or refuses to answer questions, one can obtain a wealth of information through careful observation. One standard mental status examination format is outlined in Table A.2–6.

General Description

Appearance.   This part is a description of the patient's appearance, degree of self-care or self-neglect, and overall physical impression conveyed to the interviewer as reflected by the patient's posture, poise, clothing, and grooming. In an emergency setting the patient's appearance can provide crucial clues about the ability to care for self and about judgment. A patient who is disheveled or virtually naked is a patient with a decreased ability to care for self and is, thus, at risk.

Behavior and psychomotor activity.   This category refers to both the quantitative and the qualitative aspects of the patient's motor behavior, including mannerisms, gestures, twitches, stereotyped behavior, echopraxia, hyperactivity, agitation, combativeness, wringing of hands, pacing, and other physical manifestations. Psychomotor retardation or generalized slowing down of body movements should be noted. Any aimless, purposeless activity should be described. In an emergency, that information can point a clinician in the direction of a particular diagnosis and alert the clinician to increasing agitation and potential loss of control. For instance, a patient who is agitated and repeatedly picks at clothing in an aimless, purposeless way may be suffering from amphetamine intoxication, and a patient who is mute and immobile may be depressed or catatonic or experiencing a toxic reaction to some drug.

Attitude toward examiner.   The patient's attitude toward the examiner can be described as uncooperative, friendly, seductive, defensive, evasive, or guarded; any number of other adjectives can be used. The level of established rapport should be recorded. Many patients in an emergency setting are unable to establish any rapport because of their agitation, paranoia, hallucinations, depression, and other interfering factors.

Mood and Affect

Mood.   Mood is defined as a pervasive and sustained emotion that colors the person's perception of the world. Statements about the patient's mood should include its depth, intensity, duration, and fluctuations. Common adjectives used to describe mood include depressed, despairing, irritable, anxious, angry, expansive, euphoric, empty, frightened, and perplexed. Mood may be labile, meaning that it fluctuates or alternates rapidly between extremes (for example, laughing loudly and being expansive one moment, tearful and despairing the next). Lability of mood often reflects the patient's

Table A.2–6
Outline of the Mental Status Examination

I.   General description
    A. Appearance
    B. Behavior and psychomotor activity
    C. Attitude toward examiner

II.   Mood and affect
    A. Mood
    B. Affect
    C. Appropriateness

III.   Speech

IV.   Perceptual disturbances

V.   Thought
    A. Process or form of thought
    B. Content of thought

VI.   Sensorium and cognition
    A. Alertness and level of consciousness
    B. Orientation
    C. Memory
    D. Concentration
    E. Abstract thinking
    F. Fund of information and intelligence

VII.   Impulse control

VIII.   Judgment and insight

IX.   Reliability

---

general lack of control, which can contribute to the patient's being at increased risk.

Affect. Affect may be defined as the patient's external expression of emotional responsiveness. Affect is what the examiner observes as the patient's facial expression, including the amount and the range of expressive behavior. Affect may or may not be congruent with mood. Affect is described as being within normal range, constricted, blunted, or flat. To diagnose flat affect, one should find virtually no signs of affective expression, the patient's voice should be monotonous, and the face should be immobile. The examiner should note the patient's difficulty in initiating, sustaining, or terminating an emotional response; in an emergency setting that information can provide clues to the patient's level of emotional control.

Appropriateness. The appropriateness of the patient's emotional responses can be considered in the context of the subject matter the patient is discussing. For example, paranoid patients who are describing a delusion of persecution should be angry or frightened about the experiences they believe are happening to them. Inappropriateness of affect is a quality of response found in some schizophrenic patients; their affect is incongruent with what they are saying (for example, they have a flattened affect when speaking about murderous impulses). Inappropriateness may also reflect the degree to which an impaired patient is unable to exercise judgment or control with regard to an emotional response.

Speech

Speech is described in terms of its rate, volume, rhythm, and amount. Speech may be rapid, slow, pressured, hesitant, dramatic, monotonous, loud, whispered, slurred, staccato, or mumbled. Impairments of speech, such as stuttering, are included in this section. Unusual rhythms (termed *dysprosody*) and any accent that may be present should be noted. A patient whose speech is loud and pressured may be a patient who is losing or has already lost control. A patient whose speech is slow, inaudible, or monosyllabic may also be at increased risk because of such factors as severe depression and interference from internal stimuli.

Perceptual Disturbances

Hallucinations and illusions may be experienced in reference to the self or the environment. The sensory system involved (auditory, visual, olfactory, or tactile) and the content of the hallucinatory experience should be described. Visual and tactile hallucinations, for instance, may raise suspicions about a possible underlying organic condition. Command hallucinations may be telling the patient to hurt others or the self. The patient's capacity for resisting the demands of command hallucinations should be assessed. The circumstances surrounding any hallucinatory experiences are important because hypnagogic hallucinations (occurring as a person falls asleep) and hypnopompic hallucinations (occurring as a person awakens) are of much less serious significance than other types of hallucinations. Feelings of depersonalization and derealization (extreme feelings of detachment from one's self or the environment) are other examples of perceptual disturbances. Patients who are actively hallucinating may not be able to state directly that they are hallucinating. For instance, a patient's hallucinations may be telling the patient not to speak, or the hallucinations may be so distracting that the patient cannot even hear the questions.

Thought

Thought is divided into process or form and content. Process refers to the way in which a person puts together ideas and associations—that is, the form in which a person thinks. Process of thought may be logical and coherent or completely illogical and even incomprehensible. Content refers to what a person is actually thinking about—ideas, beliefs, preoccupations, obsessions. Table A.2–7 lists common disorders of thought, divided into process and content.

Thought process (form of thinking). Disturbances in the continuity of thought include statements that are tangential, circumstantial, loose, rambling, evasive, or perseverative. Thought process impairments may be reflected in incoherent or incomprehensible connections of thoughts (word salad), clang associations (association by rhyming), punning (association by double meaning), and neologisms (new words created by the patient through the combination or the condensation of other words).

Content of thought. Disturbances in the content of thought that are particularly relevant to a psychiatric emergency patient include delusions,

Table A.2–7
Examples of Disorders of Thought

Process or Form of Thought

Loosening of associations or derailment
Flight of ideas
Racing thoughts
Tangentiality
Circumstantiality
Word salad or incoherence
Neologisms
Clang associations
Punning
Thought blocking
Vague thought

Content of Thought

Delusions
Paranoia
Preoccupations
Obsessions and compulsions
Phobias
Suicidal or homicidal ideas
Ideas of reference and influence
Poverty of content

preoccupations (which may involve the patient's illness), obsessions, compulsions, plans, intentions, recurrent ideas about suicide or homicide, and specific antisocial urges. Specific questions should always be asked about suicidal ideation. Does the patient have thoughts of doing harm to himself or herself? Is there a plan? A major category of disturbances of thought content involves delusions. Delusions are fixed, false beliefs out of keeping with the patient's cultural background. The content of any delusional system should be described, and the examiner should attempt to evaluate its organization and the patient's conviction as to its validity. The manner in which it affects the patient's life is appropriately described in the history of the present illness. For instance, are the patient's delusions driving the patient to act in a potentially dangerous or impulsive way? Delusions may be bizarre and may involve beliefs about external control. Delusions may have themes that are persecutory, paranoid, grandiose, somatic, guilty, nihilistic, or erotic.

Sensorium and Cognition

In general, this portion of the mental status examination seeks to assess organic brain function and the patient's intelligence, capacity for abstract thought, and level of insight and judgment. In the emergency setting the clinician must be particularly concerned with the patient's level of consciousness and orientation in order to rule out any underlying organic pathology. The presence of a significant disorientation or a diminished level of consciousness must be presumed to represent organic pathology until proved otherwise. The Mini-Mental State Examination can be used to quickly and concisely assess the patient's sensorium.

Alertness and level of consciousness. Disturbances of consciousness usually indicate organic brain impairment. The term "clouding of consciousness" describes an overall reduced awareness of the environment. A patient may be unable to sustain attention to environmental stimuli or to sustain goal-directed thinking or behavior. The patient who has an altered state of consciousness often shows some impairment of orientation as well, although the reverse is not necessarily true. Some terms used are clouding, somnolence, stupor, coma, lethargy, alertness, and fugue state.

Orientation. Disorders of orientation are traditionally separated according to time, place, and person. Any impairment usually appears in that order (that is, the sense of time is impaired before the sense of place); similarly, as the patient improves, the impairment clears in the reverse order. The clinician must determine whether patients can give the approximate date and time of day. Do the patients behave as though they are oriented to the present? In questions about the patients' orientation to place, it is not sufficient that they be able to state the name and the location of the hospital correctly; they should also behave as though they know where they are. In assessing orientation for person, the interviewer asks patients whether they know the names of the people around them and whether they understand their roles in relationship to them. Do they know who the examiner is? Do they know their own birthday? It is only in the most severe instances that patients do not know who they themselves are.

Memory. The examiner must try to assess whether the process of registration, retention, or recollection of material is involved. Specific data can be addressed under specific categories of memory: *remote memory:* childhood data, important events known to have occurred when the patient was younger or free of illness, personal matters, neutral material; *recent past memory:* the past few months; *recent memory:* the past few days, what the patient did yesterday and the day before; what the patient had for breakfast, lunch, and dinner; *immediate retention and recall:* digit-span measures of the ability to repeat six figures after the examiner dictates them—first forward, then backward (patients with unimpaired memory can usually repeat six digits backward).

In organic mental syndromes, recent or short-term memory is often impaired first, and remote or long-term memory is impaired later. If there is impairment, what efforts does the patient make to cope with or to conceal impairment? Is denial, confabulation, catastrophic reaction, or circumstantiality used to conceal a deficit? Reactions to the loss of memory can give important clues about underlying disorders and coping mechanisms. For instance, a patient who appears to have memory impairment but, in fact, is depressed is more likely to be concerned about the memory loss than is someone with memory loss secondary to dementia. Confabulation (unconsciously making up false answers when the memory is impaired) is most closely associated with organic mental syndromes.

Concentration. A patient's concentration may be impaired for a variety of reasons. For instance, organic brain disease, anxiety, depression, and such internal stimuli as auditory hallucinations—all may contribute to impaired concentration. Subtracting serial 7s from 100 is a simple task that requires intact concentration and intact cognitive capacities. If patients cannot subtract 7s, they should be asked to subtract 3s. The examiner must always assess whether anxiety or some disturbance of mood, thought, or consciousness or a learning deficit is responsible for the difficulty.

Abstract thinking. The ability of patients to deal with concepts is the focus of attention here. Can patients explain similarities, such as those of an apple and a pear or those of truth and beauty? Do patients understand the meanings of simple proverbs, such as, "A rolling stone gathers no moss?" The appropriateness of the answers and the manner in which the answers are given should be noted. In a catastrophic reaction, brain-damaged patients become extremely emotional and cannot think abstractly.

Fund of information and intelligence. If a possible organic mental impairment is suspected, the physician can inquire whether the patient has trouble with mental tasks, such as counting the change from $10 after a purchase of $6.37. If that task is too difficult, easier problems (such as how many nickels are in $1.35) may be substituted. The patient's educational level (both formal education and self-education) and socioeconomic status must be taken into account. A patient's handling of difficult or sophisticated concepts can be reflective of intelligence, even in the absence of formal education or an extensive fund of information. Patients who are extremely agitated, paranoid, or delusional or who are actively hallucinating may appear to have a lower fund of information or intelligence than they do under less dramatic circumstances.

Impulse Control

Is the patient capable of controlling sexual, aggressive, and other impulses? An assessment of impulse control is critical in an emergency setting to ascertain the patient's awareness of socially appropriate behavior, and it is a critical measure of the patient's potential danger to self and others. Some patients are unable to control impulses secondary to organic mental diseases, others secondary to psychoses, and others as the result of chronic characterological defects, as observed in the personality disorders. Impulse control can be estimated from information in the patient's recent history and from behavior observed during the interview. For example, a patient who walks up to a woman on the street and spits at her when she refuses to give him money is a patient with poor impulse control. A patient who, on entering the emergency room, embraces and kisses the psychiatrist is evincing a poor control of impulses. A patient who is suicidal or homicidal, with markedly impaired judgment, and who also has diminished impulse control is a true psychiatric emergency.

Judgment and Insight

Judgment. During the course of the history taking, the examiner should be able to assess many aspects of patients' abilities to make social judgments. Do the patients understand the likely outcome of their behavior, and are they influenced by that understanding? If not, patients with a significant degree of impairment in judgment may be at markedly increased risk to harm themselves or others. Tests of judgment may involve the patients' predictions of what they would do in imaginary situations. For instance, a patient may be asked, "What would you do if you smelled smoke in a crowded movie theater?" In most emergency situations the clinician should have a sense of the patient's level of judgment without having to ask judgment questions. For instance, a patient who is brought in by the police after being found naked on the street or wandering on the subway tracks has grossly impaired judgment and is at markedly increased risk to self. Patients whose judgment is impaired by intrusive paranoid delusions and hallucinations may walk the streets with an iron club, waiting to defend themselves against imagined threats, and are obviously at increased risk to hurt others. A patient with organic brain impairment may be disinhibited because of damage to the frontal lobes and, thus, may act in a manner that shows poor judgment (for example, masturbating in public).

Insight. Insight refers to patients' degree of awareness and understanding of what is happening to them and why. Patients may exhibit a complete denial of their illness or may show some awareness that they are ill but place the blame on others, on external factors, or even on organic medical, rather than psychological, factors. They may acknowledge that they have an illness but ascribe it to something unknown or mysterious in themselves. Most patients in an emergency situation have some degree of diminished insight. Impaired insight, especially when coupled with impaired judgment, can lead a patient to act out behaviors that are potentially dangerous. For instance, patients with no insight into the delusional nature of their paranoid beliefs may act in aggressive ways toward others.

Reliability

The mental status part of the report concludes with the examiner's impressions of the patients' reliability and capacity to report the situation accurately. It includes an estimate of the examiner's impression of the patient's truthfulness or veracity. For instance, if the patient is open about significant active substance abuse or about circumstances that the patient knows may reflect badly (for example, trouble with the law), the examiner may estimate the patient's reliability to be good. A patient who denies having pushed a person on the street, even though the incident was observed by several people, is judged not to be reliable.

FURTHER DIAGNOSTIC STUDIES

When the examiner has completed a comprehensive psychiatric history and mental status examination, the question of what further diagnostic studies should be performed can be specifically addressed. Further investigations that are necessary to fully work up the psychiatric emergency patient include (1) a full physical examination; (2) additional psychiatric diagnostic interviews; (3) interviews by a social worker with the patient's family members, friends, or neighbors; and (4) psychological, neurological

(Table A.2–8), or laboratory tests as indicated (for example, an electroencephalogram [EEG], a computed tomography [CT] scan, tests of other medical conditions, reading comprehension and writing tests, tests for aphasia, projective psychological tests, a dexamethasone-suppression test [DST], and drug screens).

Table A.2–8
Basic Neurological Testing
(Appropriate in assessment of psychiatric emergency patient as indicated)

I. High cortical functions

A. Observation
Behavior
Mood and affect
Speech and use of language
Quality of articulation
Choice of words
Coherence of thought
Attention
Response time
Memory for events

B. Specific bedside tests

1. Orientation	Person:	What is your name?
		Your current location?
		Are you married?
		Type of work?
	Place:	Where are you now?
		How did you get here?
	Time:	What is the date today?
		(year, month, day of week, and month)
		What are the season's recent holidays?
2. Attention	Repetition of digits, forward and reverse	
Concentration	Serial subtracting of 7s or 3s from 100	
General memory	Tests of simple arithmetic	
	Recall of three items after five minutes	
	Listing of last six presidents	
3. Specific memory	Remote:	Names of children, birthdates, dates of marriage, mother's maiden name
	Recent past:	Recall of events over past few months
	Recent:	Breakfast, tests performed yesterday, newspaper headlines, examiner's name
	Immediate:	Repetition digits forward and reverse
4. Speech and language	Name the parts of a wristwatch	
Choice of words	Follow two- and three-step commands	
Articulation	Read out loud	
	Write a paragraph	
5. Visual-spatial	Draw a clock face	
Visual-motor	Copy figures	
	Bisect a line	

II. Motor, sensory, and reflex functions

(Note speed, strength, and coordination of movements)

A. Observation
Gait
Stance

Table A.2–8—*continued*

A. Observation—*continued*

Presence or absence of tremor
Involuntary movements
Abnormalities of muscle tone
Coordination

B. Specific bedside tests

1. Holding up both arms or legs against gravity
2. Rapid alternating movements
3. Alternating touching the patient's nose and the examiner's finger
4. Buttoning clothes
5. Opening and closing a safety pin
6. Standing on toes and heels
7. Running heel down shin
8. Reflex testing: biceps, triceps, supinator, patellar, achilles, plantar

III. Cranial nerves and special senses

A. Observation

Symmetry of facial muscles
Facial expression
Abnormal movements of tongue, mouth, jaw, eyes, face
Eye movements and pupil size
Ability to hear spoken words or sounds
Ability to smell commonplace odors

B. Specific bedside tests

1. Smell	Determine odor of soap, coffee, tobacco, and vanilla in each nostril		
2. Sight	Visual fields:	Confrontation testing	
	Pupils:	Size, reactivity to light, accommodation	
	Ocular movements:	Range and quality	
	Optic fundi:	Careful inspection	
3. Hearing	Tuning fork tests		
	Formal audiograms		
4. Face	Sensation:	Pin and wisp of cotton	
		Corneal reflexes	
	Musculatare:	Wrinkle forehead, show teeth, forcibly close eyes and lips	
5. Tongue	Inspection for discoloration, loss of papillae, atrophy, fasiculations		
6. Jaw	Jaw jerk, buccal and sucking reflexes		

3 / Medical Conditions in the Psychiatric Emergency Room

A primary responsibility of the emergency psychiatrist is to rule out the possibility of organic disease masquerading as functional illness. Also, medical conditions may coexist with recognized psychiatric problems. Studies have shown that 5 to 30 percent of all patients presenting to emergency rooms with self-referred psychiatric complaints and patients already screened by clinical staff members and referred for psychiatric evaluation have physical problems serious enough to affect the clinical picture and require treatment. The identification of such problems often leads to rapid, definitive, and sometimes lifesaving treatment. The failure to consider those possibilities in making a differential diagnosis may lead to unnecessary delays in appropriate treatment, inappropriate treatment, unacceptable patient suffering, or even death. At a minimum, the implications for cost effectiveness, medicolegal concerns, and stigmatization associated with psychiatric labeling are enormous.

The emergency psychiatrist must remain up-to-date regarding general medical knowledge and maintain good working relationships with other specialists. A psychiatric diagnosis should be made only after all possible organic causes have been considered. The medical evaluation—including the patient's history, physical examination, and appropriate ancillary testing—is a fundamental component of a comprehensive psychiatric assessment. The medical evaluation should not be deferred except in rare cases when the patient's or the clinician's safety is at stake—for example, in cases of catatonic excitement. Deferral of the medical evaluation only delays the implementation of the most appropriate treatment plan and may decrease the likelihood of identifying important clinical conditions. The validity of certain tests, such as toxicology screening tests, diminishes rapidly over the course of several hours.

MEDICAL EVALUATION

The emergency evaluation is not expected to be definitive. However, every effort should be made to gather as much information as possible about the patient, the acute phase of the illness, and any underlying medical problems. Generally, the psychiatric evaluation is conducted before the medical examination, but the emergency psychiatrist or a proxy—such as an internist, a physician's assistant, or a nurse practitioner—must be flexible, pragmatic, and sensitive in the approach to the patient. The triage psychiatrist can quickly determine which patients require the most urgent attention and whether psychiatric or medical evaluation should be the initial focus. The psychiatrist should decide on the most appropriate treatment setting—the psychiatric emergency room, the medical emergency service, the doctor's office, or a clinic.

The comprehensive emergency evaluation may include input from a variety of disciplines and specialists, but the psychiatrist has ultimate responsibility for the patient. Referrals are often made to the psychiatrist after the patient has been medically cleared by another physician. Medical clearance generally refers to the relative condition of the patient—that is, whether the patient is stable enough to be transferred or needs a definitive physical assessment. Because of an unfortunate tendency of many nonpsychiatrists to ascribe complaints of patients labeled psychiatric to psychological causes, the emergency psychiatrist must maintain a high index of suspicion for organic disease, especially in the evaluation of acute psychotic states. "Psychotic" is not synonymous with "psychiatric." Regardless of how frightening or uncooperative the patient may be, the physician must consider the possibility of a medical cause.

Similarly, some psychiatrists are not interested in medical problems or comfortable in treating them. The psychiatrist, the physician of record, must continue to assess the patient for possible organic pathology throughout the patient's stay in the emergency room.

As always, diagnosis is most accurate when it is made on the basis of a thorough history, a complete physical examination, and corroborating laboratory tests. The constraints of the emergency room setting and the confusing picture of the patient in extremis complicate the task of the diagnostician. Patients may be unable or unwilling to give a history. A patient confined in physical restraints is difficult to examine. Paranoia may need to be addressed before a patient consents to give a blood sample.

Recommendations

1. All patients coming from other treatment settings—a medical emergency room, an emergency medical service in the field, a private office—should be sent with copies of their evaluations and findings. The referring clinician is expected to call ahead to discuss the case and the reasons for the referral.

2. Request old records, including nonpsychiatric hospital admissions and clinic visits, on the patient's arrival in the emergency room.

3. Make translators available as needed.

4. Have male and female clinicians on duty to make the patient as comfortable as possible and to minimize possible charges of sexual impropriety during the physical examination.

5. Perform whatever measures are necessary to make an adequate assessment, while respecting the patient and the patient's wishes. Include emergency diagnostic testing and the control of violent behavior. Laws and legal precedents are clear, as the measures pertain to the medical evaluation of the emergency service patient.

Mental Status Examination

The mental status examination is an invaluable part of the medical assessment, as well as of the psychiatric evaluation. When a patient is unable or unwilling to give a medical or psychiatric history, the mental status examination is crucial. Many physical problems—for example, thyroid disease and brain tumors—may be suspected on the basis of a good mental status examination.

Consultation

Consultation with other medical specialists should be available to the emergency psychiatrist. A consultation can clarify or complete the initial evaluation of the patient and allow for the most comprehensive treatment to be started as early as possible. The consultant may also delineate whatever further diagnostic work is required.

Vital Signs

Vital signs, at intervals of every two to eight hours, can be helpful in monitoring the patient's physical condition. They may also have diagnostic significance. Tracking a pattern of changing vital signs over the course of several hours often confirms an initial impression of acute intoxication or withdrawal.

LABORATORY AND OTHER ANCILLARY TESTS

The mental and physical condition of the patient in acute distress and the busy condition of the emergency room often make a traditional evaluation of the patient difficult. Therefore, laboratory and other ancillary tests may take on added importance in the emergency setting. To heighten the probability of diagnostic accuracy and to address the less emergent but often undertreated medical problems of the patient who is chronically mentally ill and who uses the emergency room as a de facto primary care office, the psychiatrist should consider the following battery of initial screening tests, supplemented by additional tests ordered on the basis of the physician's clinical judgment:

1. Blood tests: sequential multichannel autoanalyzer (SMA) 12; complete blood count (CBC) with differential; toxicology screening, especially for alcohol, cocaine, and opiates; pregnancy test for all women of childbearing age; thyroid function studies; liver enzyme studies
2. Urinalysis
3. Chest X-ray at least every 6 to 12 months
4. Electrocardiogram (ECG)

The clinical usefulness of most of those tests is obvious, but several points as they pertain to the delivery of psychiatric care must be stressed. Infection control—as a public health concern for the individual patient, the inpatient unit patient population, and health care workers—cannot be overemphasized. In addition to such high-profile infectious diseases as acquired immune deficiency syndrome (AIDS), hepatitis B, and treatment-resistant strains of tuberculosis, less publicized illnesses, such as chicken pox and measles, and such infestations as lice and scabies are on the rise. Outbreaks of even isolated cases of such diseases can lead to a quarantine and an increased length of stay for otherwise healthy patients or the closure of the entire inpatient unit, with a resulting reduction in hospital bed capacity. The effects on lost work time for staff members may also be serious.

Not all tests need be repeated each time a patient presents in the emergency room. In view of the high percentage of repeat visitors coming to the emergency room (in some populations up to 66 percent), the value of reviewing previous records is clear. Checking for documentation of a positive varicella titer can reduce costs, save time, and allow for a safe assignment to an inpatient bed. However, chest X-rays to monitor tuberculosis, chronic obstructive pulmonary disease, and lung cancer, for example, should be repeated every six months to a year. It makes sense to think of the emergency room as a public health station, since many patients use it in that way.

It is not necessary to delay a patient's hospital admission until all test results are obtained, especially in nonemergency cases. However, it is advantageous to perform all tests as early in the hospital course as possible.

The number of pregnant women, including those with previously unconfirmed pregnancies, presenting to psychiatric emergency rooms is usually low, but blood pregnancy testing should be performed on all girls and women of childbearing age. The public health concerns regarding unmanageable or unwanted pregnancies, unfit parents, and babies addicted to alcohol and drugs justify that relatively inexpensive test. Treatment decisions, especially the need to delay treatment in cases of suspected pregnancy, can be made with confidence once the pregnancy issue has been confirmed either way.

COMMON ORGANIC CONDITIONS

The most common organic conditions diagnosed in the psychiatric emergency room are listed in Table A.3–1. Cases of alcohol and drug abuse, presenting as acute intoxications and states of withdrawal, are far and away the most common conditions and are often the most difficult ones to diagnose. Of all hospital patients, 40 to 60 percent suffer from substance abuse as a primary or secondary diagnosis. A commonly used method of tracking the number of substance-abusing patients in the general population is based on the frequency of overdose presentations in the emergency room. The emergency psychiatrist must be vigilant to the possible causative and complicating effects of those problems on the patient. Acute intoxications and withdrawal states are potential medical emergencies and are best managed in the medical emergency room. After a six-to-eight-hour period of observation in the medical emergency room, most patients can be safely managed in a psychiatric setting.

Endocrine disease and other multiorgan system conditions, because of their confusing symptom pictures and shifting areas of acuity, are often prematurely and inaccurately diagnosed as functional illness. The emergency psychiatrist must consider all possibilities during the initial assessment.

Depression is the most common psychiatric disorder and the one most often confused with medical illness. It is usually a component of a serious physical illness or a reaction to it. All physicians should be aware of the possibility of depression and prepared to treat the patient as needed.

Organic Conditions Associated with Chronic Mental Illness

A significant number of emergency room visits are made by a relatively stable group of persons with chronic mental illnesses. They are often elderly, treatment-resistant, and homeless or living on the margins of society and were previously institutionalized. They may be dually afflicted with chronic substance-abuse problems, such as alcoholism and cigarette smoking, and the physical sequelae of those problems. In addition to those risk factors for chronic medical problems, their psychiatric symptoms often cause them to be unable or unwilling to live their lives at even the most basic level of

TABLE A.3–1
Organic Conditions Presenting in the Psychiatric Emergency Room

Disease	Common Medical Symptoms	Psychiatric Symptoms and Complaints	Impaired Performance and Behavior	Laboratory Tests and Findings	Diagnostic Problems
Hyperthyroidism	Heat intolerance Excessive sweating Diarrhea Weight loss Tachycardia Palpitations Vomiting	Nervousness Excitability Irritability Pressured speech Insomnia May express fear of impending death Psychosis	Fine tremor Impaired cognition Decreased concentration Hyperactivity Intrusiveness	Free T_4 increased T_3 increased TSH decreased T_3 uptake decreased ECG: Tachycardia Atrial fibrillation P and T wave changes	Full range of symptoms may not be present Hyperthyroidism and anxiety states may coexist Rule out occult malignancy, cardiovascular disease, amphetamine intoxication, cocaine intoxication, anxiety states, mania
Hypothyroidism	Cold intolerance Dry skin Constipation Weight gain Brittle hair Goiter	Lethargy Depressed affect Personality change Maniclike psychosis Paranoia Hallucinations	Muscle weakness Decreased concentration Psychomotor slowing Apathy Unusual sensitivity to barbiturates	TSH increased TSH low if pituitary disease Free T_4 ECG: Bradycardia	More common in women Associated with lithium carbonate therapy Rule out pituitary disease, hypothalamic disease, major depression, bipolar disorder
Hypoglycemia	Sweating Drowsiness Stupor Coma Tachycardia	Anxiety Confusion Agitation	Tremor Restlessness Seizures	Hypoglycemia Tachycardia	Excess insulin often complicated by exercise, alcohol, decreased food intake Rule out insulinoma, postictal states, agitated depression, paranoid psychosis
Hyperglycemia	Polyuria Anorexia Nausea Vomiting Dehydration Abdominal complaints	Anxiety Agitation Delirium	Acetone breath Seizures	Hyperglycemia Serum ketones Urine ketones Anion gap acidosis	Almost always associated with brittle diabetes in young juvenile diabetics and elderly non-insulin-dependent diabetics Rule out depressive states, anxiety states

Brain neoplasms	Headache Vomiting Papilledema Focal findings on neurology examination	Personality changes		Lumbar puncture: increased CSF pressure, skull X-ray, CT scan, EEG	40–50% gliomas most common in 40–50-year age group Cerebellar tumors most common in children Rule out intracranial abscess, aneurysm, subdural hematoma, seizure disorder, cerebrovascular disease, reactive depression, mania, schizophreniform disorder, dementia
Frontal lobe tumor		Mood changes Irritability Facetiousness Impaired judgment Impaired memory Delirium	Seizures Loss of speech Loss of smell	Angiogram: space-occupying lesion	
Parietal lobe tumor	Hyperreflexia Babinski's sign Astereognosis		Sensory and motor abnormalities Contralateral hemiparesis Focal seizures Visual problems Seizures		
Occipital lobe tumor	Headache Papilledema Homonymous hemianopsia Contralateral homonymous field cut Early evidence of increased intracranial pressure Papilledema	Aura Visual hallucinations			
Temporal lobe tumor			Psychomotor seizures Aphasia		
Cerebellar tumor			Disturbed equilibrium Disturbed coordination		
Head trauma	History or evidence of head trauma Headache Dizziness Bleeding from ear Altered level of consciousness Loss of consciousness Focal neurological findings	Confusion Personality changes Memory impairment	Seizures Paralysis	Lumbar puncture, skull X-rays, CT scan show evidence of bleeding or increased intracranial pressure Cerebral angiogram EEG	History of blow to head or bleeding confirms cause of ALS Rule out cerebrovascular disease, seizure disorder, alcoholism, diabetes mellitus, hepatic encephalopathy, depression, dementia

TABLE A.3-1—*continued*

Disease	Common Medical Symptoms	Psychiatric Symptoms and Complaints	Impaired Performance and Behavior	Laboratory Tests and Findings	Diagnostic Problems
AIDS	Fever Weight loss Ataxia Incontinence Focal findings on neurological examination	Progressive dementia Personality changes Depression Loss of libido Psychosis Mutism	Impaired memory Decreased concentration Seizures	HIV testing CT, MRI, lumbar puncture, CSF, and blood cultures	>60% of patients have neuropsychiatric symptoms; always consider in high-risk populations and young patients with signs of dementia Rule out other infections, brain neoplasms, presenile dementia, depression, schizophreniform disorder
Injuries requiring ambulatory surgical evaluation and treatment (for example, wrist slashing)	Alcoholism and other substance abuse Recent surgery Chronic pain Chronic illness Terminal illness	>90% have major psychiatric disease History of prior suicide attempts Depressed mood Postpartum psychosis in women	Frequent accidents Repeated emergency room visits Eager to leave emergency room prior to full evaluation		Suicidal behavior is a symptom of underlying psychiatric illness Knowledge of risk factors is helpful but not a substitute for good clinical judgment Prediction is best done through assessment of current risk projected into the immediate future

Hyponatremia	Excessive thirst Polydipsia Stupor Coma	Confusion Lethargy Personality changes	Seizures Speech abnormalities	Decreased serum Na$^+$ Serum Na$^+$ and osmolalities to document syndrome of inappropriate secretion of antidiuretic hormone (SIADH)	Caused by excessive free water for level of total body Na$^+$ Often abnormal SIADH May be psychogenic Rule out nephrotic syndrome, liver disease, congestive heart failure, schizophreniform disorder, schizotypal personality disorder
Pancreatic carcinoma	Weight loss Abdominal pain	Depression Lethargy Anhedonia	Apathy Decreased energy	Elevated amylase	Always consider in depressed middle-aged patients Rule out other GI illness, major depression
Cushing's syndrome	Central obesity Purple striae Easy bruising Osteoporosis Proximal muscle weakness Hirsutism	Depression Insomnia Emotional lability Suicidality Euphoria Mania Psychosis Delirium	Disturbed sleep Decreased energy Agitation Difficulty in concentrating	Elevated blood pressure Poor glucose tolerance Dexamethasone-suppression test (may be falsely positive)	Must distinguish other causes—for example, cancer from exogenous steroid excess Suicide rate in untreated cases is about 10% Rule out major depression, bipolar disorder
Adrenocortical insufficiency	Nausea Vomiting Anorexia Stupor Coma Hyperpigmentation	Lethargy Depression Psychosis Delirium	Fatigue	Decreased blood pressure Decreased Na$^+$ Increased K$^+$ Eosinophilia	May be primary (Addison's disease) or secondary Rule out eating disorders, mood disorder
Seizure disorder	Sensory distortions Aura	Confusion Psychosis Dissociative states Catatoniclike state	Violence Motor automatisms Belligerence Bizarre behavior	EEG, including NP leads	Consider complex partial seizures in all dissociative states Rule out postictal states, catatonic schizophrenia

TABLE A.3–1—*continued*

Disease	Common Medical Symptoms	Psychiatric Symptoms and Complaints	Impaired Performance and Behavior	Laboratory Tests and Findings	Diagnostic Problems
Hyperparathyroidism	Constipation Polydipsia Nausea	Depression Paranoia Confusion		Increased Ca^{++} PTH variable ECG: shortened QT interval	Causes hypercalcemia Rule out major depression, schizoaffective disorder
Hypoparathyroidism	Headache Paresthesias Tetany Carpopedal spasm Laryngeal spasm Abdominal pain	Anxiety Agitation Depression Confusion	Impaired memory	Low Ca^{++}, normal albumin Low blood pressure ECG: QT prolongation, ventricular arrythmias	Causes hypocalcemia Rule out anxiety disorder, mood disorder
Systemic lupus erythematosus	Fever Photosensitivity Butterfly rash Joint pains Headache	Depression Mood disturbances Psychosis Delusions Hallucinations	Fatigue	Positive ANA Positive lupus erythematosus test Anemia Thrombocytopenia Chest X-ray: pleural effusion, pericarditis	Multisystemic autoimmune disease most frequent in women Psychiatric symptoms are present in 50% of cases Steroid treatment can cause psychiatric symptoms Rule out depression, paranoid psychosis, psychotic mood disorder
Multiple sclerosis	Sudden transient motor and sensory disturbances Impaired vision Diffuse neurological signs with remissions and exacerbations	Anxiety Euphoria Mania	Slurred speech Incontinence	CSF may show increased gamma globulin CT: degenerative patches in brain and spinal cord	Onset usually in young adults Rule out tertiary syphillis, other degenerative disease, hysteria, mania (late)

Condition	Physical Findings	Psychiatric/Mental	Symptoms	Laboratory	Comments
Acute intermittent porphyria	Abdominal pain Fever Nausea Vomiting Constipation Peripheral neuropathy Paralysis	Acute depression Agitation Paranoia Visual hallucinations	Restlessness Diaphoresis Weakness	Leukocytosis Elevated δ-aminolevulinic acid Elevated porphobilinogen Tachycardia	Autosomal dominant More common in women in the 20–40 age group May be precipitated by a variety of drugs Rule out acute abdominal disease, acute psychiatric episode, schizophreniform disorder, major depression
Hepatic encephalopathy	Asterixis Hyperreflexia Spider angiomata Palmar erythema Ecchymoses Liver enlargement and atrophy	Euphoria Disinhibition Psychosis Depression	Restlessness Decreased activities of daily living (ADL) Impaired cognition Impaired concentration Ataxia Dysarthria	Abnormal liver function test results Abnormal albumin EEG: diffuse slowing	May be acute or chronic depending on cause Rule out intoxication, mania, depression, dementia
Injuries requiring inpatient surgical evaluation and treatment (for example, suicide attempts, self-mutilation)	Alcoholism and other substance abuse Serious injury Major blood loss Damage to genitals, eyes, face, etc	99% have severe psychiatric disease associated with psychosis, psychotic depression Impaired mental status secondary to intoxication Bizarre, inappropriate affect	Remain at great risk for suicide		Must assess and treat the underlying psychiatric condition on a priority basis Maintain a high index of suspicion for suicide risk
Pheochromocytoma	Paroxsysmal hypertension Headache	Anxiety Apprehension Feeling of impending doom	Panic Diaphoresis Tremor	Hypertension Elevated VMA in 24-hr. urine Tachycardia	Adrenal medulla secreting catecholamines Rule out anxiety, panic disorder

TABLE A.3-1—*continued*

Disease	Common Medical Symptoms	Psychiatric Symptoms and Complaints	Impaired Performance and Behavior	Laboratory Tests and Findings	Diagnostic Problems
Wilson's disease	Kayser-Fleischer corneal ring Hepatitislike picture	Mood disturbances Delusions Hallucinations	Choreoathetoid movements Gait disturbance Clumsiness Rigidity	Decreased serum ceruloplasm Increased copper in urine	Hepatolenticular degeneration Autosomal recessive disorder of copper metabolism Often presents in adolescence, early adulthood Rule out extrapyramidal reactions, schizophreniform disorder, mood disorder
Huntington's chorea	Family history	Depression Euphoria	Rigidity Choreoathetoid movements		Autosomal dominant Rule out mood disorder, mania, schizophrenia
Vitamin deficiencies Thiamine	Neuropathy Cardiomyopathy Wernike-Korsakoff syndrome Nystagmus Headache Amnesia	Confusion Confabulation	General malaise Inability to sustain a conversation Poor concentration	Low thiamine level	Most common in alcoholics Rule out hypomania, depression, presenile dementia
Nicotinamide	Diarrhea Stocking-glove dermatitis	Confusion Irritability Insomnia Depression Psychosis Dementia	Memory disturbances		Rule out mood disorder, mania, schizophreniform disorder, presenile dementia

Pyridoxine		Apathy Irritability	Memory disturbance Muscle weakness Seizures		Often caused by medication: isoniazed Rule out mood disorder, presenile dementia
Vitamin B_{12}	Pallor Dizziness Peripheral neuropathy Dorsal column signs	Irritability Inattentiveness Psychosis Dementia	Fatigue Ataxia	Low B_{12} level Schilling test Megaloblastic anemia	Often due to pernicious anemia Rule out presenile dementia, mania, mood disorder
Tertiary syphilis	Skin lesions Leukoplakia Periostitis Arthritis Respiratory distress Progressive cardiovascular distress	Personality changes Irritability Confusion Psychosis	Irresponsible behavior Decreased attention to activities of daily living (ADL)	VDRL, Treponema antibody test CSF abnormal	General paresis Rule out neoplasias, meningitis, presenile dementia, psychotic mood disorder, schizophrenia

Table A.3–2
Organic Conditions Associated with Chronic Mental Illness

Hypertension
Diabetes mellitus
Malnutrition
Vitamin deficiencies
Exposure: Hypothermia
            Hyperthermia
Stasis ulcers
Tuberculosis
Venereal diseases
Gynecological disease
Occult malignancies: breast cancer
Infestations

personal hygiene. They often lack routine general medical care. They are often the victims of rape and other assaults. They are subject to malnutrition, exposure to the elements, and overcrowding.

The emergency physician must be alert to the likelihood that acutely decompensated patients with chronic mental illnesses are afflicted by one or more of the conditions listed in Table A.3–2. The physician must consider those conditions as important parts of the differential diagnosis of such common conditions as major depression, chronic anemia, presenile dementia, senile dementia, and vitamin deficiencies. The physician must be prepared to treat such illnesses as hypertension and active tuberculosis. Most often, the physician should be prepared to recommend further evaluation or treatment while the patient is on an inpatient unit or in a clinic. Such diagnoses as venereal disease, hypertension, and breast disease, if overlooked during the initial medical evaluation, may go untreated for the remainder of the patient's hospitalization.

Psychiatrists are prone to consider the patient designated medically cleared as physically sound. And there is the risk of countertransference reactions and resultant inadequate evaluations in working with such patients. The emergency physician is challenged by the complex and confusing picture of physical problems that are often not mentioned by the patient or detected by other clinicians, as well as by the full range of psychiatric symptoms. It is the doctor's duty to meet both challenges in work with all patients.

4 / Telephonic Emergency Psychiatric Medicine

The telephone has become an increasingly important tool in emergency psychiatric medicine. The patient's first contact with a psychiatrist frequently takes place over the telephone. The nature of such encounters runs the gamut from the mildly anxious or depressed person who is taking the first step toward psychotherapy to desperate calls for help from psychotic or suicidal persons. The management of the initial encounter may have profound effects on the outcome of the crisis. The emergency physician may also receive calls from patients who are not genuinely in crisis. Those calls may be a dependent patient's attempts to receive reassurance from the therapist, a hostile patient's attempts to annoy or intimidate the therapist, or frank malingering.

Hotlines are 24-hour telephone services, usually staffed by trained nonprofessionals, that provide support, counsel, or referral for persons in a wide range of crisis situations. Suicide hotlines field calls from persons who are thinking of killing themselves or who have already initiated an attempt. Similar hotlines have been set up to help the victims and the perpetrators of abuse, the victims of natural disasters, persons with substance abuse problems, persons with fears and questions about acquired immune deficiency syndrome (AIDS), and many others (Table A.4–1).

Telepsychiatry is the use of conventional telephones and the new videotelephone technology in the diagnosis and the treatment of psychiatric illness. It is especially useful in rural areas where a single psychiatrist serves a large or difficult-to-reach area. In such settings, evaluation, treatment planning, and even brief psychotherapy may take place over the telephone. The psychiatrist may advise a nonpsychiatric physician by telephone how to manage an emergency.

GUIDELINES FOR TELEPHONE ASSESSMENT

Regardless of the setting—private office, hospital emergency room, telephone hotline, or telephonic psychiatric emergency service—certain basic principles should guide the physician who is evaluating a patient over the telephone.

Identifying Data

The physician should obtain identifying data—name, age, telephone number, number the patient is calling from, and address—as early as possible. Many patients readily comply with requests for information about themselves, but some patients resist revealing basic information. Some psychiatrists advocate terminating the telephone contact if patients refuse to reveal their identities in the belief that the callers are not genuinely seeking help but are using the telephone service in a hostile or manipulative way. However, that may not always be the case. Patients who are ashamed of their symptoms may try to conceal their identities, as may paranoid patients. Patients who are ambivalent about their urges to harm themselves or others reveal that ambivalence in their refusal to identify themselves.

If the caller refuses to provide identifying data, the emergency psychiatrist should try to establish rapport by eliciting the reasons for the call and the source of the caller's distress. If callers present a clear and present danger to themselves or to others, the physician must persist in trying to obtain the name, telephone number, and location. The clinician should ask the patients why they feel they must conceal their identities, and address the patients' concerns promptly. Some common concerns center on issues of

Table A.4-1
Selected Hotlines for Psychiatric Emergencies*

AIDS Hotline	1-800-342-2437
Alcohol 24 hour National Helpline	1-310-983-8383
Alzheimer's Disease and Related Disorders Association	1-800-272-3900
Child Abuse and Neglect Information Prevention Resource Center	1-800-342-7472
Child Abuse Hotline	1-800-422-4453
Council on Compulsive Gambling	1-800-426-2537
800 Cocaine Information	1-800-262-2463
Epilepsy Foundation of America	1-800-332-1000
National Council on Compulsive Gambling	1-800-522-4700
National Food Addiction Hotline	1-800-872-0088
National Runaway Switchboard	1-800-621-4000
Parents Anonymous	1-800-421-0353
Runaway Hotline	1-800-231-6946
Suicide Prevention Center	1-310-983-8383

*These phone numbers are subject to change at any time.

confidentiality, involuntary hospitalization, and being forced to take medication.

Reason for Call

The physician should give patients an opportunity to tell the reason for the call and to describe their present state. As in any evaluation, the psychiatrist elicits a chief complaint and a history of the present illness. In the emergency setting the most obvious dangers are suicidality and outwardly directed aggression. If the patient does not spontaneously discuss those thoughts, the psychiatrist should ask about suicidal and homicidal ideation. If such ideation is elicited, a thorough assessment must be completed: Does the patient have a plan? Does the patient have the means—a gun, poison, hoarded pills? Does the patient have lethal intent? Does the patient want to die? Has the patient already taken action on suicidal or aggressive ideation? Has the patient made any past attempts?

Patients who have suicidal ideation without a plan or intent frequently respond to support, reassurance, and suggestions to follow up their telephone call with a visit to a clinic to see a psychiatrist.

If patients have suicide plans or if they have already made suicide attempts, the physician must contact the police right away. If possible, the psychiatrist should ask a colleague to make the call to the police so that the psychiatrist can keep the caller on the line. If that is not possible, tell patients that you will call them back shortly, and then call the police. Afterward, remain in continuous telephone contact with the patients until the police arrive.

Expectations

What are the patient's expectations—the underlying reason for the call? What kind of help is the patient asking for? Are the expectations realistic? Some patients want the clinician to keep them from acting on dangerous impulses. Conflicts—largely unconscious—regarding dependence and autonomy may be acted out in the crisis situation, and the physician should keep that in mind so as not to be drawn into such enactments.

Support System

The physician should determine if the patient has a support system and, if so, how to contact those people. If the situation warrants, tell the patient that you or a colleague will contact the persons named. If the patient has no support system, ask if there is a neighbor or someone in the vicinity who can be contacted to help the patient get to a hospital or a doctor's office. Similarly, find out if the patient has a regular psychiatrist or psychotherapist and the name and telephone number of that person.

If the patient is neither suicidal nor homicidal but is in a life crisis, the psychiatrist can sometimes provide significant aid by allowing the patient to talk about the crisis over the telephone and exploring different behavioral options.

Patients with chronic psychiatric illnesses, such as schizophrenia and bipolar disorder, are often able to detect an incipient decompensation. They may call the emergency service complaining of an exacerbation or a resurgence of psychotic or depressive symptoms. Some of those patients may use the telephone contact to obtain immediate relief; others may be fearful of coming to the hospital because of previous negative experiences with involuntary hospitalizations. Ask the patient about any recent life events that may have precipitated the decompensation. Ask the patient about as-required (PRN) medications, and try to determine if the patient has been compliant with treatment.

Severely ill psychiatric patients have impaired coping skills, and it may be both appropriate and necessary to offer concrete advice in many instances. The patient may need help in obtaining social services or entitlements—finding low-fee or no-fee psychiatric care, for example. The psychiatrist may make small alterations in the patient's medications. Patients who are taking low-dose maintenance antipsychotics can be instructed to increase their dosage or to take an extra dose until they can be reevaluated by their regular physician.

Some patients use a telephone emergency service to help with overwhelming anxiety, panic attacks, and phobias. Most of those patients respond to simple reassurance and appreciate empathic support and referral to outpatient treatment.

NONEMERGENCIES

Legitimate Nonemergencies

Patients with no other resources may call the emergency service with fairly straightforward questions. They may have questions about their medications, about side effects, or about drug interactions. Other patients may call with a request for a referral to a clinic or a private practitioner. Such questions can be answered factually with information or an appropriate referral.

Annoyance Calls

Some patients use the telephone emergency service for gratification of other needs, rather than for seeking help. Lonely, socially isolated patients may repeatedly call hotlines and emergency rooms just to talk. Patients with telephone paraphilias have been known to make obscene phone calls to psychiatrists, hospitals, and hotlines. Patients with severe personality disorders may call with empty suicide threats, attempting to drag the psychiatrist into enactments of their chaotic inner lives. Most psychiatrists agree that there is little benefit to the patient in prolonging those contacts. Such patients should be told that they are in need of psychiatric help and told to go to the hospital or clinic.

DOCUMENTATION

As with patient contacts in the hospital, telephone evaluations must be documented. The caller's name, address, telephone number, age, and sex and the date and the time of the call should be recorded. The physician should then write a brief synopsis of the conversation, carefully documenting the assessment of the patient's dangerousness to self or to others. The treatment plan should also be placed in the record.

---

5 / Legal Issues In Emergency Psychiatric Medicine

Psychiatric emergencies require immediate intervention to prevent death or serious harm to the patient or to others and usually occur in seconds or minutes (rarely, hours), rather than days or weeks. Elements of both time and severity are involved. Therefore, the legal system gives clinicians considerable leeway and the benefit of doubt for their customary interventions in genuine emergencies. The physician practicing in an emergency room can be reassured that the law is neither capricious nor counter to common sense in that setting.

ELEMENTS OF MALPRACTICE

A given intervention is an example of malpractice only if the patient can prove that the four elements—the "four Ds"—of malpractice are present. The four Ds are Dereliction (negligence) of a Duty Directly causing Damages. Thus, a patient must prove (1) a provider's duty of care, (2) the breaching of that duty, (3) an injury to the patient, and (4) that the injury was the direct result of the duty's being breached.

Dereliction or Negligence

Dereliction is a failure to do something that would normally be done under similar circumstances by other reasonable persons. A typical standard is the level of care practiced by the average psychiatrist under the same or similar circumstances. For example, if patients in the emergency room state that they have plans to kill themselves and they are not admitted to the hospital, that would be dereliction.

Duty

The element of duty raises both factual and legal issues. For instance, did the specific provider owe a duty of care to the particular patient; if the answer is yes, what is the standard of care by which that duty should be measured? In general, the physician's duty is to provide appropriate care to the patient; a common requirement is that the care provided be given in good faith, with the patient's best interests in mind. A duty is created whenever care is offered, explicitly or implicitly, and it persists until treatment is formally terminated. A patient who enters the emergency room but who is never seen or evaluated has not been treated in a dutiful manner by the physician.

Direct Causation

For malpractice to be proved, a direct cause-and-effect relation must exist between the physician's actions or nonactions and the patient's injuries. Giving an already intoxicated patient a large dose of a benzodiazepine, resulting in respiratory depression, is an example of direct causation.

Damages

For malpractice to exist, actual damage—that is, harm—must occur. Examples of damages or harm are physical injury, emotional harm, and death.

COMMON FORMS OF MALPRACTICE

Suicide

Suicide is by far the most common reason for a malpractice claim. The emergency room psychiatrist must be vigilant for signs and symptoms indicative of suicidal risk. A number of questions arise about the psychiatrist's ability to determine the likelihood of suicide. For instance, what are the absolute criteria necessary to make the decision to civilly commit or otherwise abridge a person's civil liberties, based on the probability of dangerousness to self? How apparent must the danger be for a psychiatrist to be held liable for missing it? What measures are the mental health staff members required to take to prevent a suicide? When in doubt, admit the patient to the hospital.

Misdiagnosis

The psychiatrist need not make a final diagnosis in the emergency room, but a thorough differential diagnosis must be considered. The failure to discover suicidal or homicidal intent, to diagnose an underlying medical condition, to recognize the side effects of medication, to consider toxic levels of medication or intoxication with a drug of abuse—all are examples of misdiagnosis.

Negligent Treatment

Negligent treatment means insufficient, excessive, or inappropriate treatment.

Inappropriate Involuntary Hospitalization

Involuntary hospitalization is hospitalizing patients against their will when they are dangerous to themselves or to others. Those are the only conditions for which patients can be hospitalized against their will. The legal principle of least restrictive alternative requires that the least restrictive and intensive means of handling a situation be used whenever patients' rights are limited. Thus, if patients do not pose significant risks to themselves or to others, the psychiatrist has no legal basis for hospitalizing them against their will.

Sexual Relations with Patients

It is illegal and unethical to have sexual relations with a patient under any conditions. Impaired psychiatrists have been known to do unnecessary and inappropriate genital examinations in the emergency room.

INFORMED CONSENT

Informed consent implies three basic elements: the patient's consent is informed, voluntary, and competent.

Informed

Information is the data base that the patient uses to make a decision about treatment. The physician is required to give the patient information about the risks and the benefits of the proposed treatment and information about alternative treatments and the risks of not treating the condition. The degree to which a patient is thought to be adequately informed has been judged to be different from court to court and state to state, although the recent trend is toward providing as much information as possible.

Voluntary

Consent requires the patient's voluntary agreement to follow a given course of treatment as prescribed by the physician. It is not always clear when legitimate persuasion becomes coercive enough to negate the consent. In emergencies a clinician may treat against the patient's will if the treatment prevents harm to the patient or to others. If the patient, for a variety of reasons, cannot give valid consent (for example, when the patient is unconscious or incompetent) and the risk to the patient's life for not intervening is significant, the concept of *implied consent* applies, and the physician can administer treatment. In other situations, such as in the emergency room, an agitated, out-of-control patient can be told, "If you do not take this pill, you will be given an injection"; the patient's consent to take the pill is an emergency response, rather than informed consent. A patient who takes medication as the result of such a verbal interaction cannot be construed to have given legal, voluntary consent, although the action may still be construed as defensible under the circumstances.

Competent

Competence is defined in both a legal context and an actual context. Legally, in almost all states a person who has reached the age of 18 years is considered competent. A court of law must pass judgment to decide that the patient is incompetent. Actual competence, however, is assessed by an evaluation of the person's mental status. Actual competence is the capacity of the patient to understand the information provided, to recognize the presence of an illness, and to make reasoned decisions about treatment. For example, patients in the emergency room who have an impairment of consciousness are not able to make competent decisions.

LIABILITY PREVENTION

Documentation

In malpractice litigation the rule of thumb is, "If you didn't write it down, it didn't happen." The physician should include a description of the patient's clinical condition (for example, the results of the mental status examination) and the elements in the decision-making process, such as the risks and the benefits of alternative treatment plans.

Often, obtaining a signed consent form is prudent. The form should contain as much information as possible about the proposed treatment plan, written in layperson's language. If written consent is not possible, documentation is still possible with the use of a witnessed oral consent that describes the amount of information provided to the patient and the patient's agreement to the proposed plan. You should note whether the patient was able to participate in the decision-making process; if the patient was not able to participate, you should note the reasons why, such as severe agitation, psychosis, and decreased level of consciousness. All treatments rendered should be written down, especially dosages, responses to medications, and the times that medications were given.

Consultation

Obtaining a consultation provides the clinician with a second opinion on the specific case and provides information on the usual standard of care. Consultations may be formal or informal, but in either case the primary clinician should document the opinion of the consultant and the effects of the consultation on the treatment decisions. Medical and neurological consultations must always be obtained if underlying organic conditions are suspected.

INVOLUNTARY HOSPITALIZATION

Involuntary hospitalization entails depriving the patient of liberty. Failure to hospitalize, however, may result in harm to the patient or to society or to both. The physician in the emergency room has a responsibility toward patients and a duty to care for patients who are unable to care for themselves. In addition, the emergency psychiatrist has a duty to protect others from potentially dangerous patients. Although commitment criteria vary from state to state, almost all criteria refer to danger to self, danger to others, and the inability to care for oneself.

In discussing hospitalization with a potentially dangerous patient, the clinician should emphasize the benefits to the patient of emergency hospitalization. Many patients—especially those with schizophrenia or suicidal depression—are ambivalent about hospitalization. Despite their protests, they may welcome admission to a safe place. Paranoid patients may find comfort in the idea that the hospital is a place where they will be safe from their persecutors; manic patients may be relieved to find a place where dangerous impulses can be contained; suicidal patients may be relieved that they cannot give in to suicidal impulses. Many patients accept hospitalization if you discuss frankly the potential for the relief of their most distressing symptoms.

In weighing the risks and the benefits of involuntary hospitalization, most clinicians opt for a conservative approach, especially in emergency situations. When you are in doubt, it is more prudent to admit a patient to the hospital than to treat and release the patient from the emergency room.

INVOLUNTARY DISCHARGE

Just as some patients must be admitted to the hospital against their will, some patients may have to be involuntarily discharged from the emergency room. Persons who neither need nor want true psychiatric treatment sometimes come to the emergency room requesting or demanding services. Patients without significant psychopathology may feign symptoms to obtain food, shelter, or protection. Such patients often vehemently refuse to leave the emergency room and may have to be forcibly evicted from the premises.

Clinicians are vulnerable to charges of abandonment in those situations unless they safeguard against such charges by careful documentation of the reasons for discharge. The physician should make suitable referrals for the patients, make sure that those referrals are available, and (when appropriate) leave the door open for the patients' return to the emergency room.

Similarly, malingering patients may be involuntarily discharged from the emergency room if the clinician can document that the patients are not dangerous to themselves or to others, that they are not grossly psychotic, and that they are able to care for themselves outside the hospital.

When a patient is genuinely in crisis—suicidal, threatening violence, or grossly psychotic—treatment may not be terminated until the situation has been adequately managed.

RIGHT TO REFUSE TREATMENT

Psychiatric patients have the right to refuse treatment under ordinary circumstances, and that right is predicated on the informed-consent requirement before treatment. Most state courts maintain that even civil commitment does not necessarily deprive a patient of the right to refuse treatment. However, a physician may override patients' refusal in emergency situations, such as when patients pose immediate threats to other people or to themselves. The Massachusetts Supreme Judicial Court, in *Rogers v. Commissioner,* held that in an emergency a patient may be treated "against his will . . . to prevent the 'immediate, substantial, and irreversible deterioration of a serious mental illness.' "

OTHER CIVIL RIGHTS OF PATIENTS

The patient's other civil rights include (1) the right to receive the least restrictive treatment, (2) the right to receive visitors, and (3) the right to have free communication with the outside world by telephone. Those rights should be safeguarded in the emergency room, provided patients are not in danger of harming themselves or others.

Because patients have the right to the least restrictive alternative, the clinician, when undertaking seclusion or restraint, must hold the patient's health and well-being as the first concern. Seclusion and restraint should not be used for the convenience of the staff and should never be used punitively. The least-restrictive-alternative premise applies to the use of seclusion and restraint in the sense that the least amount of time in seclusion and restraint that is possible to control a crisis situation is what is legally justifiable. The clinician need not hesitate to use seclusion and restraint in genuine emergencies. As in other situations, consultation and documentation are the psychiatrist's best protection against negative repercussions resulting from the use of seclusion or restraint. The symptoms and the behaviors that are determined to justify seclusion and restraint should be frequently assessed.

CONFIDENTIALITY AND PRIVILEGE

Confidentiality concerns the clinician's obligation not to reveal information about the patient to others without the patient's specific permission to do so. Breach of confidentiality is a major cause of legal action against psychiatrists. Privilege is a legal term that is applied only in legal proceedings; it exists in most but not all state jurisdictions. *Privilege* concerns the patient's right to exclude information given to the psychiatrist from testimony in a judicial setting. Two exceptions to the rule of privilege are civil commitment hearings and situations in which the patients themselves raise the issue of a mental condition, such as in the use of an insanity defense.

The emergency room has a circle of confidentiality, within which the revelation of material does not require the patient's permission. Included within that circle are all members of the treatment team, supervisors, and consultants.

Exceptions to Confidentiality

Emergencies.   In bona fide emergencies, information may be released for the sake of emergency interventions, but efforts should be made to obtain the patient's permission. The need to obtain a history—especially a drug, medical, or medication history—from family members, friends, or other treating physicians takes precedence over the rule of confidentiality in emergency situations.

Reportable conditions. Child abuse and certain communicable diseases entail mandatory reporting to government agencies. Examples of potentially reportable conditions include gunshot and stab wounds, motor vehicle accidents, encephalitis, meningitis, food-borne diseases, tuberculosis, venereal disease, acquired immune deficiency syndrome (AIDS), and animal bites. The clinician must know the specific statutes from state to state, as they vary widely in terms of what, who, and how much must be reported.

Duties to inform third parties. Therapists have a new duty not simply to their patients but also to parties who may be harmed by their patients. Since the 1976 *Tarasoff v. Regents of University of California* decision, a number of states have mandated that confidentiality must be breached when there is a threat against a third party. That duty involves the same implied responsibility of preventing future harm that is inherent in the requirement that physicians report suspected cases of child abuse and neglect. However, although most state jurisdictions have not enacted specific laws with regard to that duty, it is generally thought advisable for physicians to act as though the law existed. There have been two Tarasoff decisions. In the first Tarasoff decision (Tarasoff I), the court held that, because of an alleged special relationship between therapists and their patients, therapists have a special duty toward potential victims. That special duty was interpreted in Tarasoff I solely as a duty to *warn* a probable victim. Later, however, the court broadened the reading of Tarasoff (Tarasoff II), holding that therapists have a duty to take reasonable steps to *protect* endangered third parties (conceivably by means that include both warnings and commitment of the patient).

In short, when a patient makes a threat to seriously harm a specific person and when there is a clear and present danger that the patient will carry out that threat, a therapist is generally thought to have an obligation to breach confidentiality and to warn and protect the potential victim.

---

6 / Psychiatric Emergencies in Children

Few children or adolescents seek psychiatric intervention on their own, even during a crisis; thus, the majority of their emergency evaluations are initiated by parents, relatives, teachers, therapists, physicians, and child protective service workers (Table A.6–1). Some referrals are for the evaluation of life-threatening situations for the child or for others, such as suicidal behavior, physical abuse, and violent or homicidal behavior. Other urgent but non-life-threatening referrals pertain to children and adolescents with exacerbations of clear-cut serious psychiatric disorders, such as mania, depression, florid psychosis, and school refusal. Less diagnostically obvious situations occur when children and adolescents present with a history of a wide range of disruptive, aberrant behaviors and are accompanied by overwhelmed, anxious, and distraught adults who perceive the child's actions

Table A.6–1
Referral Sources of Child Psychiatric Emergencies

Parents and guardians
Schools (Schools may request an immediate psychiatric evaluation for a problem child before
    allowing the child to return to school.)
Therapists and physicians, especially if the child may require hospitalization
Child protective services

as an emergency, despite the absence of life-threatening behavior or an obvious psychiatric disorder. In those cases, the spectrum of contributing factors is not immediately clear, and the emergency psychiatrist must assess the entire family or system involved with the child. Familial stressors and parental discord may contribute to the evolution of a crisis for a child. For example, immediate evaluations are sometimes legitimately indicated for a child caught in the crossfire of feuding parents or in a seemingly irreconcilable conflict between a set of parents and a school, therapist, or protective service worker regarding the needs of the child (Table A.6–2).

An emergency setting is often the site of an initial evaluation of a chronic problem behavior. For example, an identified problem—such as severe tantrums, violence, and destructive behavior in a child—may have been present for months or even years. Yet the initial contact with the mental health system in the emergency room or private office may be the first opportunity for the child or adolescent to disclose underlying stressors, such as physical or sexual abuse.

In view of the integral relation of severe family dysfunction to childhood behavioral disturbance, the emergency psychiatrist must make an assessment of familial discord and of psychiatric disorder in family members during an urgent evaluation. One way to make the assessment is to interview the child and the individual family members both alone and together and to obtain a history from informants outside the family whenever possible. Noncustodial parents, therapists, and teachers may add valuable information regarding the child's daily functioning. Many families, especially those with mental illness and severe dysfunction, may have little or no inclination to seek psychiatric help on a nonurgent basis; therefore, the emergency evaluation becomes the only way to engage them in an extensive psychiatric treatment program.

LIFE-THREATENING EMERGENCIES
Suicidal Behavior

Assessment.   Suicidal behavior is the most common reason for an emergency evaluation in adolescents. Despite the minimal risk for a completed suicide in a child under 12 years of age, suicidal ideation or behavior in a child of any age must be carefully evaluated, with particular attention to the psychiatric status of the child and the ability of the family or the guardians to provide the appropriate supervision. The assessment must determine the circumstances of the suicidal ideation or behavior, its lethality, and the persistence of the suicidal intention. An evaluation of the family's

Table A.6–2
Familial Risk Factors

Physical and sexual abuse
Recent family crisis: loss of a parent, divorce, loss of job, family move
Severe family dysfunction, including parental mental illness

sensitivity, supportiveness, and competence must be done to assess their ability to monitor the child's suicidal potential. Ultimately, during the course of an emergency evaluation, the psychiatrist must decide whether the child may return home to a safe environment and receive outpatient follow-up care or whether hospitalization is necessary. A psychiatric history, a mental status examination, and an assessment of family functioning helps establish the general level of risk.

Risk factors for suicide in adolescents include prior attempts, being male, a history of aggressive behavior, a severe depressive disorder, access to a lethal method (such as a gun), and alcohol and drug abuse. In girls, additional risk factors include teenage pregnancy and being a runaway. The risk is high in adolescents whose parents or other relatives have attempted suicide. In young children the lethality of their suicide attempts is usually low, but suicidal ideation and behavior often reflect intolerable stressors in the environment, including neglect and physical and sexual abuse. In addition, young children with suicidal behavior often live with exceedingly high levels of parental discord and psychopathology and with pervasive maladjustment, including school failure. In some cases a suicidal youngster has learned that it takes an extreme, though misguided, measure to attract the attention of a dysfunctional family.

Management.   When self-injurious behavior has occurred, the adolescent is likely to require hospitalization on a pediatric unit for treatment of the injury or for the observation of medical sequelae after a toxic ingestion. If the adolescent is medically clear, the psychiatrist must decide whether the adolescent needs psychiatric admission. If the patient persists in suicidal ideation and shows signs of psychosis, severe depression (including hopelessness), or marked ambivalence about suicide, psychiatric admission is indicated. An adolescent who is taking drugs or alcohol should not be released until an assessment can be done when the patient is in a nonintoxicated state. Patients with high-risk profiles—such as late-adolescent males, especially those with substance abuse and aggressive behavior disorders, and those who have severe depression or who have made prior suicide attempts, particularly with lethal weapons—warrant hospitalization. Young children who have made suicide attempts, even when the attempt had a low lethality, need psychiatric admission if the family is so chaotic, dysfunctional, and incompetent that follow-up treatment is unlikely.

When a child or an adolescent reports no further suicidal ideation, there is no flagrant exacerbation of psychiatric illness, and both the child and the family seem to be responsible, outpatient follow-up care can be arranged. A follow-up psychiatric appointment must be set up before the child leaves the emergency setting; both the child and the other family members must be willing to participate, and the family must agree to support the child by removing any potentially lethal items from the home. Children and adolescents should sign an agreement before going home indicating that they will not engage in suicidal behavior and that they will tell a responsible adult if they again feel suicidal. Even when an adolescent denies persistent suicidal ideation, the family can be instructed to bring the child back to the emergency setting if suicidal ideation reemerges before outpatient treatment begins.

Violent Behavior and Tantrums

Assessment.   The first task in an emergency evaluation of a violent child or adolescent is to make sure that both the child and the staff members are physically protected so that nobody is hurt. If the child appears to be calming down in the emergency area, the clinician may indicate to the child that it would be helpful if the child recounted what happened and may ask whether the child feels in control enough to do so. If the child agrees and the clinician judges the child to be in good control, the clinician may approach the child with the appropriate backup close at hand. If not, the clinician may either give the child several minutes to calm down before reassessing the situation or, with an adolescent, suggest that a medication may help the adolescent relax.

If the adolescent is clearly combative, physical restraint may be necessary before anything else is attempted. Some rageful children and adolescents brought to an emergency setting by overwhelmed families are able to regain control of themselves without the use of physical or pharmacological restraints. Children and adolescents are most likely to calm down if approached calmly in a nonthreatening manner and given a chance to tell their side of the story to a nonjudgmental adult. At this time, the psychiatrist should look for any underlying psychiatric disorder that may be mediating the aggression. The psychiatrist should speak to family members and others who have been witnessing the episode to understand the context in which it occurred and the extent to which the child has been out of control.

Management.   Prepubertal children, in the absence of major psychiatric illness, rarely require medication to keep them safe, since they are generally small enough to be physically restrained if they begin to hurt themselves or others. It is not immediately necessary to administer medication to a child or an adolescent who was in a rage but is in a calm state when examined. Adolescents and older children who are assaultive, extremely agitated, or overtly self-injurious and who may be difficult to subdue physically may require medication before a dialogue can take place. During the assessment the psychiatrist must determine whether the violent behavior is typical for the patient, is the first such episode, is part of a cyclic mood disorder, heralds a psychotic break, or is a product of intoxication with drugs or alcohol.

Medication selected for the control of aggression is chosen on the basis of the presumptive underlying disorder and the factors influencing the patient's current state, such as drug or alcohol intoxication. If the adolescent is able to cooperate and is not an immediate threat to self or others but is still felt to be at high risk, a medication by mouth may be considered; otherwise, a parenteral route is necessary. For adolescents who are violent secondary to a psychotic condition, antipsychotics are generally used to decrease their agitation. Intramuscular injections of a number of antipsychotics—including haloperidol (Haldol), chlorpromazine (Thorazine), and fluphenazine (Prolixin)—are available. For patients who are suspected of acute drug or alcohol intoxication or who have an organic cause of the aggression, intravenous or intramuscular use of a short-acting benzodiazepine, such as lorazepam (Ativan), is recommended. Antipsychotics are not the first choice for the above patients, since the antipsychotics may lower the seizure threshold, have potentially adverse anticholinergic properties, and impair thermoregulation. Sodium amobarbital (Amytal), given intramuscularly, has also been effective in the short-term management of aggression (Table A.6–3).

Children who have a history of repeated, self-limited, severe tantrums may not require admission to a hospital if they are able to calm down during the course of the evaluation. Yet the pattern will, no doubt, reoccur unless ongoing outpatient treatment for the child and the family is arranged. For adolescents who continue to pose a danger to themselves or others during the the evaluation period, admission to a hospital is necessary.

Fire Setting

Assessment.   A sense of emergency and panic often surrounds the parents of a child who has set a fire. Parents or teachers often request an emergency evaluation, even for a very young child who has accidently lit a fire. Many children, during the course of normal development, become interested in fire, but in the majority of cases a school-age child who has set a fire has done so accidently while playing with matches and seeks help to put it out. When a child has a strong interest in playing with matches, the level of supervision by family members must be clarified, so that no further accidental fires occur. The clinician must distinguish between a child who accidently or even impulsively sets a single fire and a child who engages in repeated fire setting with premeditation and subsequently leaves the fire without making any attempt to extinguish it. In repeated fire setting, the risk is obviously higher than in a single occurrence, and the psychiatrist must determine whether underlying psychopathology exists in the child or in the family members. The psychiatrist should also evaluate family interactions, since any factors that interfere with effective supervision and communication—such as high levels of marital discord and harsh, punitive parenting styles—may impede appropriate intervention.

Fire setting is one of a triad of symptoms—enuresis, cruelty to animals, and fire setting—that were believed, some years ago, to be typical of children with conduct disorders; however, no evidence indicates that the three symptoms are truly linked, although conduct disorder is the most frequent psychiatric disorder that occurs with pathological fire setting.

Management.   The critical component of management and treatment for fire setters is to prevent further incidents while treating any underlying psychopathology. In general, fire setting alone is not an indication for hos-

Table A.6–3
Short-Term Pharmacological Treatment of Violent Children and Adolescents

Drug	Pediatric Dose (6–12 years)	Adolescent and Adult Dose (>12 years)
Haloperidol	0.5–1 mg oral IM not established as safe	1–5 mg oral 2–5 mg IM, may repeat in 1 hour
Chlorpromazine	0.25 mg/kg oral 0.5 mg/kg IM	50–100 mg oral 25 mg IM, may repeat 1 hour
Fluphenazine	Not approved<12 yrs.	1–5 mg oral 2–5 mg IM
Lorazepam	Not approved<12 yrs.	1–2 mg oral, may repeat in 1 hour 2–4 mg IM, may repeat in 1 hour
Sodium amobarbital	Not approved<12 yrs	250 mg IM

pitalization, unless there is a continued direct threat that the patient will set another fire. The parents of children with a pattern of fire setting must be emphatically counseled that the child must not be left alone at home and should never be left to take care of younger siblings without direct adult supervision. Children who exhibit a pattern of concurrent aggressive behaviors and other forms of destructive behavior are likely to have a poor outcome. Outpatient treatment should be arranged for children who repeatedly set fires. Behavioral techniques that involve both the child and the family are helpful in decreasing the risk for further fire setting, as is positive reinforcement for alternate behaviors.

Child Abuse: Physical and Sexual

Assessment. Physical and sexual abuse occurs in girls and boys of all ages, in all ethnic groups, and at all socioeconomic levels. The abuses vary widely with respect to severity and duration, but any form of continued abuse constitutes an emergency situation for the child. No single psychiatric syndrome is a sine qua non of physical or sexual abuse, but fear, guilt, anxiety, depression, and ambivalence regarding disclosure commonly surround the child who has been abused.

Young children who are being sexually abused may exhibit precocious sexual behavior with peers and present a detailed sexual knowledge that reflects exposure beyond their developmental level. Children who endure sexual or physical abuse often display sadistic and aggressive behaviors themselves. Children who are abused in any manner are likely to have been threatened with severe and frightening consequences by the perpetrator if they reveal the situation to anyone. Frequently, an abused child who is victimized by a family member is placed in the irreconcilable position of having to either silently endure continued abuse or defy the abuser by disclosing the experiences and be responsible for destroying the family and risk being disbelieved or abandoned by the family.

In cases of suspected abuse, the child and other family members must be interviewed individually to give each member a chance to speak privately. If possible, the clinician should observe the child with each parent individually to get a sense of the spontaneity, warmth, fear, anxiety, or other prominent features of the relationships. However, one observation is generally not enough to make a final judgment about the family relationships; abused children almost always have mixed emotions toward abusive parents.

The assessment of physical abuse includes looking for scars and suspicious injuries, such as symmetrical bruises, especially on the face, the back, the buttocks, and the thighs; looking for burns, including those made by cigarettes and immersion in hot water (glove or socklike distribution); looking for multiple unexplained fractures; and looking for head injuries, such as hematomas and areas of missing hair. Children who are physically handicapped or mentally retarded or who have difficulty in communicating verbally may be at higher than usual risk for abuse. Parents who have been abused, lack a support system, have unrealistic expectations of their children, and are stressed themselves by debts, illness, unemployment, and substance abuse may be at high risk of physically abusing their children.

Physical indicators of sexual abuse in children include sexually transmitted diseases (for example, gonorrhea); pain, irritation, and itching of the genitalia and the urinary tract; and discomfort while sitting and walking. In many instances of suspected sexual abuse, however, physical evidence is not present. Thus, a careful history is essential. The physician should speak directly about the issues without leading the child in any direction, since already frightened children may be easily influenced to endorse what they think the examiner wants to hear. Furthermore, children who have been abused often retract all or part of what has been disclosed during the course of an interview.

The psychiatrist must establish a level of suspicion regarding physical and sexual abuse from an initial evaluation. Factors that complicate the assessment of sexual and physical abuse include custody disputes between the parents in which the parents develop an intense mistrust of each other and coerce the child into believing that abuse has or has not taken place.

The use of anatomically correct dolls in the assessment of sexual abuse can help the child identify body parts and show what has happened, but no conclusive evidence supports sexual play with dolls as a means of validating abuse.

Management. When physical or sexual abuse is suspected, the child's protection and safety are the primary concerns. A report to the local child protective agency is required by law. If the doctor doubts that the child will be safe at home or with a reliable relative, the child must be admitted to a hospital until the investigation by the protective service agency is completed.

Children may take a long time to build up enough trust in an adult to reveal much of their abusive experience and their inner world, so treatment of the sequelae of abuse cannot be completed on an urgent basis. Abused children are vulnerable to many psychiatric symptoms and subject to additional family crises once the abuse has been disclosed. Therefore, the child needs an outpatient therapist to act as an advocate for the child in dealing with family members and to support the child as the inner experiences of child abuse are explored.

Neglect: Failure to Thrive

Assessment.   In child neglect a child's physical, mental, or emotional condition has been impaired because of a parent's or caretaker's inability to provide adequate food, shelter, education, or supervision. Similar to abuse, any form of continued neglect is an emergency situation for the child. Parents who neglect their children range widely and may include parents who are very young and ignorant about the emotional and concrete needs of a child, parents with depression and significant passivity, substance-abusing parents, and parents with a variety of incapacitating mental illnesses.

In its extreme form, neglect can contribute to failure to thrive—that is, an infant, usually under a year old, becomes malnourished in the absence of an organic cause. Failure to thrive typically occurs under circumstances in which adequate nourishment is available yet a disturbance within the relationship between the caretaker and the child results in a child who does not eat enough to grow and develop. A negative pattern may exist between the mother and the child in which the child refuses feedings and the mother feels rejected and eventually withdraws. She may then avoid offering food as frequently as the infant needs it. Observation of the mother and the child together may reveal a nonspontaneous, tense interaction, with withdrawal on both sides, resulting in a seeming apathy in the mother. Both the mother and the child may seem depressed.

A rare form of failure to thrive in children who are at least several years old and are not necessarily malnourished is the syndrome of psychosocial dwarfism. In that syndrome, marked growth retardation and delayed epiphyseal maturation accompany a disturbed relationship between the parent and the child, along with bizarre social and eating behaviors in the child. Those behaviors sometimes include eating from garbage cans, drinking toilet water, binging and vomiting, and diminished outward response to pain. Half of the children with the syndrome have decreased growth hormone. Once the children are removed from the troubled environment and placed in another setting, such as a psychiatric hospital with appropriate supervision and guidance regarding meals, the endocrine abnormalities normalize, and the children begin to grow at a more rapid rate.

Management.   In cases of child neglect, as with physical and sexual abuse, the most important decision to be made during the initial evaluation is whether the child is safe in the home environment. Whenever neglect is suspected, it must be reported to the local child protective service agency. In mild cases the decision to refer the family for outpatient services, as opposed to hospitalizing the child, depends on the clinician's conviction that the family is cooperative and willing to be educated and to enter into treatment and that the child is not in danger. Before a neglected child is released from an emergency setting, a follow-up appointment must be made.

Education for the family must begin during the the evaluation; the family must be told, in a nonthreatening manner, that failure to thrive can become life-threatening, that the entire family needs to monitor the child's progress, and that they will receive some help in overcoming the many possible obstacles interfering with the child's emotional and physical well-being.

Anorexia Nervosa

Assessment.   Anorexia nervosa occurs in females about 10 times as often as in males. It is characterized by the refusal to maintain body weight, leading to a weight at least 15 percent below the expected, by a distorted body image, by a persistent fear of becoming fat, and by the absence of at least three menstrual cycles. The disorder usually begins after puberty, but it has occurred in children of 9 or 10 years, in whom expected weight gain does not occur, rather than a loss of 15 percent of body weight. The disorder reaches medical emergency proportions when the weight loss approaches 30 percent of body weight or when metabolic disturbances become severe. Hospitalization then becomes necessary to control the ongoing process of starvation, potential dehydration, and the medical complications of starvation, including electrolyte imbalances, cardiac arrhythmias, and hormonal changes.

An important variable in the management of the disorder is the patient's reliability and ability to cooperate; a denial of the need for treatment is often inherent in the disorder. That denial may make hospitalization a requirement even before it is a medical emergency. In addition, the patient's history must be elicited from family members, as well as from the patient, since patients with anorexia nervosa tend to minimize their dysfunction.

Although no laboratory tests confirm the diagnosis, the psychiatrist must assess the severity of the metabolic disruption. An electrocardiogram (ECG); a complete blood count (CBC); an electrolyte panel, including kidney and liver function tests; and a urinalysis are useful. Anemia, leukopenia, proteinuria, hypercholesterolemia, and a host of endocrinological abnormalities may be present.

Management.   Anorexia nervosa requires a lengthy and multifaceted treatment approach to address the nutritional needs of the patient, as well as the psychological issues. In an urgent evaluation, however, the physician must decide whether the patient is in medical danger and requires hospitalization.

During the evaluation, the family must begin to be educated regarding the serious sequelae of the disorder and the patient's likely denial and possible secrecy about the symptoms; an immediate appreciation of the severity of the disturbance may be masked. Follow-up care must be arranged if hospitalization is not planned. The family members must understand that, although issues of autonomy may be active components of the patient's psychological life, an adolescent with anorexia nervosa is not likely to be the best judge of the need for treatment.

Acquired Immune Deficiency Syndrome (AIDS)

Assessment.   Acquired immune deficiency syndrome, which is caused by the human immunodeficiency virus (HIV), occurs in neonates through perinatal transmission from an infected mother, in children and adolescents secondary to sexual abuse by an infected person, and in adolescents through intravenous drug abuse with infected needles and through sexual activities with infected partners. Child and adolescent hemophiliac patients may contract AIDS through tainted blood transfusions.

Children and adolescents may present for emergency evaluations at the urging of a family member or a peer; in some cases they take the initiative themselves when they are faced with anxiety or panic about high-risk behavior. Early screening of high-risk persons may lead to the treatment of asymptomatic infected patients with such drugs as azidothymidine (AZT) and possibly other new medications that may slow the course of the disease. During the assessment of the risks for HIV infection, an educational process can be initiated with both the patient and the rest of the family so that an adolescent who is not infected but exhibits high-risk behavior can be counseled about that behavior and about safe-sex practices.

In children the brain is often a primary site for HIV infection; encephalitis, decreased brain development, and such neuropsychiatric symptoms as impairment in memory, concentration, and attention span may be present before the diagnosis is made. The virus may be present in the cerebrospinal fluid before it shows up in the bloodstream. Changes in cognitive function, frontal lobe disinhibition, social withdrawal, slowed information processing, and apathy constitute some common symptoms of the AIDS dementia complex. Organic mood disorders, organic personality disorder, and frank psychosis may also occur in HIV-infected patients.

Management.   Whenever an HIV test is under consideration, the physician should explain to the patient and the family the reasons the patient is thought to be at high risk. Ways of decreasing high-risk behavior should be addressed, as well as the ramifications of a positive or negative test result. The patient must have an appointment in person to discuss the test result when it comes back.

For children and adolescents who are infected with the virus or who have AIDS, the quality of their lives will be determined by the support system that can be established for them and their families. The support system includes a medical team that is sensitive to the child's needs, psychotherapists who understand the natural history of the illness, and a supportive school environment. The Centers for Disease Control recommends that children with AIDS attend school unless they have open skin lesions or problems with secretions or exhibit biting behavior. The emergency evaluation can be a beginning point to introduce and refer families to the various components of the medical-psychiatric support team that they will need over the course of the disease.

Adolescents who are sexually active must be strongly encouraged to actively protect their partners. Currently, no law mandates verification that adolescents have informed their sexual partners of their HIV status and now practice safe sex. Hospitalization, voluntary or involuntary, may be used when a patient discloses a purposeful plan or intention to infect a partner. Since adolescents tend to indulge in magical thinking, especially with regard to being immune to danger, a simple description of the risks for HIV infection, given to an adolescent during an emergency evaluation, probably will not go far. Adolescents who are at high risk for exposure to HIV infection should be referred for ongoing counseling, psychotherapy, or a community group in which decreasing high-risk behaviors can be discussed and, it is hoped, adopted.

URGENT NON-LIFE-THREATENING SITUATIONS

School Refusal

Assessment. Refusal to go to school may occur in a young child who is first entering school or in an older child or adolescent who is making a transition into a new grade or school, or it may emerge in a vulnerable child without an obvious external stressor. In any case, school refusal requires immediate intervention, since the longer the dysfunctional pattern continues, the more difficult it is to interrupt.

School refusal is generally associated with separation anxiety, in which the child's distress is related to the consequences of being separated from the parent, so the child resists going to school. School refusal may also occur in children with school phobia, in which the fear and the distress are targeted on the school itself. In either case, a serious disruption of the child's life occurs. Although mild separation anxiety is universal, particularly among very young children who are first facing school, treatment is required when a child actually cannot attend school. Severe psychopathology, including anxiety and depressive disorders, is often present when school refusal occurs for the first time in an adolescent. Children with separation anxiety disorder typically present extreme worries that catastrophic events will befall their mothers or attachment figures or themselves as a result of the separation. Separation-anxious children may also exhibit many other fears and symptoms of depression, including such somatic complaints as headaches, stomachaches, and nausea. Severe tantrums and desperate pleas may ensue when one tries to separate the child from the mother. Among young children the preoccupation that a parent will be harmed during the separation is frequently verbalized; in adolescents the stated reasons for refusing to go to school are often physical complaints.

As part of an urgent assessment, the psychiatrist must ascertain the duration of the patient's absence from school and must assess the parents' ability to participate in a treatment plan that will undoubtedly involve firm parental guidelines to ensure the child's return to school. The parents of a child with separation anxiety disorder often exhibit excessive separation anxiety or other anxiety disorders themselves, thereby compounding the child's problem. When the parents are unable to participate in a treatment program from home, hospitalization should be considered.

Management. When school refusal caused by separation anxiety is identified during an emergency evaluation, the underlying disorder can be explained to the family, and an intervention can be started immediately. In severe cases, however, a multidimensional, long-term family-oriented treatment plan is necessary. Whenever possible, a separation-anxious child should be brought back to school the next school day, despite the distress, and a contact person within the school (counselor, guidance counselor, or teacher) should be involved to help the child stay in school while praising the child for tolerating the school situation.

When school refusal has been going on for months or years or when the family members are unable to cooperate, a treatment program to move the child back to school from the hospital should be considered. When the child's anxiety is not diminished by behavioral methods alone, tricyclic antidepressants, such as imipramine (Tofranil), are helpful. Medication is generally prescribed not at the initial evaluation but after a behavioral intervention has been tried.

Munchausen Syndrome by Proxy

Assessment.   Munchausen syndrome by proxy is, essentially, a form of child abuse in which a parent, usually the mother, or a caretaker repeatedly fabricates or actually inflicts injury or illness in a child for whom medical intervention is then sought, often in an emergency setting. Although it is a rare scenario, mothers who inflict injury often have some prior knowledge of medicine, leading to sophisticated symptoms; the mothers sometimes engage in inappropriate camaraderie with the medical staff regarding the treatment of the child. Careful observation may reveal that the mothers often do not exhibit appropriate signs of distress on hearing the details of the child's medical symptoms. Prototypically, such mothers tend to present themselves as highly accomplished professionals in ways that seem inflated or blatantly untrue.

The illnesses appearing in the child can involve any organ system, but certain symptoms are commonly presented: bleeding from one or many sites, including the gastrointestinal tract, the genitourinary system, and the respiratory system; seizures; and central nervous system depression. At times, the illness is simulated, rather than actually inflicted.

The syndrome is sadly paradoxical in that the mother acts overtly overprotective of the child yet is the direct instigator of harm to the child. To make matters worse, the child may collude with the mother's untrue assertions regarding the origins of the illnesses. Factors that increase the index of suspicion for the syndrome include a child who has been seen in many emergency rooms for many unrelated symptoms yet does not have a regular physician or adequate follow-up care, symptoms that seem to flare up only when the mother has been present, unusual symptoms that are not consistent with the clinical history given, and recurrent identical symptoms that are reported to be unresponsive to treatment.

Management.   The syndrome is difficult to identify, particularly when the child exhibits obvious medical signs and symptoms and strongly supports the mother's history. A definitive diagnosis is not likely during a single emergency evaluation. When suspicion is aroused, however, the scenario must be dealt with on several levels: reporting the suspected child abuse to a child protective agency, taking steps to keep the child safe, and ensuring the appropriate medical treatment.

The emergency team must refrain from direct accusation of the mother, so that a rapport can be established and follow-up arrangements made. The mother is likely to agree to a follow-up appointment if she feels that she is a respected member of the treatment team who is being enlisted to help deal with the child's complex medical problems. If possible, the child should be hospitalized to closely monitor the interactions of the mother and the child and to consider the dangers posed by the child's return to the mother. The cases are difficult to validate because of the mother's pathological role in creating the disorder, yet, when suspician is repeatedly documented and especially when suspected abuse is reported from many settings, a pattern becomes apparent that points to the syndrome.

OTHER CHILDHOOD DISTURBANCES

Posttraumatic Stress Disorder

Assessment. Children who have been subjected to a severe catastrophic or traumatic event may present for a prompt evaluation because they have extreme fears of the specific trauma occurring again or sudden discomfort with familiar places, people, or situations that previously did not evoke anxiety. Within weeks of a traumatic event, a child may re-create the event in play, in stories, and in dreams that directly replay the terrifying situation. A sense of reliving the experience may occur, including hallucinations and flashback (dissociative) experiences, and intrusive memories of the event come and go. Many traumatized children, over time, go on to reproduce parts of the event through their own victimization behaviors toward others, without being aware that those behaviors reflect their own traumatic experiences.

The reenactment may not be easily recognized by a clinician in an initial evaluation, especially if the specifics of the trauma have not been disclosed. The psychiatrist must find out the details of the traumatic events to determine the child's degree of posttraumatic stress, as opposed to another anxiety disorder, such as separation anxiety disorder. Children without preexisting psychopathology often experience severe anxiety symptoms after exposure to a tramatic event, and children whose coping mechanisms are already compromised by psychopathology are likely to have poorer outcomes. The clinician should directly ask the child to recount the events as they are remembered.

Management. Once posttraumatic stress disorder is recognized, the typical symptoms can be discussed with the child and the family to reassure them that the child's feelings are natural consequences of the experiences. The family can be advised that outpatient treatments of various kinds can be helpful. When avoidance and depressive symptoms are prominent, tricyclic antidepressants may be helpful, usually as an adjunct to psychotherapy. Psychotherapy of various types—including behavioral methods, play techniques, and supportive interventions—can be useful in controlling fears and in helping the child develop a feeling of mastery over the traumatic events.

Dissociative Disorders

Assessment.   Dissociative states—including the extreme form, multiple personality disorder—are believed to be most likely to occur in children who have been subjected to severe and repetitive physical, sexual, or emotional abuse. Children with dissociative symptoms may be referred for evaluation because family members or teachers observe that the children sometimes seem to be spaced out or distracted or act like different persons. Dissociative states are occasionally identified during the evaluation of violent and aggressive behavior, particularly in patients who truly do not remember chunks of their own behavior.

The ability to spontaneously drift into a trancelike state during severe episodes of stress seems to be the basis of the disorders. Over time, psychological triggers that induce trance states may generalize to other situations, and eventually the trances may occur in an unpredictable fashion. When the experiences of a patient during one or more trance states evolve into distinct internal identities, multiple personality disorder can arise.

Dissociative disorders often include psychotic phenomena, such as hearing voices that converse, feeling controlled by external forces, disorientation, and an inability to recount or remember events or periods of time. An important clue is a history of multiple incidents in which others have witnessed unusual behaviors, yet the patient does not have any recall of the behaviors.

Children without dissociative disorders who have been traumatized may experience transient phobic hallucinations that are self-limited or develop imaginative self-comforting techniques. Yet children who persistently converse with imaginary companions beyond 5 years old, who are known to have been abused, who have auditory hallucinations, who refer to different internal identities by name, and who seem to display variable identities should be evaluated further for a dissociative disorder.

Management.   Since dissociative states in children seem to be closely linked to a history of traumatic events and abuse, the clinician must determine whether a child with dissociative symptoms is currently being abused or is in danger. A child with dissociation who remains in an abusive situation is likely to deteriorate. Dissociative states, including multiple personality disorder, are not simple diagnoses to make; any child with dissociative phenomena requires ongoing outpatient evaluation and treatment.

When a child who dissociates is violent or self-destructive or endangers others, hospitalization is necessary. A variety of psychotherapy methods have been used in the complex treatment of children with dissociative disorders, including play techniques and, in some cases, hypnosis.

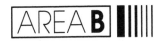

Clinical Problems in Emergency Psychiatric Medicine

1 / Abuse: Child, Elder, and Spouse

I. CHILD ABUSE

Child abuse is defined as physical or psychological damage to a child under the age of 18 that is sustained as a result of neglect or maltreatment, usually by a parent, a parent surrogate, or a relative. The typical child abuser is a single, unemployed mother under age 30, although the abuser may also be another caretaker, such as the father, a babysitter, or a friend. Many victims of physical abuse are also abused sexually. About 500,000 new cases of physical and sexual abuse are reported each year, and more than 4,000 abused children die. An estimated 2 to 4 million children (out of 30 million children in the United States) have been abused. The most serious injuries have been reported in children under the age of 3 years.

Victims, family, and health care professionals tend to deny, underreport, and misdiagnose cases of abuse, especially in patients from upper socio-economic groups. Physical and sexual abuse often occurs when the abuser is using drugs or alcohol. The perpetrators of abuse are likely to have personal histories of having witnessed abuse or have been abused themselves.

Abuse occurs most often in the context of volatile and dysfunctional interpersonal relationships, violent marital relationships, and heightened stress in the environment. The abused child is viewed in some way as different or special. The difference may involve such issues as mental retardation, high intelligence, hyperactivity, prematurity, serious illness, or physical or neurological abnormalities.

CLINICAL FEATURES AND DIAGNOSIS
Physical Abuse

Obvious cases of abuse may present with bruises, fractures, dislocations, burns, lacerations, focal neurological deficits, signs of intracranial bleeding, or abdominal injury. Malnutrition or dehydration may indicate food or water deprivation. Physical abuse is also called *battered child syndrome.*

Munchausen syndrome by proxy is a form of child abuse in which a caretaker (usually the child's mother) brings a child with a fabricated illness to medical attention. The caretaker may report nonexistent symptoms in the child (for example, reporting apneic episodes), alter laboratory tests (for example, putting blood in the child's urine sample), or induce illness by various methods (for example, administering a symptom-inducing medication). Children are then subjected to multiple unnecessary medical work-ups and treatments. The diagnosis should be suspected in cases involving children whose symptoms disappear when separated from their caretakers, who are often medically knowledgeable and overinvolved. The child usually presents as treatment-refractory or a diagnostic dilemma with ailments that include apnea, vomiting, failure to thrive, sepsis, and bleeding.

Sexual Abuse

Sexual abuse is difficult to diagnose reliably, since false allegations by parents occur, especially in child-custody cases. The physician should suspect sexual abuse of a child with evidence of genital injury or irritation, foreign bodies in the vagina or the rectum, excessive masturbation, venereal disease, or pregnancy.

Acute conditions may also present with a variety of symptoms and syndromes, from evidence of posttraumatic stress disorder to sleep disorders and somatic complaints. Regressive behaviors (thumb sucking, enuresis) often occur. Depression with suicidal ideation may be present.

Chronic conditions may involve a picture of hypersexuality on the child's part (preoccupation with sexual words and ideas, compulsive masturbation, seductive behavior), generalized low self-esteem, and a sense of isolation from peers and parents. Child victims are usually unable to give a reliable history.

The sexual abuser is usually male. The physician should consider whether an older sibling, cousin, uncle, or friend with whom the child has contact is a possible perpetrator. Sexual abuse can also occur in child-care centers.

Child victims can be of any age; even infants are abused. The use of children in—or the exposure of children to—pornography, talking about sex with young children, and allowing children to witness sex between adults are other forms of sexual abuse. Girls are sexually abused approximately twice as often as boys.

Emotional Abuse

Grossly abnormal care can be the result of conscious cruelty, lack of parenting skills, or unwanted parenthood. There is an increased incidence of emotional abuse when the parent is mentally retarded. The most typical picture is a failure to thrive in a young child. The physician should look for hypokinesis, apathy, an unhappy facial expression, delayed responsiveness, malnutrition, and fearfulness.

See Table B.1–1 for indicators of child abuse and neglect.

INTERVIEWING AND PSYCHOTHERAPEUTIC GUIDELINES

Interviews should be conducted in a manner that conveys respect and allows for the utmost privacy. When interviewing a child, do not suggest answers or press for accusatory responses. Several interviews may be necessary before a child feels safe enough to reveal specific information. Do not display strong emotions to the child, even if the abuse is personally abhorrent. Gently ask the child to describe what happened. Drawings and dolls can be helpful. Tell the parents that you are required by law to make a report to a child protective service when abuse is confirmed or even suspected. When the parents suspect that another adult has abused their child, reassure the parents that an honest, supportive, and direct approach with the child will lessen any further emotional trauma. Use open-ended questions with caretakers, such as, "How do you deal with the stress of being a parent?" and "How is Johnny punished when he is bad?" Interview

Table B.1-1
Physical and Behavioral Indicators of Child Abuse and Neglect

Type of Abuse	Physical Indicators	Behavioral Indicators

Physical abuse	Unexplained bruises and welts
	  on face, lips, mouth
	  on torso, back, buttocks, thighs
	  in various stages of healing
	  clustered, forming regular
	    patterns like articles used to
	    inflict (e.g., electric cord, belt
	    buckle)
	  on several surface areas
	  regularly appear after absence,
	    weekend, or vacation
	Unexplained burns
	  cigar or cigarette burns, especially
	    on soles, palms, back, or
	    buttocks
	  immersion burns (socklike,
	    glovelike, doughnut-shaped on
	    buttocks or genitalia)
	  patterned like electric burner,
	    iron, etc.
	  rope burns on arms, legs, neck,
	    or torso
	  infected burns, indicating delay
	    in seeking treatment
	Unexplained fractures or
	  dislocations
	  to skull, nose, or facial structure
	  in various stages of healing;
	  multiple or spinal fractures
	Unexplained lacerations
	  to mouth, lips, gums, eyes
	  to external genitalia in various
	    stages of healing
	Bald patches on scalp
		Feels deserving of punishment
		Wary of adult contacts
		Apprehensive when other
		  children cry
		Behavioral extremes:
		  aggressiveness or withdrawal
		Frightened of parents
		Afraid to go home
		Reports injury by parents
		Vacant or frozen stare
		Lies very still while surveying
		  surroundings
		Does not cry when approached
		  by examiner
		Responds to questions in
		  monosyllables
		Inappropriate or precocious
		  maturity
		Manipulative behavior to get
		  attention
		Capable of only superficial
		  relationships
		Indiscriminately seeks affection
		Poor self-concept

Physical neglect	Underweight, poor growth pattern,
	  failure to thrive
	Consistent hunger, poor hygiene,
	  inappropriate dress
	Consistent lack of supervision,
	  especially in dangerous activities
	  or long periods
	Wasting of subcutaneous tissue
	Unattended physical problems or
	  medical needs
	Abandonment
	Abdominal distention
	Bald patches on the scalp
		Begging, stealing food
		Extended stays at school (early
		  arrival and late departure)
		Rare attendance at school
		Constant fatigue, listlessness, or
		  falling asleep in class
		Inappropriate seeking of affection
		Assuming adult responsibilities
		  and concerns
		Alcohol or drug abuse
		Delinquency (e.g., thefts)
		States there is no caretaker

Sexual abuse	Difficulty in walking or sitting
	Torn, stained, or bloody
	  underclothing
	Pain, swelling, or itching in genital
	  area
	Pain on urination
	Bruises, bleeding, or lacerations in
	  external genitalia, vaginal or anal
	  areas
	Vaginal or penile discharge
	Venereal disease, especially in
	  preteens
	Poor sphincter tone
	Pregnancy
		Unwilling to change for gym or
		  participate in physical
		  education class
		Withdrawal, fantasy, or infantile
		  behavior or knowledge
		Poor peer relationships
		Delinquent or runaway
		Reports sexual assault by
		  caretaker
		Change in performance in school

Table B.1-1—*continued*

Type of Abuse	Physical Indicators	Behavioral Indicators
Emotional maltreatment	Speech disorders Lag in physical development Failure to thrive Hyperactive or disruptive behavior	Habit disorders (sucking, biting, rocking, etc.) Conduct or learning disorders (antisocial, destructive, etc.) Neurotic traits (sleep disorders, inhibition of play, unusual fearfulness) Psychoneurotic reactions (hysteria, obsession, compulsion, phobias, hypochondria) Behavior extremes (compliant, passive; aggressive, demanding) Overly adaptive behavior (inappropriately adult, inappropriately infantile) Developmental lags (mental, emotional) Attempted suicide

Table from J W Lauer, I S Laurie, M K Salus, et al: *The Role of the Mental Health Professional in the Prevention and Treatment of Child Abuse and Neglect.* US Department of Health, Education and Welfare, National Center on Child Abuse and Neglect, Washington, 1979.

the child and each parent alone and together. Note any change in behavior in each setting. Does the child become fearful in the presence of a parent? Does a parent appear threatening to the child? If any history of violence is presented, other questions can be gently directed toward other potential problem areas, such as drug and alcohol involvement, wife battering, and financial or legal problems.

EVALUATION AND MANAGEMENT

1. The emergency physician who suspects child abuse is legally required to refer all such cases to the local child protection agency.

2. Always consider abuse in a child brought to the emergency room with any signs or symptoms listed in Table B.1-1.

3. Almost a third of all abused children are under the age of 5 years and are unable to give a history. Children older than 5 years may feel too frightened, guilty, loyal, or anxious to give a reliable history. Take the history from the person bringing the child to the emergency room. Obtain old records, if they are available, to identify a pattern of abuse.

4. Use the physical examination to obtain evidence of abuse or sexual trauma. Look for genital irritations, trauma, and discharges; also look for minor bruises, welts, fractures, lacerations, abrasions, abdominal injuries, and central nervous system injuries. Have a nurse present during the examination. Do not force the child to submit to an examination. In sex-abuse cases, check for sexually transmitted diseases. Hospitalize the victim if necessary.

5. Carefully document any evidence of abuse. It is sometimes impossible to make a definitive diagnosis of abuse on one visit, so any documentation

may be used in the future to identify a pattern. Complete a detailed physical examination, and obtain X-rays and a medical or surgical consultation, even if the patient is hesitant. Look for burns, head-injury fractures, and bruises. Photograph visible injuries.

6. Many centers have specific rape protocols that require the collection of specimens and physical evidence. Those protocols should be carefully followed.

7. In cases of suspected sexual abuse, obtain oral, anal, and vaginal cultures to rule out the presence of gonorrhea.

8. Identify and treat other psychiatric disorders, such as depression, anxiety, insomnia, and substance abuse.

9. Evaluate the dangerousness of returning the child to the home. Although it is usually undesirable to separate a child from a parent, the child must be removed and protected if the situation presents a persistent danger. That is a physician's legal responsibility. Children can be placed in foster homes or with relatives or friends. The possible abuser should not be confronted until the safety of the child has been assured by removing the child or the suspected abuser from the home. The arrival of the child victim in the emergency room may be a rare opportunity for intervention.

10. Report the case to an appropriate protective service agency (for example, Child Protective Services), which will initiate the legal process.

11. Intervention includes an evaluation of the abuser, the victim, and the family. Try to determine the duration and the pattern of abuse. Organize follow-up and monitoring plans that include the possibility of legal action to protect the victim.

12. Support groups may be helpful, especially for adolescent victims. Local and national programs can aid parents and children, such as the National Committee for the Prevention of Child Abuse.

13. Victims of child abuse often grow up to be child abusers themselves. Ask the parents about their personal histories of child abuse, and check for the presence of a mental disorder, especially substance abuse and alcohol dependence.

DRUG TREATMENT

Psychotropic medication is not used in the treatment of abused children. The psychiatric sequela of abuse, such as depression or anxiety, may require appropriate medication; however, psychosocial approaches are preferred.

II. ELDER ABUSE

Elder abuse is defined as the physical, sexual, or psychological mistreatment of elderly persons. Abuse is most likely to occur to men over age 75 who are bedridden or who have a chronic illness that requires constant nursing attention.

An estimated 1 million elders (out of 32 million elderly people in the United States) have been mistreated. The highest risk of abuse is by a family member (for example, a grown child who has no relief from caretaking activities). The typical abuser is a white middle-class man between 40 and 60 years old who is under financial or mental stress.

CLINICAL FEATURES AND DIAGNOSIS

Physical Manifestations

The patient may show evidence of dehydration, malnutrition, bedsores, fecal impaction, dermatitides, lice infestation, bruises, welts, burns, punctures, hair pulling, or ammoniacal odor from urinary incontinence. Look for anogenital injuries as manifestations of sexual abuse.

Psychosocial Manifestations

On the mental status examination, look for confusion, psychomotor retardation or agitation, depression, suicidal ideas or attempts, anger or generalized apathy, and the need for excessive sleep or insomnia.

Look for overt anger by a family member or a caretaker that is directed toward the patient and for inconsistencies between the histories given by a family member and the patient. Insistence by a family member that the patient be hospitalized or placed in a nursing home immediately or a refusal to have the physician see the patient alone should arouse suspicion of abuse.

INTERVIEWING AND PSYCHOTHERAPEUTIC GUIDELINES

Always interview the patient and the family members alone and together. Note any changes in behavior in each setting. Ask the patient: "Have you ever been hurt by a family member?" "Do they feed you?" "Do you get out of the house?" "Do you get a bath?" "Are you given any medicine?" Inquire about any observed physical signs: "How did you get that black-and-blue mark?"

EVALUATION AND MANAGEMENT

1. Report elder abuse to an appropriate health agency. Reporting is mandatory in most states (for example, California and New Jersey); it is voluntary in other states (for example, New York and Pennsylvania).

2. During the physical examination, look for fractured bones, contusions, and abrasions. Evidence of venereal disease and unusual genital infection suggest sexual abuse. Attend to the patient's immediate medical needs. Hospitalize the patient if necessary. Photograph visible injuries.

3. Try to create a good working relationship with the elderly patient. If the patient is cognitively alert, explain to the patient that you believe he or she is being abused. Reassure the patient that help is available.

4. Develop a comprehensive, interdisciplinary plan—medical, psychological, and legal. If the patient is returned to the home, give the patient an emergency phone number and make a follow-up appointment.

5. Tell the family members that support services will be made available to help them provide care. Elder neglect (a form of abuse) may be unintentional. Family members may be overwhelmed by their responsibilities.

6. Plans depend on circumstances. The patient may be kept at home with a home worker and visiting nurse services or may be placed in a nursing home. Remember that most elderly abuse victims fear institutionalization more than the possibility of continued abuse.

7. Provide programs for abusers who may require psychiatric treatment. Support services are available locally and nationally (for example, National Coalition Against Domestic Violence).

DRUG TREATMENT

Medication in the elderly abused population should be used with extreme caution because confusion is often present and medication may mask physical or psychiatric signs and symptoms.

Patients with a clear sensorium who are extremely agitated may be sedated with a single small dose of diazepam (Valium) 2.5 mg by mouth.

III. SPOUSE ABUSE

Spouse abuse is defined as physical assault within the home (domestic violence) in which one spouse is repeatedly assaulted by the other. The victim is the wife in almost every case (battered wives) and is most commonly a woman under 35 years of age. Husband abuse occurs rarely and almost always in response to the wife's having been beaten or when a frail elderly man is married to a very young woman. Spouse abuse is reported in about 1.8 million households, but it is thought to be an underreported phenomenon. Between 2,000 and 5,000 deaths each year are attributed to spouse abuse.

The typical abuser is a man between 18 and 24 years who is unemployed and suffering from alcoholism, substance abuse, or some other mental disorder. He is often extremely possessive and jealous. The typical wife beater came from a violent home where he witnessed his mother's being beaten. He may also have been abused by his own father or mother as a child, and he may frequently abuse his own children. Most spouse abuse occurs repeatedly in a consistent pattern that is set up early in a marriage or a relationship. The abuse may increase in violence around the holidays. Violence often occurs when the husband sees his wife as less available than in the past because of her pregnancy, relationships with friends, going to school, or taking a job.

CLINICAL FEATURES AND DIAGNOSIS

Look for multiple injuries at various sites—contusions, lacerations, and abrasions, particularly around the face. Look for ecchymoses in the neck area, indicating a stranglehold.

Look for bathing-suit-pattern injuries—bruises over the chest, the breasts, the abdomen, and the pelvis that are not readily visible to observers.

Pregnant women are often victims; look for injuries on the abdominal wall over the uterus.

A medical workup is essential, especially X-rays for fractures. Always consider head injuries, especially if the patient is confused or lethargic. Somatic symptoms—such as headaches, chronic pain, and gastrointestinal distress—are common. Depression, anxiety, insomnia, and suicidal gestures and attempts are also common.

INTERVIEWING AND PSYCHOTHERAPEUTIC GUIDELINES

The abused person often appears very guarded or depressed, and the abuser may appear nervous and possessive. Separate the victim from the abuser to get an accurate history, but remember that the victim may be too frightened to reveal the truth. The victim may initially describe problems in the marriage, issues of infidelity, or financial and legal problems without mentioning abuse. In fact, the victim may initially deny being abused. Be courteous and respectful of the patient, and show concern for her safety. Assure the patient that she is not to blame. Many women feel that they provoked the abuse—for example, by not making dinner. The patient may be frightened of her husband. Do not confront her or pressure her to lodge a complaint, but allow her to ventilate her anger. Explain that abuse is a common problem, that she is not alone, and that help is available.

The batterer may intimidate the patient, but the patient must be handled tactfully, as she may flee into denial and guilt if she feels that her husband is being confronted and exposed. Try to ask the patient if she has ever been hit by her husband. If he drinks, ask if he gets drunk and how he acts then. Does he curse or lose his temper? Is he jealous for any reason? Ask about her suicidal ideas and attempts; they are often seen in battered women.

EVALUATION AND MANAGEMENT

1. Admit the patient to a general hospital if there is a medical or surgical need or to a psychiatric hospital if the patient is actively suicidal. Make a diagnostic evaluation of any associated drug or alcohol abuse. Photograph the injuries for possible legal documentation, even if the patient does not wish to press charges at the time. Old hospital charts should be reviewed for evidence of prior abuse or trauma.

2. Refer the woman to a shelter if she is unwilling to return home.

3. Give her an emergency number to call if she feels threatened at any time after returning home or if she feels that her husband is menacing her.

4. Schedule a follow-up appointment, or refer the patient to a support group for battered wives—for example, National Woman Abuse Prevention Center.

DRUG TREATMENT

Extremely agitated patients may require sedation with a single dose of a benzodiazepine in the emergency room or your office—for example, diazepam 2.5 to 5 mg intramuscularly (IM) or by mouth or lorazepam (Ativan) 1 to 2 mg IM or by mouth.

Psychiatric complications of spouse abuse, such as depression, may require antidepressant medication at a later date as part of a comprehensive treatment plan.

Cross-References:

Incest, rape and sexual abuse, violence.

---

2 / Acquired Immune Deficiency Syndrome (AIDS)

According to the Centers for Disease Control (CDC), acquired immune deficiency syndrome (AIDS) is a "disease, at least moderately predictive of a defect in cell-mediated immunity, occurring in a person with no known cause for diminished resistance to that disease." Human immunodeficiency virus (HIV) is transmitted through infected bodily fluids—in particular, semen and blood. AIDS is lethal and has reached epidemic proportions.

High-risk groups include (1) male homosexuals who have been sexually active since 1977, (2) intravenous drug users, (3) recipients since 1977 of blood transfusions (for example, hemophiliac patients) that were not screened for HIV, (4) sexual partners of any persons in any high-risk group, (5) persons with open wounds that were exposed to HIV-contaminated blood. In addition, persons requesting an HIV test may have a high-risk factor that they are unwilling to reveal. An estimated two thirds of people with AIDS have associated neuropsychiatric symptoms, and one third of those patients have neuropsychiatric symptoms as the initial and presenting symptoms.

CLINICAL FEATURES AND DIAGNOSIS

A diagnosis of AIDS is made in an HIV-positive patient with findings of decreased cell-mediated immunity and subsequent opportunistic infections (such as *Pneumocystis carinii* pneumonia) or neoplasms (such as Kaposi's sarcoma). In addition, the expanded AIDS surveillance case definition includes all HIV-infected persons who have less than 200 CD4+ T-lymphocytes/μL or a CD4+ T-lymphocyte percent of total lymphocytes less than 14 or who have received a diagnosis of pulmonary tuberculosis, invasive cervical cancer, or recurrent pneumonia. If a screening test is positive for HIV antibodies, it is confirmed by a Western blot analysis test. HIV often infects the central nervous system (CNS) directly.

Making a diagnosis of infection with HIV by blood tests is important because (1) the treatment of asymptomatic HIV-infected patients with azidothymidine (AZT) and other medications is useful and (2) behavior can be changed to avoid spreading HIV (for example, by safe sex and by not sharing needles). HIV screening is indicated in any person in a high-risk group.

Functional disorders that often develop as a consequence of having AIDS include depression, anxiety disorders, adjustment disorders, and, less commonly, psychosis or mania. HIV-infected patients can present with organic disorders as a result of direct CNS infection with HIV or an opportunistic CNS infection, such as toxoplasmosis, cryptococcosis, cytomegalovirus, and herpes. Organic mental disorders include delirium, dementia, depression, mania, psychoses, organic personality disorders, and frank neurological signs. CNS metastases of Kaposi's sarcoma and primary CNS lymphoma are common.

A full dementia syndrome in AIDS is also common. AIDS dementia may present with memory loss and other cognitive dysfunctions, psychomotor retardation, social withdrawal, and apathy. Neurological signs, motor deficits, and seizures (including temporal lobe seizures) can occur. AIDS dementia is believed to be due to a chronic encephalitis from HIV infection; it is progressive. The medical workup of an AIDS patient usually includes specific blood tests, a computed tomographic (CT) or magnetic resonance imaging (MRI) scan, a lumbar puncture, and cultures of the blood and the cerebrospinal fluid (CSF).

INTERVIEWING AND PSYCHOTHERAPEUTIC GUIDELINES

Ask all patients whether they have been tested for HIV. Any patient in a high-risk group should be counseled about possible HIV testing and about changing behavior to reduce risk. Major psychological implications surround the HIV test. Extensive pretest and posttest counseling and a written informed consent are required (Tables B.2–1 and B.2–2).

EVALUATION AND MANAGEMENT

1. When treating a known or suspected HIV-positive patient, protect staff members, family members, and other patients from possible exposure. Staff members should be immediately instructed to practice universal precautions, especially when invasive procedures, a physical examination, or blood tests are indicated. AIDS patients require a thorough physical examination and medical evaluation for signs of opportunistic infection. An infectious-disease consultation is often helpful.

2. Carefully evaluate the patient's cognition, which is often impaired in HIV-positive patients who have no other manifestations of AIDS. Subtle signs, such as impaired concentration and diminished memory, may be the sole initial findings.

3. Mild adjustment disorders, anxiety disorders, and depression can generally be treated with brief supportive psychotherapy. The general approach is similar to that used with cancer patients. Group therapy is sometimes helpful for the patient and for family members. Working through guilt feelings about high-risk behavior is often important. Talking about safe sexual practices and the cessation of intravenous (IV) drug use should be a priority.

4. AIDS patients present many ethical issues, including HIV testing, the seeking of experimental treatments, the duty to warn potential sexual part-

Table B.2–1
Pretest HIV Counseling

1. Discuss the meaning of a positive result, and clarify distortions (e.g., the test detects exposure to the AIDS virus; it is not a test for AIDS).
2. Discuss the meaning of a negative result (e.g., seroconversion requires time, recent high-risk behavior may require follow-up testing).
3. Be available to discuss the patient's fears and concerns (unrealistic fears may require appropriate psychological intervention).
4. Discuss why the test is necessary. (Remember, not all patients will admit to high-risk behaviors.)
5. Explore the patient's potential reactions to a positive result (e.g., "I'll kill myself if I'm positive.") Take appropriate necessary steps to intervene in a potentially catastrophic reaction.
6. Explore past reactions to severe stresses.
7. Discuss the confidentiality issues relevant to the testing situation (e.g., is it an anonymous or nonanonymous setting). Inform the patient of other possible testing options in which the counseling and testing can be done completely anonymously (e.g., in which the result would not be made a permanent part of a hospital chart). Discuss who may have access to the test results.
8. Discuss with the patient how being seropositive can potentially affect social status (e.g., health and life insurance coverage, employment, housing).
9. Explore high-risk behaviors, and recommend risk-reducing interventions.
10. Document discussions in the patient's chart.
11. Allow the patient time to ask questions.

Table from R B Rosse, A A Giese, S I Deutsch, J M Morihisa: *Laboratory and Diagnostic Testing in Psychiatry.* American Psychiatric Press, Washington, 1989, p 55. Used with permission.

Table B.2–2
Posttest HIV Counseling

1. Interpretation of test result:
   • Clarify distortion (e.g., "A negative test still means you could contract the virus at a future time; it does not mean you are immune from AIDS.")
   • Ask questions of the patient about his or her understanding and emotional reaction to the test result.
2. Recommendations for prevention of transmission (careful discussion of high-risk behaviors and guidelines for the prevention of transmission).
3. Recommendations on the follow-up of sexual partners and needle contacts.
4. If the test result is positive, recommendations against donating blood, sperm, or organs and against sharing razors, toothbrushes, and anything else that may have blood on it.
5. Referral for appropriate psychological support:
   • HIV-positive patients often need to have available a mental health team (assess need for inpatient versus outpatient care; consider individual or group supportive therapy). Common themes include the shock of the diagnosis, the fear of death and social consequences, grief over potential losses, and dashed hope for good news. Also look for depression, hopelessness, anger, frustration, guilt, and obsessional themes.
   • Active supports available to patient (e.g., family, friends, community services).

Table from R B Rosse, A A Giese, S I Deutsch, J M Morihisa: *Laboratory and Diagnostic Testing in Psychiatry.* American Psychiatric Press, Washington, 1989, p 58. Used with permission.

ners and family members, the effects on health insurance, and the potential loss of employment. Although few standardized guidelines exist for handling those ethical questions, they should be addressed directly and worked through.

DRUG TREATMENT

Psychotropic medications should be avoided if possible; if medications are necessary, use only low dosages, since AIDS patients are very susceptible to side effects. AIDS patients may have personality disorders or substance dependence disorders that antedate AIDS. Mood, anxiety, and psychotic disorders that are not responsive to psychotherapy can be treated with medication, although high dosages should be avoided. Antidepressants with strong anticholinergic effects may cause a worsening of cognitive deficits. Some depressed AIDS patients can be treated with low dosages of amphetamines. High-potency antipsychotics and benzodiazepines are sometimes indicated. Severe behavioral problems, such as agitation and assaultiveness, that do not respond to psychotherapeutic interventions can be treated with medication. Generally, benzodiazepines should be avoided because of the possibility of worsening any cognitive impairment, and high-potency antipsychotics—such as haloperidol (Haldol) in doses of 0.5 to 2 mg by mouth or intramuscularly (IM)—should be given.

Also known as zidovudine (Retrovir), azidothymidine (AZT) is an approved treatment for HIV infection. The drug blocks the replication of HIV and has brought about an improvement in CNS and other manifestations of AIDS. Many other drugs not approved by the Food and Drug Administration (FDA) are used by AIDS patients; therefore, a careful medication history is imperative.

Cross-References:

Delirium, dementia, depression, suicide.

---

3 / Adolescent Crisis

Adolescent crisis is defined as turmoil in an adolescent leading to significant behavioral, academic, social, or psychiatric problems.

CLINICAL FEATURES AND DIAGNOSIS

An estimated 30 percent of hospital emergency room (ER) visits involve patients under 18 years of age, and about 15 percent of all general hospital psychiatric emergencies involve adolescents. Most researchers agree that the two most frequently encountered adolescent emergencies are (1) suicide or severe depressions and (2) violence or other antisocial manifestations. Suicide and homicide account for the greatest number of deaths in adolescence. Teenage girls are reportedly seen more frequently in psychiatric ERs than are boys, in a ratio of 3 to 2; that ratio is attributed to the increased frequency of suicidal behavior in adolescent girls, especially girls between the ages of 12 and 14. At least one third of adolescent suicide attempts are by pill ingestion. Chronic separations and losses, including suicide in the family, are common features in suicidal adolescents' backgrounds. Runaway teenagers account for up to 13 percent of adolescent psychiatric emergency assessments, and the vast majority run away to escape an abusive or destructive home life.

Important questions include the following: What is the patient's baseline behavior? How does the adolescent's present behavior compare with adolescents of the same age and background? How is the patient doing in school? How are the patient's parents doing? How does the patient socialize? What is the patient's history of sexual activity and violence? What are the patient's peer relationships like?

Depression in children and adolescents may present with behavioral problems, rather than symptoms typically found in depressed adults. For example, acting out behavior and a drop in school performance may be signs of depression in an adolescent who sleeps well and has neither a change in weight nor anhedonia.

Other diagnostic questions and concerns include the following:

1. Is the patient psychotic?

2. Is there a history of drug or alcohol use?

3. Is the history consistent with a chronic psychotic disorder, a mood disorder, a substance abuse disorder, or a behavioral disorder, such as conduct disorder? Has there been a recent clear-cut change in mood?

4. Is there a childhood history of attention-deficit disorder? Children with attention-deficit disorder often have other mental disorders in adolescence and adulthood.

5. Is there a history of truancy, fire setting, cruelty to animals, stealing, fighting, temper tantrums, the use of a weapon, robbery, burglary, running away, forcing sexual activity, destruction of property, or other antisocial acts? If so, the patient may have a conduct disorder or an antisocial personality disorder. Homicide risk is greatly increased by any evidence of an organic mental syndrome, abnormal results on electroencephalograms (EEGs), childhood psychoses (especially schizophrenia), conduct disorders, severe mental retardation, compulsive fire setting, and a marked history of abuse or deprivation. A close association is reported between homicidal behavior and depressive phenomena.

6. Is there a history of temporal lobe or psychomotor epilepsy? A reported 18 percent of adolescents incarcerated for violent acts had probable temporal lobe epilepsy, compared with 0.5 percent of adolescents in the general population.

7. Has a recent or ongoing stressor precipitated the crisis? Is there an acute family problem? Has there been a recent loss? Has there been a change in the school or family environment? Is there an implicit or explicit family endorsement of violence?

8. Is the adolescent a victim of physical or sexual abuse? If so, the presenting problems may be those of depression, suicidal ideation and gestures, sexual acting out, truancy, running away, and alcohol and drug abuse.

9. Has the child been a participant in or a witness of any especially extreme, sudden, violent, or unusual event?

10. Is the adolescent involved with a cult?

11. Are there increased complaints of multiple vague medical symptoms, such as stomachaches, headaches, nausea, and eye problems?

INTERVIEWING AND PSYCHOTHERAPEUTIC GUIDELINES

Try to engage the patient in a nonthreatening way, and give the patient a chance to talk freely and to complain or ventilate. Many adolescents are threatened by the possibility of psychiatric intervention or hospitalization and do not know how to react.

It is often necessary to interview an adolescent alone, without the parents. The parents then may be seen separately or in conjunction with the adolescent. It may be helpful to reassure the patient that the interview is confidential and to convey the idea that you are focused on what the patient perceives as problems. Some adolescents open up at the opportunity to speak with a supportive professional in safe conditions.

Sometimes adolescents refuse to participate in interviews in an attempt to exhibit some control in situations into which they feel they have been placed against their wishes. In such a situation, it is usually not helpful to confront the adolescent's defiance directly. A common and useful technique is to reframe the defiance in positive terms, such as the adolescent's need for privacy or autonomy. A typical statement is, "I can understand your need for privacy. After all, coming here was not your idea, and you don't know me from Adam. Please, only talk when you feel it is safe to do so; I want to be able to respect your needs."

EVALUATION AND MANAGEMENT

1. Adolescents in crisis can present a complex interaction of individual, family, psychosocial, biological, and medical problems and can require time-consuming emergency evaluations. It is important to obtain information from corroborating sources, including the parents, other family members, a school counselor, and an outpatient therapist. It is also essential to rule out the presence of any underlying medical condition.

2. Try to avoid hospitalizing adolescents unless no other alternatives are possible. Hospitalization often stigmatizes the adolescent and interferes with school attendance. Furthermore, within the structure of the family, hospitalization identifies the patient as the one with the disorder when there may also be significant family pathology. Clear treatments and expected benefits of needed hospitalization should be delineated. For example, some violent patients with conduct disorders may receive only behavioral control and detention in the hospital. Often, finding an alternative living arrangement (with a relative or a friend) or arranging placement in a group home can resolve an acute crisis. However, in certain situations, such as active suicidal behavior, admission to a hospital may be the only responsible recourse.

3. The compliance rate for referrals from an emergency setting to a clinic is reportedly less than 50 percent; thus, the handling of referrals is important. The parents must be given the names of the clinic and of the therapist, and the parents should be called to determine if the appointment was kept.

4. Know the legal requirements for adolescents in your community regarding competence to consent to treatment and whether parental consent is required.

5. Consult the parents and the patient's school.

6. If an adolescent patient is psychotic, be aware of suicidal and violent behavior. In a psychotic adolescent, suicidal ideation, even without suicide attempts, is extremely serious and almost always necessitates hospitalization.

7. The potential for suicide and suicidal behavior must be monitored closely in adolescents who are acutely homicidal or violent, as the conjunction of the two behaviors is high.

8. Pay particular attention to the management of violent eruptions in the ER or your office, especially if the adolescent has a history of violence or if the adolescent is under the influence of alcohol or drugs.

DRUG TREATMENT

Specific treatment depends on the diagnosis. If the adolescent is determined to be suffering from an identifiable diagnosis that responds to medication, treat accordingly. For instance, a psychotic, agitated adolescent could be treated with an antipsychotic drug, such as haloperidol (Haldol) 1 to 2 mg by mouth or intramuscularly (IM) every 30 to 60 minutes, until the agitation is controlled. The treatment of an adolescent with medication is a decision that needs to be made by a clinician experienced in the treatment of adolescent disorders. The decision depends on a high level of clinical acumen and sensitivity.

Cross-References:

Anger, brief reactive psychosis.

---

4 / Agitation

Agitation is a state of increased mental excitement and motor activity. It may occur in a wide range of mental disorders. It can be an emergency because agitation often precedes violence.

CLINICAL FEATURES AND DIAGNOSIS

Rule out an organic mental syndrome, such as delirium or dementia. Obtain the patient's vital signs if possible. Abnormal vital signs suggesting autonomic abnormalities are the first clues of an organic disorder, such as drug or alcohol intoxication or withdrawal (Table B.4–1).

Is the patient paranoid and psychotic, with impaired reality testing? If the patient is psychotic and agitated, medication may be indicated im-

Table B.4–1
Substance-Induced Organic Mental Disorders versus Functional Disorders in Patients Presenting with Agitated Behavior[1]

Physical Examination	Probable Cause	Treatment
Agitation with blank stare,[2] anxiety, stupor, aggression, panic, bizarre behavior		
Elevated blood pressure and heart rate, vertical and horizontal nystagmus, analgesia to pinprick, muscular rigidity, salivation, vomiting	Phencyclidine (PCP)	Minimal intervention (no talking down) Sensory deprivation with observation at a distance Diazepam for intoxication Haloperidol for psychosis No phenothiazines Diazepam for seizures α-Blockers or diazoxide for severe hypertension
Agitation with persecutory delusions or euphoria with irritability		
Sympathetic signs: blood pressure elevation, tachycardia, tachypnea, mydriasis, diaphoresis, motor restlessness, tremor	Amphetamine or cocaine or other sympathomimetics	Controlled environment Acidify urine Control hyperpyrexia, seizures (diazepam), behavior (haloperidol) No sedatives
No sympathetic signs	Consider schizophrenia, schizophreniform disorder, paranoid disorder, bipolar disorder, brief reactive psychosis, atypical psychosis	
Sensory distortion, hypersensitivity of all senses, euphoria, hallucinations, pseudohallucinations		
Sympathetic excess	Epinephrine-type hallucinogens; STP, mescaline, nutmeg	Controlled environment, support and reassurance (talking down); haloperidol for behavior control
Minimal changes	Indole-type hallucinogens; LSD, psilocybin	

Undistinguishable acute delirium

Muscarinic blockade: dilated and sluggishly reactive pupils, blurred vision, flushed face, paralytic ileus, constipation, urinary retention, fever, and hyperreflexia

Muscarinic blockade not present

Pilocarpine or methacholine

Reclassify patient by physical examination; if the findings are not clear, consider mixed or unusual presentation; consider polydrug ingestion when psychological and physical presentations are contradictory or confusing

Physostigmine

Conservative, with observation and protection as needed

Table from E L Bassuk, A E Skodol: The first few minutes: Identifying and managing life-threatening emergencies. In *Emergency Psychiatry: Concepts, Methods, and Practices*, E L Bassuk, A W Birk, editors, p 26. Plenum, New York, 1984. Used with permission.

[1]Adapted from A DiSclafani, R C Hall, E R Gardner: Drug-induced psychosis: Emergency diagnosis and management. Psychosomatics 22: Oct, 1981.

[2]The patient with moderate-dose or high-dose PCP ingestion may present with stupor or coma and later exhibit low-dose signs and symptoms.

mediately. Has there been recent violence? Is the patient impulsive, with poor judgment? If so and if agitation persists, more violence may occur. Is there a treatable medical cause? Many medical conditions (for example, hypoxia, hyperthyroidism, acidosis) and medications (for example, sympathomimetics, anticholinergics, digitalis) can precipitate episodes of agitation. Does the patient suffer from a personality disorder that may make the patient prone to impulsivity or to excessive anxiety in response to stress?

Make a definitive diagnosis, so that a treatment plan can be developed. Distinguishing between an organic and a psychological cause has implications for the subsequent treatment and course of action.

INTERVIEWING AND PSYCHOTHERAPEUTIC GUIDELINES

If conversation is possible, try to quiet the patient. It is important not to express overt anger or hostility. Do not be punitive. It is also important to remain nonconfrontational and to let the patient know that you will listen empathically to angry complaints and concerns and that you will be honest with the patient about limits and treatment. Be reassuring, saying that the interview is confidential and that the patient is in a safe place and that everyone there is trying to help. Stay as calm and straightforward as possible. If talking is not effective, isolate the patient, and avoid excessive stimulation from staff members and other patients. If the patient appears to be at risk of losing control, let the patient know that the staff will maintain control decisively and emphatically. Even if a patient requires medication for sedation, try to determine the psychological issues involved in the agitation. If possible, correct the distortions and diminish the irrational fears to decrease panic, anxiety, and agitation. Patients using phencyclidine (PCP) cannot be quieted or reassured and should be isolated immediately.

EVALUATION AND MANAGEMENT

1. Protect yourself and the staff. Do not place yourself in a situation in which you may be assaulted (for example, in a small office with the door closed). Have a sufficient number of staff members present to restrain the patient if necessary.

2. Physical restraint should be used if medications are ineffective and if violence or flight is impending. Be sure to have sufficient staff members who are trained in physical restraint. Caveat: If phencyclidine (PCP) intoxication is suspected, avoid restraints if possible; instead, isolate the patient in a nonstimulating environment. If restraints are absolutely necessary, do not use limb restraints, since PCP has anesthetic effects, and the patients may injure themselves by fighting against the restraints while feeling no pain (Table B.4–2).

3. Pay attention to any clues of impending violence. In particular, maintain vigilance for any changes in behavior, mood, speech, or affect—any of which may signal an impending loss of control.

4. Maintain consistency among the staff members with regard to the treatment plan. Give the patient a clear and unconflicted message about

Table B.4–2
Physical Management

---

1. Develop specific protocols, describing methods of restraint.
2. Determine the composition of the team (optimally, six persons, although five is usually safe).
    a. One person directs the restraint procedure and controls the patient's head.
    b. One person restrains a limb (four persons in all).
    c. One person administers the medication.
3. Review the specific plan for restraint, including the assignment of roles.
4. Have the necessary equipment and medication available.
5. Inform the patient about the treatment options.
6. Ask the patient to lie down so that you can apply the restraints.
7. Apply the restraints and, perhaps, medicate the patient.
8. Continue to talk with the patient about feelings and procedural issues.
9. Never leave the patient alone.
10. Convene a meeting of caretakers to discuss continuing patient observation and subsequent plans, including removal of the restraints, medication, and disposition.
11. Remove the restraints, one limb at a time.

Table from E L Bassuk: Management of the acutely ill psychiatric patient. In *Textbook of General Medicine and Primary Care,* J Noble, editor, p 27. Little, Brown, Boston, 1984. Used with permission.

what behavior can and cannot be tolerated in the emergency room or your office; but first the staff members must be in agreement among themselves.

5. If the patient is threatening to sign out of the hospital against medical advice (AMA), the clinician must decide if the patient is capable of making that decision and whether leaving the hospital would pose a life-threatening danger to the patient. The patient's capacity depends on whether a psychotic, dementing, or delirious process is occurring. If the patient's capacity is deemed to be significantly impaired and if there is increased risk, the patient must be prevented from leaving. Full documentation is warranted. Consultation with hospital counsel may be helpful in borderline cases. When the patient's capacity is not impaired but a serious medical risk is evident, the clinician must make every effort to try to convince the patient to remain in the hospital. A nonconfrontational, sympathetic stance that involves helping the patient feel in control is generally the most effective approach.

DRUG TREATMENT

For escalating or severe agitation, tranquilization may be necessary. Usually, either sedative-hypnotics (for example, benzodiazepines or barbiturates) or antipsychotics are used.

First, check the patient's vital signs if possible. Low-potency antipsychotics (for example, chlorpromazine [Thorazine]) should be avoided if the patient is hypotensive. If fever is present, avoid antipsychotics, since they cause poikilothermia and can interfere with a fever workup.

If intoxication or withdrawal from alcohol or sedative-hypnotics is suspected, benzodiazepines are the drugs of choice, since antipsychotics may precipitate withdrawal seizures.

If stimulant intoxication is suspected, benzodiazepines are indicated.

If the patient is not psychotic, benzodiazepines are indicated to avoid the risk of antipsychotic side effects.

If the patient is psychotic, consider antipsychotics. Although psychotic patients can be tranquilized with benzodiazepines, that is not considered a definitive treatment for psychosis. However, using benzodiazepines to tranquilize a psychotic patient in the emergency room or your office has the advantage of allowing the hospital inpatient treatment team to evaluate the patient free of antipsychotics the next day.

Drug Choice

If the patient is taking a specific drug or has a history of responding to a specific drug, use that drug again. If there is no available history of drug response, any benzodiazepine is as effective as any other, and the same is true for the antipsychotics.

Benzodiazepines. The drug choice is based on the available routes of administration (for example, intramuscularly [IM]), the metabolic pathway, the rate of onset of the effects, and the elimination half-life. Lorazepam (Ativan), 1 to 2 mg orally or IM, is the usual choice because it has an intermediate elimination half-life, is available in a parenteral form with rapid delivery to the central nervous system (CNS), and is metabolized by hepatic conjugation that is not delayed by liver disease. The dose may be repeated hourly as needed unless signs of toxicity (for example, ataxia, dysarthria, cerebellar signs, nystagmus) are present. Benzodiazepines can reportedly cause disinhibition, which may be difficult to differentiate from worsening agitation. If disinhibition or benzodiazepine side effects are present, the benzodiazepine must be discontinued and an antipsychotic started.

Antipsychotics. The drug choice is based on the available routes of administration, potency, and the side-effect profile. High-potency antipsychotics are the usual drugs of choice, even though they often cause extrapyramidal side effects; those effects are easily treated with anticholinergic drugs (for example, benztropine [Cogentin] 2 mg IM). Low-potency antipsychotics, although more sedating, can cause anticholinergic side effects and hypotension, which is more of a problem. The usual choice is haloperidol (Haldol), 5 mg orally or IM, which may be repeated if necessary in one hour. Akathisia (restlessness) is a common side effect of high-potency antipsychotics and may be indistinguishable from worsening agitation.

Combined benzodiazepine-antipsychotic. A combination of the two drugs is safe and is often used. Typically, the combination is lorazepam 2 mg and haloperidol 5 mg given together intramuscularly, although thiothixene (Navane) 5 mg may be used instead of haloperidol. Those combinations are safe and may be more effective than either drug alone, although that has not been conclusively proved. Furthermore, antipsychotics may reduce the risk of benzodiazepine disinhibition, and benzodiazepines may reduce the risk of akathisia. The disadvantage of such a combination is that, if the patient responds, it is impossible to tell which drug was effective or whether only the combination was effective.

Barbiturates. Although sodium amobarbital (Amytal), 250 to 500 mg orally or IM, is a traditional treatment for agitation, the barbiturates have been largely replaced by the benzodiazepines, which are less likely to cause hypotension, have a wider therapeutic index, cause less hepatic enzyme induction, and are less likely to cause dependence.

Cross-References:

Akathisia, alcohol intoxication, chronic schizophrenia in acute exacerbation, confusion, delirium, intoxication, mania, panic disorder, paranoia, phobia, restraints, violence.

---

5 / Agoraphobia (Fear of Open Places)

Agoraphobia is the fear of suffering severe anxiety in places where the possibilities for escape are perceived to be limited.

CLINICAL FEATURES AND DIAGNOSIS

Agoraphobic patients are fearful of open places and of leaving the home. (Table B.5–1). Agoraphobia is most often (in at least two thirds of patients) associated with panic attacks or panic disorder. Patients often give childhood histories of shyness, separation anxiety, and school phobia and give a family history of anxiety, panic, and phobias. Most patients describe experiencing anticipatory anxiety in the face of situations deemed potentially threatening, such as thinking about or going to a restaurant or other public places. The anxiety then intensifies into a full-blown panic attack. The patient seldom goes to a hospital with complaints of agoraphobia but may call the hospital or a psychiatrist on the telephone. The patient is more likely to go to a hospital or a psychiatrist with a panic attack. Agoraphobia seldom requires hospitalization, although it can be severely incapacitating, as the patient becomes increasingly unable to function. Untreated, panic disorder with agoraphobia has a high rate of depression and places the affected person at risk for suicide. Patients may present with symptoms that can be mistaken for borderline personality disorder, such as intense anger, feelings of isolation, suicidal gestures, and manipulativeness. Borderline personality disorder can coexist with a diagnosis of agoraphobia, so it is important not to miss either diagnosis.

INTERVIEWING AND PSYCHOTHERAPEUTIC GUIDELINES

Explore prior attempts to seek help. Agoraphobic patients may have made numerous unsuccessful attempts to get treatment and may become progressively frustrated and hopeless. Be calm and reassuring. Inform the patient that, although the symptoms are treatable, some time may pass before they are eliminated and that the treatment process is a gradual but

Table B.5–1
Diagnostic Criteria for Panic Disorder with Agoraphobia

A. Meets the criteria for panic disorder.

B. Agoraphobia: Fear of being in places or situations form which escape might be difficult (or embarrassing) or in which help might not be available in the event of a panic attack. (Include cases in which persistent avoidance behavior originated during an active phase of panic disorder, even if the person does not attribute the avoidance behavior to fear of having a panic attack.) As a result of this fear, the person either restricts travel or needs a companion when away from home, or else endures agoraphobic situations in spite of intense anxiety. Common agoraphobic situations include being outside the home alone; being in a crowd or standing in a line; being on a bridge; and traveling in a bus, train, or car.

Table from DSM-III-R, *Diagnostic and Statistical Manual of Mental Disorders*, ed 3, revised. Copyright American Psychiatric Association, Washington, 1987. Used with permission.

effective one. If the patient comes to the emergency room or your office with a companion, interview that person as well, both individually and with the patient. Any successful treatment of an agoraphobic patient requires the close cooperation of trusted people in the patient's life. Evaluate the suicide risk and the use of alcohol or other drugs.

EVALUATION AND MANAGEMENT

1. Determine whether panic attacks are present; if they are, determine their frequency and severity. Eliciting a history of frequent, severe, recurrent panic attacks essentially confirms the diagnosis and is critical in helping to establish the treatment.

2. Rule out organic conditions (for example, thyrotoxicosis, hypoglycemia, pheochromocytoma, temporal lobe epilepsy, stimulant intoxication, and withdrawal from alcohol or sedative-hypnotics). Obtain an electrocardiogram (ECG). Mitral valve prolapse is present in about half of all patients with panic disorder. ECGs are also helpful in reassuring patients that they are not having a heart attack during the panic attack.

3. Generally, panic attacks must be treated with medications before any psychotherapeutic techniques can be used. Once the panic attacks are controlled with medication, the most effective psychotherapeutic approach is behavior therapy (desensitization or exposure). Psychodynamic issues, although important to all patients with agoraphobia, may be of particular significance in patients who experience the agoraphobia without panic attacks. Family therapy, group therapy, and insight-oriented psychotherapy may also be helpful.

DRUG TREATMENT

If panic disorder is present, treatment of the panic attacks with benzodiazepines (for example, alprazolam [Xanax] and clonazepam [Klonopin]), tricyclic antidepressants (for example, imipramine [Tofranil]), monoamine oxidase inhibitors (for example, phenelzine [Nardil]), and fluoxetine (Prozac) can be considered, although those medications should be initiated only in the context of an ongoing therapeutic relationship. An acutely anxious patient can be given lorazepam (Ativan) 1 to 2 mg by mouth or intramuscularly (IM) and a small supply of 1 or 2 mg tablets to be taken three times a day until the patient can be seen for follow-up. Caution should be taken regarding a possible history of substance abuse before carrying out such a treatment plan.

Cross-References:

Anxiety, mitral valve prolapse, panic disorder, phobia.

---

6 / Akathisia (Motor Restlessness)

Akathisia is usually defined as an uncomfortable subjective and visible motor restlessness caused by an antipsychotic medication, often accompanied by agitation and irritability.

CLINICAL FEATURES AND DIAGNOSIS

Akathisia is an extrapyramidal symptom most commonly caused by high-potency antipsychotics. An estimated 50 percent of the people with akathisia also show evidence of other extrapyramidal side effects, such as parkinsonism, dystonias, cogwheeling, rigidity, and flattened affect. The condition is difficult to treat and may not respond to any treatment. Akathisia is commonly mistaken for worsening agitation, especially since it is aggravated by stress and anxiety, and it may be mistakenly and incorrectly treated with increased dosages of antipsychotic medication. Akathisia is a common reason for noncompliance with antipsychotic medication. An estimated 20 to 50 percent of patients taking antipsychotic medications experience akathisia.

INTERVIEWING AND PSYCHOTHERAPEUTIC GUIDELINES

Reassure the patient that the drug is the cause of the symptoms, and explain that the discomfort will be relieved by lowering the dosage or taking other medications to relieve the symptoms.

EVALUATION AND MANAGEMENT

1. Obtain the patient's history of antipsychotic treatment, especially the recent history.

2. The onset of the condition varies, but it generally begins several days, sometimes weeks, after the initiation of antipsychotic medication.

3. Ask the patient about subjective restlessness, and observe the patient for motor restlessness. Typical movements include repeatedly standing and sitting, pacing, crossing and uncrossing the legs, and shuffling or tapping the feet. Incessant repetitive movements are more likely to be akathisia than to be agitation.

DRUG TREATMENT

If both akathisia and agitation are present, consider sedating the patient with a benzodiazepine—for example, lorazepam (Ativan) 2 mg intramuscularly—and then reevaluating the patient in one to two hours. A typical dosage of lorazepam is 1 mg three times a day.

If akathisia alone is present, reduce the antipsychotic dosage if the target symptoms of antipsychotic treatment allow it. β-Blockers, such as propranolol (Inderal) 10 to 40 mg three times a day, may be helpful.

Clonidine (Catapres) has also been reported to be effective. It may be given parenterally in severe cases or orally 0.1 mg three times a day.

Anticholinergic medication—for example, benztropine (Cogentin) 2 mg by mouth, intramuscularly, or intravenously—can be tried. Anticholinergic drugs are much less effective in treating akathisia than they are in treating other extrapyramidal syndromes.

Amantadine (Symmetrel), a dopamine agonist, 100 to 300 mg, may also be tried. If those interventions are not effective, akathisia may warrant changing the medication to a low-potency antipsychotic.

Cross-References:

Agitation, anxiety.

---

7 / Akinesia (Decreased Motor Activity)

Akinesia is markedly decreased motor activity, including diminished facial expressiveness and eye blinking.

CLINICAL FEATURES AND DIAGNOSIS

Akinesia may be a side effect of antipsychotic medication or a symptom of catatonia, schizophrenia, depression, or an organic disorder. When it is a side effect of medication, it may be mistaken for a symptom of one of those disorders—for example, psychomotor retardation in depression or withdrawn behavior in schizophrenia.

INTERVIEWING AND PSYCHOTHERAPEUTIC GUIDELINES

Be tolerant when conducting the interview, because the patient's responses will be slow or nonexistent. The patient may be well aware of what you are saying and doing; therefore, explain your actions. Collateral informants may be particularly useful.

EVALUATION AND MANAGEMENT

1. Obtain the patient's vital signs. Fever may indicate neuroleptic malignant syndrome or an organic disorder.

2. Obtain the patient's history of antipsychotic treatment.

3. Examine the patient for waxy flexibility. If it is present, consider catatonia as a possible diagnosis. Other features of catatonia include mutism, negativism, and posturing. Catatonia may be a sign of a functional disorder, but it may also be induced by antipsychotics, especially in patients with organic disorders.

4. If catatonia is present, consider a drug-facilitated interview with amobarbital (Amytal) or diazepam (Valium). Those or other sedative-hypnotics may reduce anxiety and allow the catatonic patient to talk. If catatonia is related to an organic disorder, cognition may worsen with the sedative-hypnotic. Although sedative-hypnotics may further sedate an akinetic patient, they are useful for diagnostic purposes.

5. Akinesia secondary to depot antipsychotics (fluphenazine [Prolixin] and haloperidol [Haldol]) may be particularly severe and may be clinically indistinguishable from catatonia. Such a severe presentation is most likely if the depot medication is given too often or at too high a dosage for the patient. A considerable length of time (for example, weeks) at a lower dosage of depot medication may be needed before improvement is seen.

DRUG TREATMENT

A decreased antipsychotic dosage may relieve the akinesia. If a decreased dosage is not possible, a different antipsychotic may be indicated. The addition of an anticholinergic medication (for example, benztropine [Cogentin] 2 mg by mouth, intramuscularly, or intravenously) may also be helpful.

Cross-Reference:

Catatonia.

---

8 / Alcohol Dementia

Although the term *alcohol dementia* is often used for any dementia in a patient with a long history of alcohol dependence, it is often confused with Wernicke's encephalopathy and Korsakoff's syndrome, which are due to thiamine deficiency. Chronic alcohol dependence is believed to be able to cause a dementia independent of thiamine deficiency. Furthermore, in the context of ongoing alcohol use, the signs of dementia may be difficult to differentiate from signs of intoxication. Alcohol withdrawal or alcohol withdrawal delirium may further complicate the clinical picture. Alcohol dementia may also be superimposed on either Alzheimer's disease or multi-infarct dementia.

CLINICAL FEATURES AND DIAGNOSIS

Proper diagnosis requires that the patient be free of alcohol for several weeks. If dementia is diagnosed (Table B.8–1), the goal is to identify the possible reversible causes.

Clinical features are marked by impairment in abstract thinking, judgment, and higher cortical functions, such as language and comprehension.

INTERVIEWING AND PSYCHOTHERAPEUTIC GUIDELINES

Orient the patient as much as possible. A calm, reassuring attitude may help assuage agitation, which is common in alcohol dementia. Obtain the patient's history of alcohol use from relatives and friends. Assess the use of other drugs (for example, cocaine and benzodiazepines). Ask about falls, head injuries, and other traumas. Assess the patient's nutritional status if possible.

EVALUATION AND MANAGEMENT

1. Obtain the patient's vital signs.

2. Do a complete dementia workup, including a complete blood count (CBC), complete chemistry panel, thyroid function tests, Venereal Disease Research Laboratory (VDRL) tests, and serum B_{12} and folate level tests. A computed tomography (CT) scan of the head and an electroencephalogram (EEG) are also indicated. Obtain routine screening tests, such as urinalysis, urine toxicology screen, electrocardiogram (ECG), and chest X-ray.

3. Conduct a thorough physical examination and workup for any medical problems.

4. Other tests—such as a lumbar puncture, magnetic resonance imaging (MRI), and neuropsychological testing—may be indicated after detoxification and stabilization.

5. Reassurance is often effective in relieving the depression and anxiety in demented patients. Support and structure are very important.

DRUG TREATMENT

Give thiamine 100 mg intramuscularly (IM) and 100 mg by mouth three times a day. Give one multivitamin (B_{12} and folate) twice a day.

Maintain the patient's sleep with benzodiazepines if needed. If the patient is dehydrated, maintain adequate hydration by encouraging the ingestion of fluids. Treat any medical problems found.

Agitation or insomnia may be treated with either benzodiazepines or antipsychotics. Benzodiazepines—for example, oxazepam (Serax) 10 to 30 mg by mouth or lorazepam (Ativan) 1 to 2 mg by mouth or IM—are suggested for patients with recent alcohol use or dependence, since benzodiazepines are not likely to precipitate withdrawal seizures. Antipsychotics—for example, fluphenazine (Prolixin) or haloperidol (Haldol), both given at 2 to 5 mg by mouth or IM—are preferable in demented patients without

Table B.8–1
Diagnostic Criteria for Dementia Associated with Alcoholism

A. Dementia following prolonged, heavy ingestion of alcohol and persisting at least three weeks after cessation of alcohol ingestion

B. Exclusion, by history, physical examination, and laboratory tests, of all causes of dementia other than prolonged heavy use of alcohol

Table from DSM-III-R, *Diagnostic and Statistical Manual of Mental Disorders,* ed 3, revised. Copyright American Psychiatric Association, Washington, 1987. Used with permission.

recent alcohol use, because antipsychotics are less likely than are benzodiazepines to worsen the patient's cognitive impairment.

Cross-References:

Alcohol intoxication, alcohol withdrawal, amnesia, dementia, Korsakoff's syndrome, Wernicke's encephalopathy.

---

9 / Alcohol Hallucinosis

Alcohol hallucinosis is defined as hallucinations that occur in an alcohol-dependent patient within two days of a decrease in drinking or a cessation of drinking and that persist after the symptoms of withdrawal have disappeared. The disorder is uncommon and occurs more often in men than in women.

CLINICAL FEATURES AND DIAGNOSIS

The hallucinations are often unpleasant buzzing sounds or voices and visual hallucinations (Table B.9–1). The patient may also have delusions and paranoid ideas of reference. The patient shows no evidence of a decreased level of consciousness, and the patient's orientation for person, place, and time is intact. The duration is variable. The symptoms may last from a few hours to a few weeks; 10 percent of all patients have symptoms that persist indefinitely.

The differential diagnosis includes schizophreniform disorder, schizophrenia, mood disorders, and organic disorders. Always consider the possibility of the concomitant abuse of drugs (for example, cocaine and hallucinogens).

INTERVIEWING AND PSYCHOTHERAPEUTIC GUIDELINES

Calmly reassure the patient. Explain the origin of the hallucinations if the patient has insight. Do not argue about the sources of the hallucinations if the patient has a delusional interpretation of their origin. Provide a quiet, safe environment.

Table B.9–1
Diagnostic Criteria for Alcohol Hallucinosis

A. Organic hallucinosis with vivid and persistent hallucinations (auditory or visual)
    developing shortly (usually within 48 hours) after cessation of or reduction in heavy
    ingestion of alcohol in a person who apparently has alcohol dependence

B. No delirium as in alcohol withdrawal delirium

C. Not due to any physical or other mental disorder

Table from DSM-III-R, *Diagnostic and Statistical Manual of Mental Disorders,* ed 3, revised.
Copyright American Psychiatric Association, Washington, 1987. Used with permission.

EVALUATION AND MANAGEMENT

1. Obtain the patient's vital signs. Rule out alcohol withdrawal, which can be accompanied by hallucinations.

2. Conduct a full medical and psychiatric evaluation, giving attention to comorbid psychiatric disorders and the physical sequelae of alcohol abuse.

3. Do a urine toxicology screen.

4. Provide a safe environment, and be alert for violent outbursts, which can result in reaction to the hallucinations. Dangerous patients may need hospitalization.

5. Refer patients for treatment of alcoholism when appropriate.

DRUG TREATMENT

Administer thiamine 100 mg intramuscularly (IM) and then 100 mg orally three times a day.

Give benzodiazepines, such as lorazepam (Ativan) 1 to 2 mg by mouth or IM every four to six hours as needed. If benzodiazepines are ineffective, consider giving antipsychotics, such as haloperidol (Haldol) 2 to 5 mg by mouth or IM every four to six hours as needed.

Cross-References:

Alcohol intoxication, alcohol withdrawal.

---

10 / Alcohol Idiosyncratic Intoxication (Pathological Intoxication)

Alcohol idiosyncratic intoxication (also called pathological intoxication) is maladaptive behavior, usually aggressive (for example, fighting), that is not characteristic of the patient and that occurs after consuming an amount of alcohol that does not cause intoxication in an average person.

CLINICAL FEATURES AND DIAGNOSIS

The onset is rapid, and the duration is usually minutes to hours, terminating in prolonged sleep characterized by impaired consciousness, disorientation, and confusion. Transient hallucinations, illusions, and delusions may be present, as well as rage, agitation, and violence. The patient is often amnestic for the episode. An underlying organic pathology—such as temporal lobe epilepsy, head trauma, or encephalitis—may make the patient susceptible to the effects of alcohol. The disorder is reportedly most common in the elderly, patients taking sedative-hypnotics, patients who feel tired, chronically anxious people, and people with impaired impulse control. The differential diagnosis includes temporal lobe epilepsy and impulse control disorders.

INTERVIEWING AND PSYCHOTHERAPEUTIC GUIDELINES

Conduct the interview in a nonthreatening, calm manner. Security guards should be present to be available as needed. The patient should not be challenged or provoked, and, if possible, an isolated, quiet area should be provided for the patient.

EVALUATION AND MANAGEMENT

1. Take immediate steps to protect patients from harming themselves or others. Restraints and sedation may be needed.
2. Conduct a full medical evaluation for underlying organic disorders and medical complications of intoxication.
3. Conduct a psychiatric reevaluation when the patient is sober to evaluate for potential dangerousness and to determine whether psychiatric disorders are present.
4. Evaluate the patient for multiple substance abuse.

DRUG TREATMENT

Severe agitation or assaultiveness can usually be controlled with low doses of a benzodiazepine (for example, lorazepam [Ativan] 1 to 2 mg by mouth or intramuscularly [IM]) or a high-potency antipsychotic (for example, haloperidol [Haldol] 2 to 5 mg by mouth or IM). Low-potency antipsychotics, such as chlorpromazine (Thorazine) and thioridazine (Mellaril), should not be used, because they pose an increased risk of postural hypotension and because they lower the seizure threshold. Long-term dosing is not indicated, because of the risk of long-term side effects.

Cross-References:

Alcohol intoxication, intermittent explosive disorder, intoxication.

11 / Alcohol Intoxication

Alcohol intoxication (simple drunkenness) is defined as maladaptive behavior after the recent consumption of an amount of alcohol adequate to produce intoxication in most people. A blood alcohol level of 30 to 60 mg/dL is generally necessary. Legal intoxication is defined as a blood alcohol level of 100 mg/dL (Table B.11-1).

CLINICAL FEATURES AND DIAGNOSIS

The physical signs of alcohol intoxication include dysarthria, incoordination, ataxia, nystagmus, and a flushed face. The condition may be associated with a variety of behavioral changes, including giddiness and disinhibition, increased talkativeness, withdrawal, and argumentativeness. The patient's judgment and recent memory are impaired.

Carefully examine the patient for signs of withdrawal, such as tremor. Look for signs of trauma, especially head injury, subdural hematoma, rib fractures (from falling), and facial hematoma (from fighting); cirrhosis, hepatitis, pancreatitis, gastritis, gastrointestinal (GI) bleeding, neuropathy, and cardiomyopathy (direct effects of alcohol); infections; and signs of exposure to the elements. See Table B.11-2 for the diagnostic criteria for alcohol intoxication and Table B.11-3 for the differential diagnosis of alcohol intoxication.

INTERVIEWING AND PSYCHOTHERAPEUTIC GUIDELINES

Conduct the interview in a quiet, nonstimulating room. Intoxicated patients are often difficult to evaluate and frustrating to interview because their mental status may change rapidly as they become sober. Patients with other mental disorders who are also intoxicated may be suicidal or homicidal while intoxicated but not after they are sober. Evaluate the patient carefully in the acute intoxicated state; however, the first goal of treatment is to maintain safety while the patient becomes clear. If the intoxicated patient is agitated or belligerent, security guards should be available. Do not challenge, provoke, or reprimand the patient. Be as nonthreatening as possible.

EVALUATION AND MANAGEMENT

1. The goal is to help the patient through acute intoxication without injury to self or others; when the patient is sober, reevaluate for a definitive treatment.

2. Evaluate the patient for other alcohol-related disorders (especially dependence and withdrawal) and for other mental disorders.

3. Consider inpatient detoxification if necessary.

Table B.11–1
Stages of Alcohol Intoxication

Blood-Alcohol Level (mg/dl)[1]	Effects on Feeling and Behavior	Time Required for All Alcohol to Leave the Body
0.02–0.03%	Absence of obvious effects; mild alteration of feelings; slight intensification of existing moods; minor impairment of judgment and memory	2 hours
0.03–0.06%	Feeling of warmth, relaxation, mild sedation; exaggeration of emotion and behavior; slight impairment of fine motor skills; slight increase in reaction time	4 hours
0.08–0.09%	Visual and hearing acuity reduced; slight speech impairment; minor disturbance of balance; increased difficulty in performing motor skills; feeling of elation or depression; desire for more to drink; speaks louder and becomes more argumentative	6 hours
0.11–0.12%	Difficulty in performing many gross motor skills; uncoordinated behavior; definite impairment of mental facilities, i.e., judgment and memory, decreased inhibitions; becomes angered if he cannot have another drink or is told he has had enough	8 hours
0.14–0.15%	Major impairment of all physical and mental functiona; irresponsible behavior; general feeling of euphoria; difficulty in standing, walking, talking; distorted perception and judgment; feels confident of driving skills; cannot recognize impairment	10 hours
0.20%	Feels confused or dazed; gross body movements cannot be made without assistance; inability to maintain a steady upright position	12 hours
0.30%	Minimum perception and comprehension; general suspension or diminution of sensibility	
0.40%	Nearly complete anesthesia, absence of perception; state of unconsciousness, coma	
0.50%	Deep coma	
0.60%	Death is possible after complete anesthesia of the respiratory center	

[1]Milligrams per deciliter.
Table from W R Cote, F D Lisnow: Alcohol use and abuse. In *Emergency Psychiatry,* E L Bassuk, A W Birk, editors, p 132. Plenum, New York, 1984. Used with permission.

Table B.11–2
Diagnostic Criteria for Alcohol Intoxication

A. Recent ingestion of alcohol (with no evidence suggesting that the amount was insufficient to cause intoxication in most people)

B. Maladaptive behavior changes (e.g., disinhibition of sexual or aggressive impulses, mood lability, impaired judgment, impaired social or occupational functioning)

C. At least one of the following signs:
   (1) slurred speech
   (2) incoordination
   (3) unsteady gait
   (4) nystagmus
   (5) flushed face

D. Not due to any physical or other mental disorder

Table from DSM-III-R, *Diagnostic and Statistical Manual of Mental Disorders,* ed 3, revised. Copyright American Psychiatric Association, Washington, 1987. Used with permission.

Table B.11–3
Differential Diagnosis of Alcohol Intoxication

1. Sedative-hypnotic intoxication
2. Hypoglycemia
3. Diabetic ketoacidosis
4. Subdural hematoma; head injury
5. Postictal states
6. Hepatic encephalopathy
7. Encephalitis
8. Other causes of ataxia (e.g., multiple sclerosis, neurodegenerative disorders)

Table adapted from S E Hyman, B E Bierer: Alcohol-related emergencies. In *Manual of Psychiatric Emergencies,* ed 2, S E Hyman, editor, p 247. Little, Brown, Boston, 1988. Used with permission.

4. Intoxicated patients who make statements about suicide or other dangerous acts may have to be admitted to an inpatient psychiatry service; however, they can be kept in the emergency room or your office for observation, since their symptoms may resolve within hours.

5. Protect the patient from falling down and accidental injury. Also, prevent the patient, if belligerent, from assaulting others.

6. Obtain the patient's vital signs. If they are elevated, treat the patient immediately for alcohol withdrawal. Intoxication and withdrawal can be present in a patient at the same time, and they suggest a long-standing pattern of heavy alcohol use that has recently decreased (typically because of the unavailability of alcohol). Anxiety, irritability, tremor, and insomnia are other signs of withdrawal.

7. Find out if the patient also abused other drugs.

8. Evaluate the patient's mental status as completely as possible, particularly focusing on current dangerousness. Identify other mental disorders if any are present. Alcohol is commonly used to self-medicate anxiety, psychotic symptoms, and depression. Suicide is common in alcohol-dependent patients, and alcohol is commonly consumed before suicide attempts. Violence and homicide attempts are also much more likely when the patient is intoxicated than when sober.

9. Decide whether withdrawal is likely from either alcohol or sedative-hypnotics, which have cross-tolerance and cross-dependence with alcohol. Withdrawal implies dependence.

10. Provide a safe environment where the patient can become sober. It may be in the emergency room, in the waiting room, in a room in your office, at a shelter, at a sobering-up station, or at home if a family member can be responsible. Ideally, monitoring for signs of withdrawal should be available.

DRUG TREATMENT

High-dose or frequent medication is not indicated, as any sedating medication would most likely interact synergistically with the alcohol already in the patient. Handle agitation with physical restraint and, in extreme circumstances, the careful use of a benzodiazepine—for example, lorazepam (Ativan) 1 to 2 mg by mouth or intramuscularly (IM), oxazepam (Serax)

10 to 30 mg by mouth, or chlordiazepoxide (Librium) 10 to 25 mg by mouth. Always carefully monitor the patient.

Cross-References:

Alcohol overdose, alcohol withdrawal, blackouts, intoxication, violence.

---

12 / Alcohol Overdose (Poisoning)

Alcohol overdose is the ingestion of a quantity of alcohol sufficient to cause severe toxicity, coma, or death.

CLINICAL FEATURES AND DIAGNOSIS

Alcohol overdose typically occurs under two conditions, either as part of a suicide attempt or as an accident (for example, after a challenge at a fraternity party). The patient has inevitably drunk a large volume of liquor rapidly. If that were not the case, the patient would have been too intoxicated to continue drinking. A blood level of 0.1 to 0.15 percent alcohol indicates intoxication, a level of 0.3 to 0.4 percent alcohol usually induces coma, and higher levels cause death. Alcohol is a central nervous system depressant, and death is due to respiratory depression or the aspiration of vomitus.

INTERVIEWING AND PSYCHOTHERAPEUTIC GUIDELINES

Prompt medical attention is essential. The patient may be comatose or too ill to interview. If so, obtain a history from collateral sources.

EVALUATION AND MANAGEMENT

1. A toxicological emergency may require gastric lavage, intubation, and admission to a medical intensive care unit.

2. In patients who overdose as part of a suicide attempt, always consider the possibility of polyoverdose, and obtain a urine toxicology screen.

3. The patient's blood alcohol level is helpful information in an overdose situation.

DRUG TREATMENT

After drawing blood samples, administer thiamine 100 mg as prophylaxis against Wernicke's encephalopathy.

Administer 50 mL of 50 percent dextrose intravenously to prevent hypoglycemia.

Administer naloxone (Narcan) because of the possibility of concomitant opioid use.

Cross-References:

Alcohol intoxication, alcohol withdrawal, alcohol withdrawal delirium, coma, opioid intoxication and withdrawal.

13 / Alcohol Seizures

Alcohol seizures occur in the context of alcohol withdrawal (rum fits). They are associated with alcohol withdrawal delirium (delirium tremens).

CLINICAL FEATURES AND DIAGNOSIS

Seizures almost always occur 24 to 72 hours after the last drink or decreased drinking and usually precede delirium. Patients who are medically compromised are especially prone to seizures. The seizures are typically generalized tonic-clonic (grand mal) seizures and are self-limited, with an average of one to four. Many patients experience multiple seizures.

INTERVIEWING AND PSYCHOTHERAPEUTIC GUIDELINES

After immediate medical intervention, a collateral history should be obtained. Be alert to postictal confusion and agitation. Reassure the patient and explain that future seizures can be controlled.

EVALUATION AND MANAGEMENT

1. If the patient is untreated, significant mortality is associated with alcohol withdrawal seizures and delirium.

2. Carefully evaluate for other medical conditions, especially head trauma.

3. Also consider withdrawal from other drugs (for example, sedative-hypnotics and anticonvulsants).

4. Evaluate for other possible causes of seizures or delirium. Usually, seizures do not indicate an underlying seizure disorder, and the electroencephalogram (EEG) after withdrawal shows no abnormalities.

5. If the seizures continue for an extended period, if status epilepticus is present, or if the seizures are focal, rather than generalized, a cause other than alcohol withdrawal must be considered.

DRUG TREATMENT

The treatment is the same as for alcohol withdrawal delirium, but also consider magnesium supplementation and anticonvulsants, in addition to benzodiazepines.

Treat the seizures aggressively with benzodiazepines—for example, chlordiazepoxide (Librium) or diazepam (Valium) (Table B.13–1).

Table B.13–1
Treatment of Alcohol Seizures

1. Diazepam 10 mg IV (stat) given slowly.[1]
2. Diazepam 5 mg IV every 5 min until calm but awake; then
3. Diazepam 5 mg IV or by mouth every 4 hours until delirium clears, then decrease dose by 50% every day until the patient is withdrawn completely.
4. Optional prophylaxis. Phenytoin loading dose 1 gm IV undiluted given slowly over 4 hours (rate no higher than 50 mg/min). ECG monitoring is helpful during IV administration.
5. IV loading followed by phenytoin 100 mg by mouth three times a day through withdrawal period. Maintain blood level between 10 and 20 mg/mL.

[1]Chlordiazepoxide 2.5 mg may be substituted for each 1 mg of diazepam.
Table from W R Cote, F D Lisnow: Alcohol use and abuse. In *Emergency Psychiatry,* E L Bassuk, A W Birk, editors, p 135. Plenum, New York, 1984. Used with permission.

The prophylactic use of anticonvulsant medications for alcohol withdrawal seizures is controversial. In patients with pure alcohol withdrawal seizures, most authorities do not recommend the use of a long-term anticonvulsant medication.

Cross-References:
Alcohol withdrawal delirium, epilepsy.

14 / Alcohol Withdrawal

Alcohol withdrawal is a syndrome associated with the cessation of or a marked decrease in alcohol consumption in a patient who is alcohol-dependent. The presence of the disorder usually implies heavy alcohol use for at least several days. Most symptoms are attributable to central nervous system (CNS) hyperirritability.

CLINICAL FEATURES AND DIAGNOSIS

The onset of withdrawal begins several hours (usually six to eight hours) after a decrease in alcohol intake (Table B.14–1). Symptoms include a mild coarse tremor and at least one of the following: nausea or vomiting, malaise or weakness, tachycardia, hypertension, sweating, anxiety, depressed mood, irritability, restlessness, transient hallucinations, illusions, headache, insomnia (Table B.14–2).

The disorder is usually self-limited in otherwise healthy patients. Alcohol withdrawal is easily identified by the patient's history and by the presence of a tremor and elevated vital signs.

INTERVIEWING AND PSYCHOTHERAPEUTIC GUIDELINES

Reassurance—coupled with a calm, specific elicitation of the patient's history—is essential.

Table B.14–1
Diagnostic Criteria for Uncomplicated Alcohol Withdrawal

A. Cessation of prolonged (several days or longer) heavy ingestion of alcohol or reduction in the amount of alcohol ingested, followed within several hours by coarse tremor of hands, tongue, or eyelids, and at least one of the following:
   (1) nausea or vomiting
   (2) malaise or weakness
   (3) autonomic hyperactivity (e.g., tachycardia, sweating, elevated blood pressure)
   (4) anxiety
   (5) depressed mood or irritability
   (6) transient hallucinations or illusions
   (7) headache
   (8) insomnia

B. Not due to any physical or other mental disorder, such as alcohol withdrawal delirium

Table from DSM-III-R, *Diagnostic and Statistical Manual of Mental Disorders,* ed 3, revised. Copyright American Psychiatric Association, Washington, 1987. Used with permission.

Table B.14–2
Signs and Symptoms of Alcohol Withdrawal

Autonomic overactivity

1. Tachycardia
2. Hypertension
3. Diaphoresis
4. Tremor
5. Fever
6. Respiratory alkalosis

Sleep disturbance

1. Sleep latency insomnia
2. Increased rapid eye movement (REM) sleep
3. Decreased deep sleep (stages 3 and 4)

Gastrointestinal

1. Anorexia
2. Nausea and vomiting

Psychological

1. Agitation, anxiety
2. Restlessness
3. Irritability
4. Distractability, poor concentration
5. Impaired memory
6. Impaired judgment
7. Hallucinosis (may be calmly tolerated; often visual, but may affect all sensory modalities)

Generalized tonic-clonic seizures

Table from R D Weiss, S M Mirin: Intoxication and withdrawal syndromes. In *Manual of Psychiatric Emergencies,* ed 2, S E Hyman, editor, p 249. Little, Brown, Boston, 1988. Used with permission.

EVALUATION AND MANAGEMENT

1. Evaluate the patient's hydration and electrolytes. Either dehydration or overhydration may be present. Correct any electrolyte deficiencies, including calcium and magnesium deficiencies. Intravenous (IV) fluids are usually not necessary.

Table B.14–3
Treatment of Alcohol Withdrawal

Stage I: Mild to moderate withdrawal

1. Regular diet as tolerated.
2. Encourage physical activity.
3. Assess hydration (i.e., skin turgor, change in normal body weight, urine specific gravity); force fluids as necessary (120 mL orange juice or milk every 30 min × 8 then 120 mL orange juice or milk every hr × 6).
4. Vital signs every 4 hr × 48 hr, then during each shift.
5. PPD intermediate strength.
6. CBC, urinalysis, prothrombin time, fasting glucose, BUN, electrolytes, alk phos., bilirubin, SGOT, CPK, LDH, uric acid, total protein, albumin, globulin, stool for occult blood, VDRL, serum calcium, magnesium, amylase.
7. Chest X-ray, ECG as soon as possible.
8. Urine toxicology screen for other drugs of abuse.
9. Chlordiazepoxide 25–100 mg by mouth on admission, repeat in 1 hr.[1]
10. Chlordiazepoxide 25–100 mg by mouth every 6 hours × 24 hr.[1]
    Day 2: Cut day 1 dose in half.
    Day 3: Cut day 2 dose in half.
    Day 4: Discontinue.
11. Thiamine HCl 100 mg IM stat and 100 mg by mouth three times a day and every night × 10 days.
12. Folic acid 1 to 5 mg IM or by mouth every day.
13. Berocca C of Solu B Forte, 2 cc IM or IV on admission, then daily × 2 days (IM administered in gluteal muscle only).
14. After third dose of Berocca, stress caps twice a day.
15. Vitamin K 5 to 10 mg IV (only if protime 3 sec control).

[1]Diazepam may be substituted for chlordiazepoxide; 1 mg diazepam = 2.5 mg chlordiazepoxide.
Table adapted from W R Cote, F D Lisnow: Alcohol use and abuse. In *Emergency Psychiatry,* E L Bassuk, A W Birk, editors, p 135. Plenum, New York, 1984. Used with permission.

2. Carefully evaluate the patient for concomitant medical problems, especially head trauma, rib fractures, infections, gastrointestinal (GI) bleeding, and hepatic disease.

3. Prevent the progression to alcohol withdrawal delirium.

4. Outpatient management is contraindicated if the patient is febrile (over 101°F), has seizures, is unable to retain fluids, shows signs of Wernicke-Korsakoff syndrome, or has a serious underlying medical disorder.

DRUG TREATMENT

Benzodiazepines (chlordiazepoxide [Librium] 25 to 100 mg by mouth four times a day is the usual dosage) relieves the withdrawal and can be tapered over several days. Lorazepam (Ativan) 1 to 2 mg is an alternative. Lorazepam may theoretically be preferable in patients with hepatic impairment, since the elimination half-life of lorazepam is more predictable than the elimination half-life of chlordiazepoxide in patients with liver disease.

Administer thiamine 100 mg intramuscularly (IM) and then 100 mg by mouth three times a day. Thiamine is mandatory, since malabsorption is common in alcohol-dependent patients, and the consequences of thiamine deficiency are serious. Multivitamins, one capsule twice a day, are also mandatory, since the patient may be deficient in vitamin B_{12} and folate.

Monitor the patient's vital signs, and adjust the benzodiazepine dosage accordingly. If signs of withdrawal are present, increase the benzodiazepine dosage. If the patient is sedated and no withdrawal signs are present, taper the benzodiazepine dosage.

If the patient is being treated in your office, instruct the patient to go to the emergency room if any serious withdrawal symptoms are noted. Ensure adequate sleep with benzodiazepines.

See Table B.14–3 for the treatment of mild to moderate alcohol withdrawal.

Cross-References:

Alcohol intoxication, alcohol overdose, alcohol withdrawal delirium.

---

15 / Alcohol Withdrawal Delirium (DTs)

Alcohol withdrawal delirium (delirium tremens [DTs]) is a severe complication of alcohol withdrawal that occurs in about 5 percent of patients withdrawing from alcohol. It usually occurs in medically compromised patients with a long history of heavy alcohol dependence who stop drinking or who markedly decrease their intake of alcohol. The condition is potentially life-threatening if untreated; the untreated mortality rate is 20 percent. Even with optimal therapy, delirium tremens has a mortality rate of 5 to 10 percent. Death generally occurs as the result of hyperthermia, volume depletion, electrolyte imbalance, infection, or, ultimately, cardiovascular collapse.

CLINICAL FEATURES AND DIAGNOSIS

In 90 percent of patients, the onset of the condition is within one week of a marked decrease in alcohol consumption, most often after 24 to 72 hours of abstinence.

The condition often develops on the third hospital day in a patient who has been admitted for other medical reasons and who is not known to be dependent.

The signs and symptoms include delirium with a severely impaired sensorium, marked autonomic hyperactivity (for example, tachycardia, hypertension, increased respiration, fever, sweating), tremor, seizures (rum fits), vivid hallucinations that are often visual or tactile, and changing levels of psychomotor activity ranging from agitation to lethargy. Nightmares and insomnia are common.

INTERVIEWING AND PSYCHOTHERAPEUTIC GUIDELINES

Use a supportive approach for those patients who are confused, bewildered, and severely anxious. Reassurance and explanations are helpful.

EVALUATION AND MANAGEMENT

1. Vigorous, intensive inpatient treatment is required. The immediate goals of treatment are to prevent exhaustion, reduce central nervous system hyperirritability, and correct life-threatening electrolyte and fluid imbalances.

2. Avoid physical restraints, since the patient may fight the restraints and cause injury.

3. Evaluate the patient's hydration and electrolytes. Dehydration is common and may warrant intravenous fluids. Electrolyte deficiencies, including those of calcium and magnesium, must be corrected.

4. Carefully evaluate the patient for concomitant medical problems, especially head trauma, rib fractures, infections, gastrointestinal bleeding, and hepatic disease.

5. Observe the patient closely for the development of possible focal neurological signs, which, if present, require a further neurological workup.

6. Institute a high-calorie, high-carbohydrate diet.

7. Administer vitamins.

8. Infections, such as aspiration pneumonia, must be suspected and, if present, treated aggressively.

DRUG TREATMENT

Benzodiazepines (chlordiazepoxide [Librium] 50 mg or lorazepam [Ativan] 2 mg is the usual choice) may be given intramuscularly (IM) if they cannot be given orally. Repeat as necessary on the basis of elevated vital signs until the withdrawal signs are no longer present. Use the total dosage given in the first day as the standing dosage for the next day. Avoid antipsychotics, as they lower the seizure threshold and lead to dystonias.

Give thiamine 100 mg IM and then 100 mg orally three times a day.

Multivitamins given twice a day are mandatory, since vitamin B_{12} and folate are often deficient.

Monitor the patient's vital signs, and adjust the benzodiazepine dosage accordingly. If signs of withdrawal are present, increase the benzodiazepine dosage. If the patient is sedated and no withdrawal signs are present, taper the benzodiazepine dosage. Ensure adequate sleep with benzodiazepines.

Maintenance with anticonvulsants is usually not indicated for seizures that develop only in the context of alcohol withdrawal.

Cross-References:

Alcohol seizures, alcohol withdrawal.

16 / Amnesia

Amnesia, an impairment in memory, can be a sign or a symptom of a variety of disorders, including organic disorders, such as brain tumors and central nervous system (CNS) infections, and functional disorders, such as posttraumatic stress disorder and dissociative disorders. Amnesia can follow a head trauma, a seizure, or a migraine headache. It may be a side effect of such substances as alcohol, sedative-hypnotics, and hallucinogens.

CLINICAL FEATURES AND DIAGNOSIS

The disorder usually begins abruptly, and the patients are usually aware that they have lost their memories. Some patients are upset about the memory loss, but others appear to be unconcerned or indifferent. Amnestic patients are usually alert before and after the amnesia occurs. A few patients, however, report a slight clouding of consciousness during the period immediately surrounding the amnestic period. Depression is a common predisposing factor and a coexisting finding on the mental status examination.

The amnesia may take one of several forms: (1) *localized amnesia*, the most common type, characterized by a loss of memory for the events of a short period of time (a few hours to a few days); (2) *generalized amnesia*, the loss of memory for a whole lifetime of experience; (3) *selective* (also known as *systematized*) *amnesia*, failure to recall some but not all events during a short period of time; and (4) *continuous amnesia*, characterized by forgetting each successive event as it occurs, although the patient is clearly alert and aware of what is happening in the environment at the time.

Amnesia may have a primary or secondary gain. The woman who is amnestic for the birth of a dead baby achieves primary gain by protecting herself from painful emotions. An example of secondary gain is a soldier who develops sudden amnesia and is removed from combat areas as a result.

The organic differential diagnostic considerations for amnesia are listed in Table B.16–1.

Is there evidence of an organic disorder? Neurological signs are common in organic disorders. Is there a history of seizures or a recent electroconvulsive therapy session with postictal amnesia? Does the patient have CNS neoplasms or infections? Brain lesions (in the brainstem, the hippocampus, the third ventricle, the hypothamic-diencephalon system, and the cortex), subarachnoid hemorrhages, and diffuse cerebral disease can present with amnesia. Does the patient have a history of head trauma? Are there metabolic problems, such as hypoglycemia, porphyria, anoxia, and hypertensive encephalopathy? Is there evidence of infection (for example, herpes encephalitis)? A careful neurological examination is necessary, and a computed tomography (CT) scan or magnetic resonance imaging (MRI) is often needed.

Is there evidence of transient global amnesia? That type of amnesia usually occurs in middle-aged or older (above 50 years) patients who present with an abrupt onset, bewilderment, and an inability to form new memories. A profound anterograde amnesia usually lasts several hours to a few days. The onset may occur during sexual intercourse, intense emotion, or physical exertion. The amnesia for the period affected may be lasting. The prominent symptoms include anxiety and repeated questioning of others about what

Table B.16–1
Differential Diagnostic Considerations in Patients with Amnesia

Anoxic amnesia
Cerebral infections (e.g., herpes simplex affecting temporal lobes)
Cerebral neoplasms (especially limbic and frontal)
Cerebrovascular accidents (especially limbic and frontal)
Drug-induced (e.g., barbiturates, benzodiazepines, phencyclidine, LSD, steroids) disorders
Electroconvulsive therapy
Epilepsy
Metabolic (e.g., uremia, hypoglycemia, hypertensive encephalopathy, porphyria) disorders
Postconcussion amnesia
Sleep-related amnesia (e.g., somnambulism)
Transient global amnesia
Wernicke-Korsakoff syndrome

happened during the amnestic period. The patient shows no loss of consciousness or of higher cognitive functions and no associated seizures. Transient global amnesia may be related to cerebrovascular events (for example, vasospasm with consequent ischemia), and it is sometimes related to a migraine headache. About 25 percent of affected patients have recurrent episodes. No treatment is required.

INTERVIEWING AND PSYCHOTHERAPEUTIC GUIDELINES

Amnestic patients may be confused or frightened; therefore, a calm, reassuring approach is needed. Do not pressure the patient into providing lost memories. Obtain a collateral history.

EVALUATION AND MANAGEMENT

1. The most important task is to thoroughly evaluate the patient for possible organic disorders, which can then be treated.

2. If a purely psychogenic amnesia is diagnosed, try to help the patient recover the lost memories to prevent the creation of an amnestic nucleus that may facilitate future amnestic episodes.

3. In psychogenic amnesia, treatment with hypnosis or sedative-hypnotics (for example, intravenous thiopental [Pentothal] or amobarbital [Amytal]) to reduce amnestic barriers can be helpful.

4. In dissociative disorders, treatment may also include hypnosis or amobarbital interviews.

5. In somnambulism, treatment involves primarily protecting the patient from possible danger during the episode (for example, falling down stairs or through a window).

DRUG TREATMENT

Drug treatment depends on the specific disorder underlying the amnesia. For instance, amnesia associated with temporal lobe epilepsy is most effectively addressed by treatment with anticonvulsants; somnambulism may be treated with benzodiazepines, as are the psychogenic and dissociative amnesias. Organic disorders underlying amnesias must be treated specifically.

Cross-References:

Alcohol seizures, fugue state, Korsakoff's syndrome.

17 / Amphetamine or Similarly Acting Sympathomimetic Intoxication and Withdrawal

I. AMPHETAMINE OR SIMILARLY ACTING SYMPATHOMIMETIC INTOXICATION

Amphetamine intoxication, a syndrome produced by amphetamine ingestion, is characterized by behavioral effects—including hypervigilance, grandiosity, euphoria, and agitation—combined with physical effects that include hypertension, tachycardia, and dilated pupils.

CLINICAL FEATURES AND DIAGNOSIS

Amphetamines are the prototypical stimulants of a pharmacologically similar class of drugs that includes cocaine; however, cocaine, specifically crack cocaine (a purified form that is smoked), is abused more often. Other drugs in the class include methamphetamine (Desoxyn), dextroamphetamine (Dexedrine), phenmetrazine (Preludin), and methylphenidate (Ritalin). All those drugs have similar pharmacological properties.

The amphetamines can be orally ingested, injected, snorted, or smoked. Cocaine is usually snorted or smoked, but it can also be injected or absorbed through the mucous membranes. Episodes of intoxication may last days or weeks, followed by a withdrawal syndrome when the drug supply is exhausted.

Many amphetamine abusers are first introduced to the drug as the result of treatment for obesity or depression. Other abusers are those most likely to use the drug to prevent fatigue, such as doctors, students, and truck drivers. Some abusers use the drug solely to get high; those abusers are usually young, tend to abuse other drugs, and often use stimulants intravenously. Significant toxic reactions occur most often in infrequent users who ingest large doses over a short period of time.

Amphetamines and other sympathomimetic drugs produce both behavioral and physical symptoms. The behavioral and emotional symptoms range from mood elevation and an increased sense of confidence and mental alertness to grandiosity, hypervigilance, fighting, psychomotor agitation, anxiety, and impaired judgment; social or occupational functioning may be markedly impaired. The physical symptoms include tachycardia, tremulousness, headaches, dizziness, pupillary dilation, hypertension, perspiration, chills, nausea, and vomiting. Chronically intoxicated users exhibit repetitive, stereotyped movements, such as picking at clothes or sheets and taking things apart and putting them back together. With severe intoxication, delirium, a delusional disorder (typically paranoid), and auditory, visual, and tactile hallucinations can be produced. With overdose, seizures and death may occur. Sudden death related to cardiac complications has been reported. Abuse of the drugs frequently leads to dependence. Unprovoked violence may occur, especially when amphetamines are combined with barbiturates.

INTERVIEWING AND PSYCHOTHERAPEUTIC GUIDELINES

Reassure the patient that the symptoms are self-limiting. Approach paranoid patients with caution; explain your actions, and keep some physical distance between you and the patient because of potential violence.

EVALUATION AND MANAGEMENT

1. The immediate goals are to reduce the central nervous system (CNS) irritability and autonomic hyperactivity, control psychotic symptoms if present, and effect rapid drug excretion.

2. The intoxication is usually self-limited, and treatment is generally supportive. However, agitation, elevated vital signs (especially an elevated temperature), status epilepticus, and potential violence warrant medication.

3. Avoid excessive stimulation by secluding the patient in a quiet, calm environment.

4. Increase the excretion of amphetamine by urinary acidification—for example, ammonium chloride (Quelidrine) 500 mg by mouth every three to four hours if no signs of liver or kidney failure are seen.

5. Obtain a history of the type and the amount of drug taken.

6. Obtain and monitor the patient's vital signs.

7. Refer the patient for psychotherapy and a drug treatment program if indicated.

DRUG TREATMENT

To treat the patient's behavioral problems, start with a benzodiazepine—for example, oxazepam (Serax) 10 to 30 mg by mouth, estazolam (ProSom) 0.5 to 1 mg by mouth, or lorazepam (Ativan) 1 to 2 mg by mouth or intramuscularly (IM)—and repeat as needed. Psychotic symptoms are well controlled with antipsychotics. Antipsychotics should be monitored closely, since they lower the seizure threshold and cause hypotension. Also, anticholinergic contaminants in the amphetamines may potentiate the anticholinergic effects of antipsychotics.

For elevated vital signs, β-blockers—for example, propranolol (Inderal)—and clonidine (Catapres) have been used effectively. However, those drugs are not effective in treating the patient's behavioral symptoms.

II. AMPHETAMINE OR SIMILARLY ACTING SYMPATHOMIMETIC WITHDRAWAL

Amphetamine withdrawal is characterized by severe fatigue, insomnia or hypersomnia, agitation, anxiety, drug craving, and depression after the discontinuation of heavy amphetamine abuse.

CLINICAL FEATURES AND DIAGNOSIS

Withdrawal generally begins within three days of a decrease in or a cessation of drug use in heavy users. The signs and symptoms peak in two to four days and include dysphoria, depression, anxiety, irritability, disturbed sleep, fatigue, and apathy. Patients may present with suicidality, which can persist with severe depressive symptoms for months.

INTERVIEWING AND PSYCHOTHERAPEUTIC GUIDELINES

Provide reassurance by explaining the cause of the symptoms and their self-limited nature. Educate and reassure the patient that dysphoria and fatigue are expected withdrawal symptoms that dissipate with time.

EVALUATION AND MANAGEMENT

1. Obtain a history of the quantity, the frequency, and the duration of drug use, including polysubstance abuse.
2. Evaluate the patient for suicidality carefully and thoroughly, and take appropriate steps, including hospitalization if needed, to protect the patient.
3. Evaluate the patient for coexisting depression that may warrant treatment.
4. Refer the patient for psychotherapy and a drug treatment program if needed.

DRUG TREATMENT

Drug treatment may not be necessary when the symptoms are self-limited, mild, or amenable to psychosocial intervention. If anxiety is prominent, consider the short-term use of a benzodiazepine—for example, lorazepam (Ativan) 1 to 2 mg by mouth three times a day. Persistent or severe depressive symptoms may require antidepressant medication. Withdrawal accompanied by psychotic symptoms should be treated with low dosages of a high-potency antipsychotic, such as thiothixene (Navane), trifluoperazine (Stelazine), fluphenazine (Prolixin), or haloperidol (Haldol), all given at 2 to 5 mg by mouth twice a day.

Cross-References:

Cocaine intoxication and withdrawal, depression, hospitalization, intoxication, psychotropic drug withdrawal, suicide.

18 / Anger

Anger is an emotion, ranging from irritability to rage, that is experienced by all. Usually, anger is in reaction to an unpleasant or threatening stimulus.

CLINICAL FEATURES AND DIAGNOSIS

Most often, the diagnosis of anger is obvious and self-evident. Sometimes, anger is masked and presents as depression, apathy, or agitation.

INTERVIEWING AND PSYCHOTHERAPEUTIC GUIDELINES

Repeatedly reassure the patient that the situation is under control and that any concerns the patient has will be listened to in an empathic, noncritical manner. Try to determine if the patient is psychotic. If the patient is delusional, do not try to convince the patient that the delusion is false.

Determine if the patient is depressed or experiencing grief. In the first six months after a significant loss, a grieving person may experience and express a tremendous amount of resentment about the loss. A depressed patient may also present with a primary picture of irritability, frustration, and apparent anger when, in fact, the primary underlying problem is depression.

If patients are intoxicated with drugs or alcohol or both, they can become emotionally disinhibited and angry. In addition, demented patients often experience confusion, disorientation, frustration, and disinhibition, which can lead to angry outbursts.

If the patient is not psychotic, depressed, grieving, demented, or using substances, try to explore the reasons for the anger, and allow the patient to express the emotions felt.

EVALUATION AND MANAGEMENT

1. The primary objective is to prevent the escalation of the patient's anger to violence or other maladaptive acts. Often, allowing the patient to verbally express anger in a safe setting may significantly relieve the affect.

2. Be sure that sufficient staff members are present to restrain the patient if the anger escalates to violence.

3. Isolate the patient from the object of the anger. For example, if the patient is angry at his or her family, have the family wait in another room.

DRUG TREATMENT

If the patient's anger is escalating or if psychotherapeutic approaches are ineffective and violence or other maladaptive behavior seems to be imminent, medicate the patient.

If the patient is already taking a tranquilizer (a benzodiazepine or an antipsychotic), increase the dosage of that drug unless the patient is elderly or demented or is abusing substances. In those cases, benzodiazepines in particular may produce a paradoxical effect, which can lead to increased agitation and anger.

For patients not already taking a tranquilizer, benzodiazepines and antipsychotics are effective. Start with benzodiazepines (for example, lorazepam [Ativan] 1 to 2 mg by mouth or intramuscularly [IM]), since they have fewer side effects than do antipsychotics. If several doses of a benzodiazepine are ineffective, use an antipsychotic (for example, haloperidol [Haldol] 2 to 5 mg by mouth or IM or chlorpromazine [Thorazine] 25 to 100 mg by mouth or 10 to 25 mg IM).

Cross-References:

Agitation, homicidal and assaultive behavior, violence.

---

19 / Anniversary Reaction

An *anniversary reaction* is a set of behaviors, symptoms, or dreams that occur on the anniversary of a significant past event. Patients with recurrent depression often become depressed at the same time of year as in previous episodes. Patients who have suffered a significant medical illness (for example, myocardial infarction) may present with symptoms of the illness on the anniversary of the first episode. Family members of a patient who died of an acute illness may have symptoms of their relative's illness on the anniversary of the death.

CLINICAL FEATURES AND DIAGNOSIS

Determine the temporal pattern of the symptoms.

Identify the events that precipitated the episode. In anniversary reactions of an acute medical illness, a wide variety of stimuli may be present; often, family members are helpful in identifying the precipitants.

Rule out organic illness. Is the relative really suffering from heart failure?

INTERVIEWING AND PSYCHOTHERAPEUTIC GUIDELINES

Reassurance and a calm exploration of the chronology of the reaction are needed. Explain to the patient that anniversary reactions are likely to recur for several years and that feelings about the event should be expressed.

EVALUATION AND MANAGEMENT

If the reaction is determined to be psychogenic, explore the possible causes with the patient, and refer the patient for psychotherapy. In many cases, however, ventilation of feelings in the emergency room or your office may be sufficient, with no other treatment necessary.

DRUG TREATMENT

Drug treatment is generally not indicated unless the reaction is so severe (for example, major depression, psychosis, or extreme agitation) that specific drug treatment is warranted.

Cross-Reference:

Grief and bereavement.

---

20 / Anorexia Nervosa

Anorexia nervosa is an eating disorder characterized by a disturbed body image and severe self-imposed dietary limitations. The condition is thought to affect up to 1 percent of adolescent girls.

CLINICAL FEATURES AND DIAGNOSIS

Symptoms of anorexia nervosa include a body weight that is 15 percent below normal for the patient's age and height, an intense fear of being fat in spite of being underweight, a distorted body perception in which patients perceive themselves as fat even though they are emaciated, and a loss of three or more consecutive menstrual periods because of starvation (Table B.20-1).

This potentially fatal disorder usually begins between the ages of 13 and 20, is 9 to 10 times more common in females than in males, and is difficult to treat. Anorexia is more common in middle and upper socioeconomic groups than in low socioeconomic groups. Women who are pursuing careers that emphasize appearance are most vulnerable to the condition. Anorectic patients are often anxious, obsessive, and rigid. The disorder often begins in the context of a conflict about independence or sexuality. It may coexist with bulimia nervosa in cycles of rigid starvation followed by the loss of control, with eating binges causing guilt that leads to induced vomiting. Anorectic patients may also abuse diuretics or laxatives in an attempt to lose weight.

Anorexia nervosa is thought to be related to depression, although antidepressant treatments are not always effective. Anorectic patients may be uncooperative when brought in by their families for medical problems caused by starvation.

INTERVIEWING AND PSYCHOTHERAPEUTIC GUIDELINES

The patient is often brought into the emergency room or your office by the family or friends. Speak to the informants separately to get a history,

Table B.20-1
Diagnostic Criteria for Anorexia Nervosa

A. Refusal to maintain body weight over a minimal normal weight for age and height (e.g., weight loss leading to maintenance of body weight 15 percent below that expected; or failure to make expected weight gain during period of growth, leading to body weight 15 percent below that expected).

B. Intense fear of gaining weight or becoming fat, even though underweight.

C. Disturbance in the way in which one's body weight, size, or shape is experienced (e.g., the person claims to "feel fat" even when emaciated, believes that one area of the body is "too fat" even when obviously underweight).

D. In females, absence of at least three consecutive menstrual cycles when otherwise expected to occur (primary or secondary amenorrhea if her periods occur only following hormone [e.g., estrogen] administration.)

Table from DSM-III-R, *Diagnostic and Statistical Manual of Mental Disorders,* ed 3, revised. Copyright American Psychiatric Association, Washington, 1987. Used with permission.

since patients may deny or at least minimize the extent of their difficulties. Control is a major issue for anorectic patients, who are afraid that you will force them to eat. Avoid any such power struggles, which are likely to be repetitions of family concerns. Concentrate on obtaining the patient's history while maintaining an empathic, supportive stance.

EVALUATION AND MANAGEMENT

1. Conduct a full medical evaluation for nutritional deficiencies and metabolic diseases. In addition to the nutritional consequences of starvation, some medical conditions—for example, cancer and gastrointestinal disorders—can present with severe weight loss, and those possibilities must be fully evaluated. Electrolyte imbalances can be caused by vomiting, diuretics, or laxatives.

2. Screen for substance abuse. Stimulant abuse can also produce weight loss, although the loss is typically not as much as that seen in anorexia nervosa. Check the patient's stool for phenolphthalein (for example, Ex-Lax) as evidence of laxative abuse.

3. Evaluate the patient for depression. Anorectic patients are often depressed. Antidepressants may be indicated.

4. If medical complications exist, forcible treatment may be needed—for example, intravenous fluids or nasogastric feedings. When there is a family crisis or a risk of suicide, hospitalization may be needed (Table B.20–2).

5. Insight-oriented psychotherapy may not be useful. Cognitive approaches to change the patient's perceptions about body image and food are often helpful. Family therapy is strongly indicated.

DRUG TREATMENT

Antidepressants are commonly used and may be of value. Cyproheptadine (Periactin) may be helpful because of the weight-gain side effect of

Table B.20–2
Indications for Hospitalization of Patients with Eating Disorders

Emergency

- Weight loss >30% over 3 months
- Severe metabolic disturbance (pulse <40 beats/minute, temperature <36°C, systolic blood pressure <70 mmHg, serum potassium <2.5 nmol/L despite oral potassium)
- Severe depression or suicide risk
- Psychosis
- Diabetes mellitus in poor control
- Failure of elective outpatient treatment

Elective

- Family crisis
- Complex differential diagnosis
- Need to confront patient or family denial

Table from J R Hillard: Other emergencies. In *Manual of Clinical Emergency Psychiatry,* J R Hillard, editor, p 275. American Psychiatric Press, Washington, 1990. Adapted from D B Herzog: *Advances in Psychiatry: Focus on Eating Disorders.* Park Row, New York, 1987. Used with permission.

the drug. Serotonergic antidepressants—such as fluoxetine (Prozac), sertraline (Zoloft), and paroxetine (Paxil)—may also be useful.

Cross-References:

Bulimia nervosa, depression, starvation.

21 / Anticholinergic Intoxication

Anticholinergic intoxication is a syndrome of specific signs and symptoms, including mydriasis, constipation, elevated temperature, tachycardia, urinary retention, flushing, dry skin, and delirium caused by parasympathetic blockade. Anticholinergic (antimuscarinic) intoxication can be caused by many psychotropic drugs. Most often, the syndrome is produced by anticholinergic drugs that are coadministered with antipsychotic drugs to prevent extrapyramidal side effects, particularly antipsychotic-induced parkinsonism and antipsychotic-induced dystonia. All antipsychotics have some anticholinergic effects, but the effects are most prominent with low-potency antipsychotics, such as chlorpromazine (Thorazine) and thioridazine (Mellaril). Clozapine (Clozaril) also has prominent anticholinergic effects. Some chronically mentally ill patients abuse anticholinergic drugs for their hallucinatory effects.

Other psychotropic drugs can also produce anticholinergic effects. The most commonly implicated are tricyclic antidepressants, such as amitriptyline (Elavil) and imipramine (Tofranil). Other heterocyclic antidepressants, antihistamines, and monoamine oxidase inhibitors can also produce anticholinergic effects. Some over-the-counter hypnotics (for example, Sominex), eye drops, and asthma preparations also have anticholinergic effects, as do some cough preparations. Elderly patients are at a higher risk of anticholinergic delirium than are young adults.

CLINICAL FEATURES AND DIAGNOSIS

The peripheral symptoms include flushing, mydriasis, dry skin, hyperthermia, urinary hesitency, acute urinary retention, and decreased bowel sounds.

The central symptoms include agitation, hallucinations (often visual), hypotension, tachycardia, fever, seizures, delirium, coma, and eventually death. A medical aphorism related to anticholinergic intoxication is: red as a beet, dry as a bone, mad as a hatter (Table B.21–1).

INTERVIEWING AND PSYCHOTHERAPEUTIC GUIDELINES

In mild cases, reassure patients by explaining the cause and the treatability of their symptoms. Delirious patients may alternate between lethargy and agitation. The interview has to accommodate those fluctuations in activity—for example, be minimally stimulating with agitated patients. Questions should be brief, simple, and repeated as needed. Reorient confused patients, and provide explanations of the procedures. Identify yourself and the other personnel as often as needed. The presence of a family member or a friend may help calm the patient.

EVALUATION AND MANAGEMENT

1. Immediately discontinue all drugs with possible anticholinergic effects.
2. Consider toxicity from other drugs (for example, alcohol and sedative-hypnotics), in addition to the anticholinergic drugs.

DRUG TREATMENT

In severely agitated patients, give oxazepam (Serax) 10 to 30 mg by mouth or lorazepam (Ativan) 1 to 2 mg by mouth or intramuscularly (IM) or by slow intravenous (IV) injection. Repeat every hour as needed. Antipsychotics should be avoided because of their anticholinergic effects.

Physostigmine (Antilirium, Eserine) inhibits acetylcholinesterase (the enzyme that breaks down acetylcholine) and reverses the syndrome. Give physostigmine 1 to 2 mg IV over a one-to-two-minute period, and repeat in 20 minutes if no response is seen. Physostigmine can also be given IM every 30 to 60 minutes, but IM absorption is unpredictable. Only give physostigmine in settings in which cardiac monitoring and life-support systems are available, since severe hypotension and bronchial constriction may be precipitated. Physostigmine is usually used either to confirm a diagnosis of anticholinergic intoxication or to reverse the dangerous symptoms of the syndrome (for example, seizures, delirium, hypotension, hallucinations). It is contraindicated in patients with cardiac abnormalities or asthma.

Physostigmine toxicity can be reversed with atropine 0.5 mg IV for every mg of physostigmine given.

Table B.21–1
Anticholinergic Syndrome Manifestations

Systemic manifestations
   Tachycardia
   Dilated, sluggishly reactive pupils
   Blurred vision
   Warm dry skin
   Dry mucous membranes
   Fever
   Reduced or absent bowel sounds
   Urinary retention
Neuropsychiatric manifestations
   Agitation
   Motor restlessness
   Confusion
   Disturbance of recent memory
   Dysarthria
   Myoclonus
   Hallucinations (including visual)
   Delirium
   Seizures

Table from S E Hyman: Toxic side effects of psychotropic medications and their management. In *Manual of Psychiatric Emergencies,* S E Hyman, editor, ed 2, p 158. Little, Brown, Boston, 1988. Used with permission.

Cross-References:

Agitation, confusion, delirium, epilepsy, hallucinations, hyperthermia, intoxication.

22 / Anticonvulsant Intoxication

Anticonvulsant intoxication is a syndrome of signs and symptoms caused by anticonvulsant ingestion. Anticonvulsants are typically prescribed as maintenance drugs for the prophylaxis of epilepsy. Toxicity can develop as a complication. All anticonvulsants are monitored by testing blood levels. Phenytoin (Dilantin) does not have linear pharmacokinetics at all blood level ranges, so a small increase in dosage may produce a marked increase in blood level.

CLINICAL FEATURES AND DIAGNOSIS

Check the patient's anticonvulsant blood level and folic acid level because many anticonvulsants produce folic acid deficiency. If the patient's folic acid level is low, check the vitamin B_{12} level, since they tend to fall together.

Look for cognitive deficits. Although controlling the seizures can produce a marked improvement in cognitive functioning, anticonvulsants can produce cognitive impairment. The symptoms include sedation, sluggishness, poor concentration, and memory impairment. They may be present even when the blood level is in the therapeutic range. Typical signs of toxicity may not be present when toxicity is manifested by psychotic symptoms.

The short-term toxic effects include nystagmus, ataxia, dysarthria, tremor, hyperreflexia or hyporeflexia, lethargy, nausea, vomiting, slurred speech, hypotension, and coma.

INTERVIEWING AND PSYCHOTHERAPEUTIC GUIDELINES

Obtain a history of the nature of the seizure disorder, including the time of the last seizure (the patient may have postictal confusion and not intoxication). Interview collateral informants. If the patient is confused, be reassuring and direct while asking simple questions in a structured interview style. Repeat any instructions or explanations, and reorient the patient as you perform the evaluation.

EVALUATION AND MANAGEMENT

1. The usual treatment for anticonvulsant toxicity is a reduction in the dosage and the remeasurement of the patient's blood levels when a normal state has been reached, usually in four to seven days.

2. Adjust the dosage, supplement the folic acid and vitamin B_{12} if needed, and arrange for a repeat blood level test in one week.

3. Always assess intoxicated patients for intentional overdoses. Take appropriate steps when dealing with suicidal patients. Since some anticonvulsants are not completely protein-bound, hemodialysis may be an alternative, in addition to the usual gastric lavage and charcoal administration.

DRUG TREATMENT

No specific antidotes are available, but reports indicate that valproic acid (Depakene) intoxication can be reversed with naloxone (Narcan), which must be used with caution, since it may induce seizures by reversing the anticonvulsant effects of valproic acid.

Cross-References:

Intoxication, suicide, temporal lobe epilepsy.

---

23 / Anxiety

Anxiety is a state characterized by a feeling of dread accompanied by somatic signs indicative of a hyperactive autonomic nervous system. Anxiety is a common nonspecific symptom that is often a normal emotion. Pathological anxiety is out of proportion to any real threat and is maladaptive.

CLINICAL FEATURES AND DIAGNOSIS

Anxiety and anxiety disorders can present with any number of physical and psychological signs and symptoms, including those outlined in Table B.23-1. Patients who present to the emergency room or your office with anxiety may have any of the disorders delineated in Table B.23-2, all of which must be considered in the differential diagnosis. The anxiety disorders are specific illnesses characterized by pathological anxiety that is not secondary to an organic factor or another psychiatric diagnosis.

Panic Disorder

Panic disorder is characterized by spontaneous panic attacks that are unexpected and consist of a symptom complex that includes shortness of breath, dizziness, palpitations, and an intense fear of dying or going crazy. Patients often go on to experience agoraphobia and anticipatory anxiety.

Generalized Anxiety Disorder

Patients with generalized anxiety disorder have ongoing worry and anxiety with associated motor tension, autonomic hyperactivity, and vigilance. A significant proportion of the patients experience panic attacks and depression.

Phobias

Phobic patients are anxious in response to social situations (social phobia) or specific objects, such as snakes (simple phobia), or situations, such as being enclosed in a small space (claustrophobia).

Obsessive-Compulsive Disorder

Patients with obsessive-compulsive disorder have obsessions (recurrent and persistent intrusive ego-dystonic ideas, thoughts, or impulses) or compulsions (repetitive purposeful behaviors or rituals designed to neutralize anxiety or prevent discomfort or some fantasied dreaded event that the patient recognizes as unreasonable) or both that interfere with the patient's functioning.

Posttraumatic Stress Disorder

Posttraumatic stress disorder occurs in response to an extraordinary trauma (for example, rape). The event is reexperienced (for example, through flashbacks), stimuli associated with the event are avoided (for example, avoiding elevators after an attack in an elevator), or the patient has a generalized numbing of responsiveness (for example, a restricted range of affect) and persistent symptoms of arousal (hypervigilance). The disorder can be complicated by substance abuse.

INTERVIEWING AND PSYCHOTHERAPEUTIC GUIDELINES

Anxious patients often feel helpless, frightened, and out of control. Remain calm and reassuring, and encourage patients to express their ideas and concerns. Reassure patients about the nature of their symptoms (for

Table B.23–1
Signs and Symptoms of Anxiety

Physical Signs	Psychological Symptoms
Trembling, twitching, feeling shaky	Feeling of dread
Backache, headache	Difficulty in concentrating
Muscle tension	Hypervigilance
Shortness of breath, hyperventilation	Insomnia
Fatigability	Decreased libido
Startle response	Lump in the throat
Autonomic hyperactivity	Butterflies in the stomach
Flushing and pallor	
Tachycardia, palpitations	
Sweating	
Cold hands	
Diarrhea	
Dry mouth (xerostomia)	
Urinary frequency	
Paresthesia	
Difficulty in swallowing	

Table B.23–2
Medical Disorders Associated with Anxiety

Gastrointestinal system
  Colitis
  Crohn's disease
  Irritable bowel syndrome
  Peptic ulcer disease

Cardiovascular system
  Cardiac arrhythmias
  Cardiomyopathies
  Congestive heart failure
  Coronary insufficiency
  Mitral valve prolapse
  Postmyocardial infarction

Respiratory system
  Asthma
  Chronic obstructive pulmonary disease
  Hyperventilation syndrome
  Pneumothorax
  Pulmonary edema
  Pulmonary embolism

Neurological system
  Acquired immune deficiency syndrome
    (AIDS)
  Dementia and delirium
  Epilepsy
  Essential tremor
  Huntington's chorea
  Lupus cerebritis
  Multiple sclerosis
  Parkinson's disease
  Vestibular dysfunction
  Wilson's disease

Endocrine system
  Adrenal insufficiency
  Carcinoid syndrome
  Cushing's syndrome
  Hyperparathyroidism
  Hyperthyroidism
  Hypoglycemia
  Hypokalemia
  Hypothyroidism

Table from W R Dubin, K J Weiss: *Handbook of Psychiatric Emergencies,* p 157. Springhouse, Springhouse, Pa, 1991. Used with permission.

example, tell panic disorder patients that they are not having a heart attack or going insane).

When obtaining the patient's history, focus on precipitants, avoidance behavior, medical problems, obsessions, compulsions, and the time, course, and nature of the symptoms.

Discuss your diagnostic formulation in a clear and realistically hopeful fashion. Anxious patients may take comfort in hearing about the cause of their anxiety and the available treatment options.

EVALUATION AND MANAGEMENT
General Principles

1. Organic disorders must be ruled out before considering other diagnoses. Does the patient with classic panic attacks have a cardiac arrhythmia or hyperthyroidism? Obtain a full medical history. Is the patient taking medications that cause anxiety? Does the patient drink large quantities of caffeinated beverages? Consider a thorough neurological examination; blood and urine screening tests, including a toxicology screen; a computed tomography (CT) scan of the head; and a neurological consultation.

2. Precipitating events, the severity and the duration of the anxiety, the patient's past history of anxiety, such associated symptoms as insomnia and depression, and the anxiety's diurnal variation must be determined. Does the patient have an impairment caused by the anxiety?

3. Before making a definitive diagnosis, consider the following questions: Does the patient have a major depressive disorder, a psychotic disorder, or a panic disorder? Is the disorder situational anxiety? Does the patient have a substance abuse problem, a personality disorder, or an organic disorder? Does the patient have hyperventilation syndrome?

Management of Specific Disorders

Situational disorders. Anxiety is common in situational disorders. Any life stress can produce anxiety. Supportive and cognitive psychotherapies are helpful.

Depression. Anxiety is a common symptom of depression. If other symptoms—such as depressed mood, changes in appetite and sleep, diurnal variation, anhedonia, feelings of hopelessness and helplessness, guilt feelings, death thoughts, psychomotor agitation or retardation, and impaired concentration—are present, depression with anxiety is the appropriate diagnosis. Cognitive and supportive psychotherapies are useful.

Anxiety disorders. Panic disorder (with or without agoraphobia), agoraphobia without a history of panic disorder, simple phobia, social phobia, obsessive-compulsive disorder, posttraumatic stress disorder, and generalized anxiety disorder—all have anxiety as a prominent symptom. The definitive treatment of those disorders includes psychotherapy, usually behavior and cognitive therapy.

Obsessive-compulsive disorder. Many clinicians consider behavior therapy to be the treatment of choice for obsessive-compulsive disorder. It is successful in 60 to 75 percent of all patients. Family therapy is also very useful. Insight-oriented therapy and supportive psychotherapy can also be of help.

Panic disorder. Behavior therapy, particularly desensitization, is often effective in the treatment of panic disorder. Family therapy and insight-oriented psychotherapy can also be of use.

Phobias. Behavior therapy is often effective in the treatment of phobias. Some patients benefit from insight-oriented psychotherapy.

Posttraumatic stress disorder. Psychotherapeutic approaches in posttraumatic stress disorder include behavior therapy, cognitive therapy, and hypnosis—all with an emphasis on short-term treatment.

Generalized anxiety disorder. Treatment approaches include insight-oriented psychotherapy, cognitive therapy, biofeedback, and relaxation techniques.

Psychotic disorders. Psychotic patients often experience anxiety in association with their psychotic symptoms.

Psychotherapy is critical in helping patients to understand and to deal with their psychotic experiences. Supportive therapy, which may include advice, reassurances, education, modeling, limit setting, and reality testing, is generally the therapy of choice. Behavior therapy, group therapy, and family therapy can also be of use.

DRUG TREATMENT

General Principles

Benzodiazepines are usually the anxiolytic drugs of choice; however evaluate the anxiety and the associated symptoms thoroughly before prescribing a benzodiazepine. For psychotic or depressed patients, an antipsychotic or an antidepressant may be more appropriate than an anxiolytic. For a substance-abusing patient, benzodiazepines may be contraindicated. For a patient with panic disorder or posttraumatic stress disorder, consider such alternatives as antidepressants. Antihistamines such as diphenhydramine (Benadryl) 25 to 50 mg or hydroxyzine (Atarax, Vistaril) 25 to 50 mg are sometimes used as an alternative to benzodiazepines.

In general, benzodiazepines should be used for short-term symptom relief—that is, not more than several months. They are not usually considered a definitive treatment, although some evidence suggests that they are effective in the long-term treatment of anxiety disorders when combined with psychotherapy. Benzodiazepines are drugs with a potential for abuse. They are the drugs often taken by cocaine abusers, who use them to come down after using cocaine. In an emergency room situation in which the patient is not well known to the treatment team, benzodiazepines should not be prescribed if there is any suspicion of malingering or substance abuse. Giving benzodiazepines in that situation may reinforce drug-seeking behavior.

When prescribing benzodiazepines, give only a several days' supply to tide the patients over until they can be seen in ongoing treatment. All benzodiazepines are effective anxiolytics, and the drug choice is based on metabolic pathway (oxidation or conjugation), desired route of administration, and elimination half-life (Table B.23–3).

Identify the diurnal pattern of the target symptoms, including both daytime and nighttime patterns. Prescribe a drug according to the desired pharmacokinetic profile. For example, daytime anxiety with insomnia at night is best treated by a long-acting benzodiazepine; daytime anxiety without insomnia suggests the use of a short-acting benzodiazepine.

Table B.23–3
Benzodiazepines

Drug	Approximate Dose Equivalents[1]	Dosage Forms	Benzodiazepines Rate of Absorption	Major Active Metabolites	Average Half-Life of Metabolites (hrs)	Short-Acting or Long-Acting[3]	Usual Adult Dosage Range (mg a day)[3]
Alprazolam (Xanax)	0.5	0.25, 0.5, 1, 2 mg tablets	Medium	α-Hydroxyalprazolam, 4-hydroxyalprazolam	12	Short	0.5–6
Chlordiazepoxide (Librium)	10	5, 10, 25 mg tablets; 5, 10, 25 mg capsules; 100 mg parenteral	Medium	Desmethylchlordiazepoxide, demoxepam, desmethyldiazepam, oxazepam	100	Long	15–100
Clonazepam (Klonopin)	0.25	0.5, 1, 2 mg tablets	Rapid	None	34	Long	0.5–10
Clorazepate (Tranxene)	7.5	3.75, 7.5, 11.25, 15, 22.5 mg tablets; 3.75, 7.5, 15 mg capsules	Rapid	Desmethyldiazepam, oxazepam	100	Long	7.5–60
Diazepam (Valium)	5	2, 5, 10 mg tablets; 15 mg capsules (extended release): 5 mg/mL parenteral: 5 mg/5 mL, 5 mg/mL solution	Rapid	Desmethyldiazepam, oxazepam	100	Long	2–60
Estazolam (ProSom)	0.33	1, 2 mg tablets	Rapid	4-Hydroxy estazolam, 1-oxo-estazolam	17	Short	1–2
Flurazepam (Dalmane)	5	15, 30 mg tablets	Rapid	Desalkylflurazepam, N-1-hydroxyethylflurazepam	100	Long	15–30
Halazepam (Paxipan)	20	20, 40 mg tablets	Medium	Desmethyldiazepam, oxazepam	100	Long	60–160
Lorazepam[4] (Ativan)	1	0.5, 1, 2 mg tablets; 2 mg/mL. 4 mg/mL parenteral	Medium	None	15	Short	2–6
Midazolam (Versed)[2]	1.25–1.7	1 mg/mL, 5 mg/mL parenteral	N/A	1-Hydroxymethylmidazolam	2.5	Short	Parenteral form only: 7.5–45

Table B.23-3—continued

Drug	Approximate Dose Equivalents[1]	Dosage Forms	Benzodiazepines Rate of Absorption	Major Active Metabolites	Average Half-Life of Metabolites (hrs)	Short-Acting or Long-Acting[3]	Usual Adult Dosage Range (mg a day)
Oxazepam[4] (Serax)	15	15 mg tablets; 10, 15, 30 mg capsules	Slow	None	8	Short	30–120
Prazepam (Centrax)	10	10 mg tablets; 5, 10, 20 mg capsules	Slow	Desmethyldiazepam, oxazepam	100	Long	20–60
Quazepam (Doral)	5	7.5, 15 mg tablets	Rapid	2 oxoquazepam, N-desalkyl-2-oxoquazepam, and 3-hydroxy-2-oxoquazepam glucuronide	100	Long	7.5–30
Temazepam[4] (Restoril)	5	15, 30 mg tablets	Medium	None	11	Short	15–30
Triazolam (Halcion)	0.1–0.03	0.125, 0.25 mg tablets	Rapid	None	2	Short	0.125–0.25

[1] High-potency drugs have an approximate dose equivalent of less than 1.0; 1.0–10—medium potency; over 10—low potency.
[2] Used only by anesthesiologists.
[3] Short-acting benzodiazepines have a half-life of less than 25 hours.
[4] Metabolized by direct conjugation. Elimination half-life is not prolonged by liver disease or in the elderly.

All benzodiazepines are well absorbed after oral administration, but diazepam (Valium) and triazolam (Halcion) are absorbed rapidly. For intramuscular injection, lorazepam is rapidly and predictably absorbed. Benzodiazepines that are oxidized can have a prolonged elimination half-life in the elderly and in those with liver disease.

Treatment of Specific Disorders

Situational disorders. Since situational disorders are usually time-limited, benzodiazepines are useful for the relief of the anxiety or insomnia. For repeated anxiety in relation to specific situations (for example, stage fright), β-blockers such as propranolol (Inderal) are useful when taken before exposure to the situation and do not have the risks of sedation and dependence.

Depression. Benzodiazepines are useful to temporarily relieve the anxiety accompanying depression, but they are not a definitive treatment. Antidepressants are indicated in depressive disorders and can be combined with cognitive and supportive psychotherapy.

Anxiety disorders. Drugs used include benzodiazepines, tricyclic antidepressants, fluoxetine (Prozac), monoamine oxidase inhibitors (MAOIs), β-blockers, and clonidine (Catapres). Benzodiazepines are indicated only for short-term treatment; however, treatment often continues for prolonged periods, which raises the question of drug dependence.

Obsessive-compulsive disorder. Clomipramine (Anafranil) and drugs that inhibit serotonin reuptake, such as fluoxetine, sertraline (Zoloft), and paroxetine (Paxil), are potentially effective drugs.

Panic disorder. MAOIs are effective drugs, but, since they require a tyramine-free diet, tricyclic antidepressants and benzodiazepines (for example, alprazolam [Xanax]) are often used first.

Phobias. Phobias can be treated with MAOIs. Tricyclic antidepressants and benzodiazepines have also been reported to be effective.

Posttraumatic stress disorder. Drugs including MAOIs, tricyclic antidepressants, and benzodiazepines have also been used with questionable success. If you suspect alcohol or drug abuse, benzodiazepines and MAOIs should be avoided.

Generalized anxiety disorder. Drugs including benzodiazepines, buspirone (BuSpar), and tricyclic antidepressants are all useful. Benzodiazepines are particularly helpful for the somatic manifestations of generalized anxiety.

Psychotic disorders. If medication is needed, the question of whether the symptoms should be treated with a benzodiazepine or an antipsychotic is controversial. In general, giving an antipsychotic represents a decision to initiate an ongoing plan to continue treatment with that antipsychotic. Antipsychotics have a relatively long elimination half-life (about one day) and are typically used in the maintenance of chronically psychotic patients.

If a chronically psychotic patient responds to an antipsychotic, the antipsychotic is usually continued. Akathesia may be the cause of anxiety in patients who are already taking antipsychotics.

Cross-References:

Amphetamine or similarly acting sympathomimetic intoxication and withdrawal; barbiturate and similarly acting sedative, hypnotic, or anxiolytic intoxication and withdrawal; caffeine intoxication; depression; hyperventilation; insomnia; intoxication; obsessions and compulsions; panic disorder; phobia; posttraumatic stress disorder; psychotropic drug withdrawal; schizophrenia.

---

24 / Aphasia (Impaired Language Comprehension and Expression)

Aphasia is a disturbance in the comprehension or the expression of language; it is caused by a brain dysfunction.

CLINICAL FEATURES AND DIAGNOSIS

Aphasia can be a symptom of lesions in the frontal, parietal, or temporal lobes that have occurred in the dominant hemisphere. Aphasia is most often caused by a discrete lesion. It always warrants a full neurological evaluation. Often, the lesions involve Wernicke's area (used in the comprehension of speech), Broca's area (used in the motor production of speech), or the arcuate fasciculus (connecting Broca's and Wernicke's areas) (Table B.24–1). The typical aphasic patient is elderly and has a cardiovascular or cerebrovascular disease.

It is important to distinguish aphasia from the confused disorganized speech sometimes presented by psychiatric patients. In addition, patients with dementia may present with poverty of speech. Dementia is usually caused by diffuse processes, rather than by discrete lesions.

Aphasias are categorized as fluent and nonfluent. *Fluent aphasia* is characterized by a normal amount and rate of speech and correctly structured sentences. However, the words or phrases are used incorrectly, making the patient's speech unintelligible. Incorrect words may be substituted in a correct sentence structure. A patient with *nonfluent aphasia* has normal comprehension but an impaired ability to name objects or repeat words. Characteristically, the patient has a minimal amount of slow speech.

Both fluent and nonfluent aphasias must be differentiated from functional psychotic disorders. Nonfluent aphasia may be confused with withdrawn, isolated behavior or elective mutism. Fluent aphasia may be confused with a thought disorder related to schizophrenia or mania. Fluent aphasia is often misdiagnosed as dementia, since the patient appears to have diffuse cognitive impairment on structured cognitive tests.

Table B.24–1
Aphasias

Type	Fluency	Comprehension	Repetition	Naming
Broca's	No*	Yes†	No	No
Wernicke's	Yes	No	No	No
Conduction	Yes	Yes	No	No
Motor transcortical	No	Yes	Yes	No
Sensory transcortical	Yes	No	Yes	No
Mixed transcortical	No	No	Yes	No
Global	No	No	No	No
Anomic	Yes	Yes	Yes	No
Thalamic	Yes	Variable	Yes	No

*No = Impaired.
†Yes = Relatively spared.

INTERVIEWING AND PSYCHOTHERAPEUTIC GUIDELINES

Be patient when evaluating aphasic patients. Empathize with patients who are frustrated secondary to the aphasia, and concentrate on the systematic evaluation of language functions. A collateral history may be needed if communication with the patient is difficult.

EVALUATION AND MANAGEMENT

1. Test various language functions. Can the patient understand simple commands, such as, "Close your eyes," either spoken or written (comprehension)? Can the patient name common simple objects, such as a pen and a watch (naming)? Can the patient repeat simple short phrases, such as, "John opened the door" (repeating)?

2. Order a complete neurological examination and computed tomographic (CT) scan or magnetic resonance imaging (MRI) of the patient's head. Look for paresis of the right arm and the right side of the face in nonfluent aphasia. Nonfluent aphasias are commonly caused by lesions of the middle cerebral artery. Fluent aphasias are less typically associated with obvious motor deficits and can be caused by cerebrovascular diseases and diseases with diffuse involvement, such as Alzheimer's disease. A lumbar puncture and an electroencephalogram (EEG) may be indicated if the diagnosis is uncertain.

3. Order screening tests for organic disorders, including a complete blood count (CBC), thyroid function tests, Venereal Disease Research Laboratory (VDRL) tests, urinalysis, urine toxicology screen, tests for B_{12} and folate, and other tests as indicated (for example, human immunodeficiency virus [HIV]).

DRUG TREATMENT

Agitation is common in aphasic patients as they try to communicate, and an anxiolytic—such as lorazepam (Ativan) 1 to 2 mg by mouth or intramuscularly (IM), estazolam (ProSom) 0.5 to 1 mg by mouth, alprazolam (Xanax) 0.5 to 1 mg by mouth, or oxazepam (Serax) 10 to 30 mg by mouth—may be useful.

Cross-References:

Delirium, dementia, dysprosody, neologisms.

---

25 / Barbiturate and Similarly Acting Sedative, Hypnotic, or Anxiolytic Intoxication and Withdrawal

I. BARBITURATE AND SIMILARLY ACTING SEDATIVE, HYPNOTIC, OR ANXIOLYTIC INTOXICATION

Intoxication by barbiturates and similarly acting drugs is an organic mental syndrome that follows the ingestion of the offending substance.

CLINICAL FEATURES AND DIAGNOSIS

The signs of intoxication include sedation, poor concentration, slurred speech, incoordination, nystagmus, ataxia, disinhibition, and poor judgment (Table B.25–1). The drugs can also cause an organic amnestic disorder (blackout). All barbiturates, benzodiazepines, other sedative-hypnotics, and alcohol produce intoxication and have cross-tolerance with each other.

Mild intoxication is relatively safe, but an overdose can be dangerous, especially with barbiturates, which have a low therapeutic index (ratio of lethal dose to effective dose) and are often taken in combination with other drugs, typically alcohol. The combination of barbiturates and alcohol produces additive effects and can be lethal. Death occurs through respiratory and central nervous system (CNS) depression with subsequent cardiovascular collapse.

Benzodiazepines are much safer than barbiturates, since benzodiazepines have a much higher therapeutic index. Sedative-hypnotics, especially benzodiazepines, are the most frequently prescribed class of psychotropic drug; therefore, they are readily available to patients attempting suicide. In addition, they are a common source of accidental overdose in children.

INTERVIEWING AND PSYCHOTHERAPEUTIC GUIDELINES

Keep the intoxicated patient under constant supervision to prevent harm to self or others. Reorient the patient as often as necessary. Try to obtain from the patient or collateral informants an accurate history of the quantity and the type of drug ingested. When the patient is no longer intoxicated, reinterview to evaluate for additional psychopathology and suicidality. Reassure and support the patient.

Table B.25-1
Diagnostic Criteria for Sedative, Hypnotic, or Anxiolytic Intoxication

A. Recent use of a sedative, hypnotic, or anxiolytic

B. Maladaptive behavioral changes (e.g., disinhibition of sexual or aggressive impulses, mood lability, impaired judgment, impaired social or occupational functioning)

C. At least one of the following signs:
   (1) slurred speech
   (2) incoordination
   (3) unsteady gait
   (4) impairment in attention or memory

D. Not due to any physical or other mental disorder

Note: When the differential diagnosis must be made without a clear-cut history or toxicologic analysis of body fluids, it may be qualified as "provisional."

Table from DSM-III-R, *Diagnostic and Statistical Manual of Mental Disorders,* ed 3, revised. Copyright American Psychiatric Association, Washington, 1987. Used with permission.

EVALUATION AND MANAGEMENT

1. Evaluate the patient for medical complications, such as pneumonia, cardiac arrhythmias, heart failure, and respiratory depression.

2. Mild intoxication can generally be treated supportively and usually leads to sleep. Evaluate the patient for possible intoxication with multiple drugs. The patient may become progressively more intoxicated with time if multiple or long-acting drugs were taken. Keep the patient from engaging in any acts that are potentially dangerous, such as driving.

3. Barbiturate overdose is a medical emergency requiring immediate attention. Identify the type and the amount of drug taken; always suspect polyoverdose. Obtain a urine toxicology screen as part of a full battery of laboratory tests. Try to keep the patient awake. Use gastric lavage and charcoal. If the patient falls asleep, admit the patient to a medical intensive care unit, and be prepared to intubate. Intravenous (IV) fluids, cardiac monitoring, and other supportive treatments are indicated. Obtain the patient's blood level of barbiturate. In any overdose case, always evaluate the patient for suicidality.

4. If taken alone (without alcohol or other CNS depressants), benzodiazepines in overdose are much safer than are barbiturates. The lethal dose of benzodiazepines in a nondependent patient may be more than 200 times the effective dose, but the therapeutic index is less if the patient is dependent. Overdose attempts with benzodiazepines usually produce a prolonged sleep. However, benzodiazepines are often taken in combination with alcohol or other CNS depressants, and the combination may be fatal, especially in patients who are medically compromised. Blood levels of benzodiazepines may help determine the level of risk. Patients who have taken an overdose of benzodiazepines should be observed at least one day in an intensive care unit (ICU), since polyoverdose is always a possibility.

DRUG TREATMENT

No medication is indicated.

II. BARBITURATE AND SIMILARLY ACTING SEDATIVE, HYPNOTIC, OR ANXIOLYTIC WITHDRAWAL

Sedative-hypnotic withdrawal is a substance-specific syndrome that follows the reduction or the termination of a psychoactive agent that had been used on a regular basis. Withdrawal from barbiturates, benzodiazepines, and other sedative-hypnotics is, like alcohol withdrawal, a potentially life-threatening emergency. Fortunately, withdrawal is easily treated with a slow taper of the drug on which the patient is dependent.

CLINICAL FEATURES AND DIAGNOSIS

Withdrawal is a state of CNS hyperactivity characterized by the following signs and symptoms: anxiety, insomnia, sensitivity to sound and light, tachycardia, mild hypertension, tremor, headache, sweating, abdominal distress, nausea, vomiting, hallucinations, and craving for the drug (Table B.25–2). Untreated, the syndrome may progress to seizures, delirium, coma, and death.

The degree of withdrawal depends on the dose, the duration of use, and the drug's pharmacokinetics. Drugs with long elimination half-lives tend to produce less severe withdrawal syndromes than do drugs with short elimination half-lives. The half-life also determines whether the onset of withdrawal occurs hours to days after sedative-hypnotic consumption has ceased. Since all sedative-hypnotics have cross-tolerance, a medically supervised detoxification can be performed with any drug of that type.

INTERVIEWING AND PSYCHOTHERAPEUTIC GUIDELINES

Withdrawal patients are likely to be agitated and uncomfortable. Empathize with their discomfort, and explain that cooperating with the interview is the quickest way for them to receive the treatment that will relieve their suffering. Emphasize the fact that accurate information regarding the type of drug used, the frequency of use, the quantity of use, and the time of the last ingestion are crucial in determining a safe, appropriate detoxification regimen. Remind the patient that underestimation of the dose can lead to inadequate detoxification doses; overestimation can lead to an overdose during detoxification. Show the patient that your primary concern is to provide effective treatment.

EVALUATION AND MANAGEMENT

1. Monitor the patient's vital signs frequently, even while the patient is asleep.

2. Determine the patient's level of dependence with a pentobarbital challenge test (Table B.25–3). If the patient is dependent on multiple sedative-hypnotics or alcohol, the method outlined here will treat withdrawal from all the drugs, since they show cross-tolerance.

Table B.25–2
Diagnostic Criteria for Uncomplicated Sedative, Hypnotic, or Anxiolytic Withdrawal

A. Cessation of prolonged (several weeks or more) moderate or heavy use of a sedative, hypnotic, or anxiolytic, or reduction in the amount of substance used, followed by at least three of the following:
  (1) nausea or vomiting
  (2) malaise or weakness
  (3) autonomic hyperactivity (e.g., tachycardia, sweating)
  (4) anxiety or irritability
  (5) orthostatic hypotension
  (6) coarse tremor of hands, tongue, and eyelids
  (7) marked insomnia
  (8) grand mal seizures

B. Not due to any physical or other mental disorder, such as sedative, hypnotic, or anxiolytic withdrawal delirium

Note: When the differential diagnosis must be made without a clear-cut history or toxicologic analysis of body fluids, it may be qualified as "provisional."

Table from DSM-III-R, *Diagnostic and Statistical Manual of Mental Disorders*, ed 3, revised. Copyright American Psychiatric Association, Washington, 1987. Used with permission.

Table B.25–3
Pentobarbital Challenge Test

1. Give pentobarbital 200 mg orally.
2. Observe for intoxication after one hour, e.g., sleepiness, slurred speech, or nystagmus.
3. If the patient is not intoxicated, give another 100 mg of pentobarbital every two hours (maximum 500 mg over six hours).
4. Total dose given to produce mild intoxication is equivalent to daily abuse level of barbiturates.
5. Substitute phenobarbital 30 mg (longer half-life) for each 100 mg of pentobarbital.
6. Decrease by about 10 percent a day.
7. Adjust rate if signs of intoxication or withdrawal are present.

3. After obtaining the patient's history and the results of a urine toxicology screen, identify the possible abuse of other drugs, including opioids, cocaine, and other stimulants.

4. After gradually detoxifying the patient from sedative-hypnotics and after evaluating the patient for any comorbid psychiatric disorders, refer the patient for outpatient drug dependence treatment and rehabilitation.

DRUG TREATMENT

No drugs are indicated, other than barbiturates at gradually reduced dosages as part of the protocol determined by the pentobarbital challenge test.

Cross-References:

Alcohol withdrawal, anxiety, blackouts, delirium, insomnia, intoxication, opioid intoxication and withdrawal, psychotropic drug withdrawal, suicide.

26 / Bed-Wetting

Bed-wetting (enuresis) is pathological if it occurs repeatedly in a patient more than 4 years old. Bed-wetting can be caused by functional and organic conditions, such as infections and anatomical abnormalities of the urinary tract. Bed-wetting typically occurs both during daytime and at night. Cultural tolerance of bed-wetting affects its reporting, but enuresis is most common in boys, institutions, and groups with a low socioeconomic status. Genetic factors exist. Bed-wetting is often precipitated by psychosocial stressors (for example, the birth of a sibling, moving, and marital discord between the parents). It is usually self-limited.

CLINICAL FEATURES AND DIAGNOSIS

Identify the duration, the course, and the precipitants of the disorder. Primary enuresis is diagnosed if no period of urinary continence has lasted for at least one year. Secondary enuresis is diagnosed for a new episode subsequent to a period of continence. Determine whether the patient voluntarily chooses to urinate.

Rule out organic causes, including anatomical defects in the urinary tract, infections, diabetes mellitus, diabetes insipidus, drug intoxication, epilepsy, sleepwalking, and the side effects of medication, such as antipsychotics. The presence of urinary frequency, urgency, pain, or residual urine suggests an organic cause.

INTERVIEWING AND PSYCHOTHERAPEUTIC GUIDELINES

Be supportive and reassuring in dealing with a child. Children often feel guilty and blamed, and they need empathy. Speak to the parents to determine whether they are punitive or humiliating. Educate them about nonpunitive behavioral approaches to enuresis.

EVALUATION AND MANAGEMENT

For functional enuresis, counsel the parents regarding appropriate toilet training, including record keeping and rewards for improvement. Behavior therapy with a bed pad attached to an alarm that sounds on wetness is often effective.

DRUG TREATMENT

Drugs are seldom indicated. Imipramine (Tofranil), which has anticholinergic side effects, has been used on a short-term basis. Desmopressin, an antidiuretic compound administered as a nasal spray, has shown some initial success.

Cross-References:
Anxiety, depression.

27 / Blackouts

Blackouts are episodes of amnesia associated with intoxication, most commonly with alcohol, during which the patient is awake.

CLINICAL FEATURES AND DIAGNOSIS

Blackouts usually last several hours, but they may persist for days. Drugs such as sedative-hypnotics, including benzodiazepines and barbiturates, produce blackouts less often than alcohol. Brain damage is a risk. During a blackout, an intoxicated person can carry out complex behaviors, such as driving and carrying on a conversation. Sometimes, complex fugue states appear, during which long-distance travel may occur. Blackouts indicate alcohol abuse and are suggestive of alcohol dependence. Blackouts are familiar experiences for many alcohol-dependent patients. In some cases, subsequent intoxication brings back the lost memory.

INTERVIEWING AND PSYCHOTHERAPEUTIC GUIDELINES

Collateral interviews with relatives, friends, or those accompanying the patient to the emergency room or your office are extremely important. Try to confirm alcohol use and patterns of drinking. Reassure the patient that alcohol is the most likely cause and that the condition is reversible and treatable.

EVALUATION AND MANAGEMENT

1. Prevent potential dangers (for example, driving and assaults).
2. Observe the patient for possible alcohol overdose.
3. Check for intoxication or overdose with other drugs by taking a history and doing urine or blood toxicology screens.
4. Evaluate the patient for other possible medical problems, including head injury and nutritional deficiencies.
5. Provide supportive treatment in a nonstimulating environment.
6. Refer the patient to an alcohol dependence and rehabilitation program.

DRUG TREATMENT

Drugs should be avoided with this disorder. However, give thiamine 100 mg intramuscularly and then by mouth three times a day to treat possible superimposed alcohol amnestic disorder (Korsakoff's syndrome) or Wernicke's encephalopathy.

Cross-References:

Alcohol dementia, alcohol hallucinosis, alcohol idiosyncratic intoxication, alcohol intoxication, alcohol overdose, alcohol seizures, alcohol withdrawal, alcohol withdrawal delirium, amnesia, fugue state, intoxication, Korsakoff's syndrome, Wernicke's encephalopathy.

---

28 / Blindness (Psychogenic)

The sudden onset of *blindness* can be a symptom of conversion disorder. The patient may be brought to your office or the emergency room because of the sudden onset of the symptom.

CLINICAL FEATURES AND DIAGNOSIS

A diagnosis of conversion disorder implies that physical symptoms, particularly losses of physical functioning and alterations in physical functioning, are the result of some psychological conflict. The symptoms are typically neurological and include paralysis, seizures, blindness, tunnel vision, aphonia, akinesia, and dyskinesia. The symptoms may achieve a primary gain by keeping a conflict unconscious or may achieve a secondary gain by causing some desired change in the environment. Patients with conversion disorder are not in conscious control of their symptoms, unlike malingering patients and those with factitious disorders.

The risk factors of blindness in conversion disorder include true medical conditions, past conversion symptoms in the patient or the family, and histrionic personality traits. A lack of concern (*la belle indifférence*) about the blindness may be present. The onset is usually rapid and in response to some acute stress.

INTERVIEWING AND PSYCHOTHERAPEUTIC GUIDELINES

Conversion symptoms stem from psychological conflicts that are actually interpersonally based (for example, arm paralysis in a wife who wants to strike her husband). The patient may be accompanied to the emergency room or your office by the person with whom the patient is in conflict. Separate them, and conduct separate interviews to determine the nature of the conflict. Providing a psychodynamic explanation for the symptoms may lead to its resolution (for example, "You don't want to see what he's doing to you.") Do not minimize the physical symptoms; declare that the symptoms are real for the patient. Begin to engage the patient in a psychotherapeutic process, focusing on working through the conflicts that led to the symptom.

EVALUATION AND MANAGEMENT

1. Rule out blindness caused by a physical condition. The signs suggesting a psychogenic origin include a failure to bump into objects, blinking or moving the head in response to the sudden appearance of a threatening object, and a loss inconsistent with neuroanatomy (for example, tunnel vision). Evaluate the patient for multiple sclerosis, systemic lupus erythematosus, and other neurological disorders. Hysterical blindness should not be confused with optic neuritis secondary to multiple sclerosis.

2. Consider the possibility of psychogenic symptoms superimposed on organically based symptoms. Patients with organic pathology often have superimposed psychogenic syndromes.

3. Identify the patient's psychological stressors.

4. Evaluate the secondary gains, including attention from the family and the avoidance of work. If secondary gains are present, try to alter the environment, or use a behavioral approach.

5. Evaluate the patient for other psychiatric diagnoses, since a significant portion of conversion disorder patients have comorbid illnesses, such as somatization disorder, depression, personality disorders, and schizophrenia.

6. Hypnosis or an amobarbital (Amytal) interview may be used to relieve the patient's anxiety.

DRUG TREATMENT

An intravenous barbiturate or benzodiazepine may relieve the patient's anxiety and symptoms. However, the relief of symptoms with an anxiolytic does not necessarily rule out the presence of an underlying medical condition.

Cross-References:

Akinesia, anxiety, aphasia, panic disorder.

---

29 / Borderline Personality Disorder

Borderline personality disorder is characterized by a long-standing pattern of instability of mood, self-image, and interpersonal relationships. Borderline patients are frequent users of psychiatric emergency rooms and can present with a range of emergencies, most commonly suicidal ideation. The patients can consume a great deal of staff time and may be exasperating for mental health care providers, especially since they often use splitting (for example, the therapist is good, and the emergency room or office staff members are bad) as a defense mechanism.

The patients can often be difficult to manage and manipulative in their suicidal gestures, which are often made to gain attention or to express anger. However, there is always the risk that a suicidal gesture will inadvertently lead to a completed suicide. In the emergency room or office setting the goal is to devise a plan that resolves the crisis without sabotaging the long-term treatment objectives.

CLINICAL FEATURES AND DIAGNOSIS

The hallmarks of the disorder are instability and an almost constant state of crisis (Table B.29–1). Under stress, borderline patients may have psychotic symptoms or major depression. They characteristically act out with manipulative, self-destructive acts or, less often, with rage directed toward others.

INTERVIEWING AND PSYCHOTHERAPEUTIC GUIDELINES

Borderline patients form an instant transference in which they may overvalue you or devalue you. Be empathic, but maintain enough objectivity to make therapeutic decisions in the patient's best interests. Set limits regarding acceptable and unacceptable behavior in the emergency room or office. Do not join in when the patient attempts to split the staff.

EVALUATION AND MANAGEMENT

1. Assess the patient's dangerousness. The most common emergency in borderline patients is a suicidal gesture, commonly by slashing the wrists or taking a drug overdose. Evaluate the potential lethality of the patient's behavior. Was the self-destructive act a genuine suicide attempt or a gesture? If the gesture is repeated, could it lead to an accidental suicide? Is the behavior a well-developed coping mechanism, with multiple similar gestures in the past, or is it new? If the patient is not admitted to the hospital, what other options are available for the patient? Can crisis intervention relieve an acute stress, or will a release simply return the patient to the same environment that led to the attempt, perhaps making the patient feel more hopeless than before?

2. Was the gesture designed to gain attention and an attempted rescue by others? If so, has that goal been achieved? Who responded? Was the response the desired one? Was the gesture designed to discharge a dysphoric affect? If so, has that affect been discharged, at least in the short term? Was the gesture designed to obtain hospitalization? If so, how does hospitalization now fit into the patient's longitudinal course? Frequent brief hospitalizations may not be desirable and may reinforce hospital dependence. Was the gesture designed to obtain control over a situation? If so, has that been achieved?

3. Evaluate the patient's related symptoms, such as drug and alcohol abuse, sexual promiscuity, binging and purging, fighting, and other signs of poor impulse control.

4. What is the patient's current treatment? If you are not the patient's therapist, get in touch with that therapist, if possible, and organize a plan for the patient that places the resolution of the immediate emergency in

Table B.29-1
Diagnostic Criteria for Borderline Personality Disorder

A pervasive pattern of instability of mood, interpersonal relationships, and self-image, beginning by early adulthood and present in a variety of contexts, as indicated by at least *five* of the following:
  (1) a pattern of unstable and intense interpersonal relationships characterized by alternating between extremes of overidealization and devaluation
  (2) impulsiveness in at least two areas that are potentially self-damaging (e.g., spending, sex, substance use, shoplifting, reckless driving, binge eating) (Do not include suicidal or self-mutilating behavior covered in [5].)
  (3) affective instability: marked shifts from baseline mood to depression, irritability, or anxiety, usually lasting a few hours and only rarely more than a few days
  (4) inappropriate, intense anger or lack of control of anger (e.g., frequent displays of temper, constant anger, recurrent physical fights)
  (5) recurrent suicidal threats, gestures, or behavior, or self-mutilating behavior
  (6) marked and persistent identity disturbance manifested by uncertainty about at least two of the following: self-image, sexual orientation, long-term goals or career choice, type of friends desired, preferred values
  (7) chronic feelings of emptiness or boredom
  (8) frantic efforts to avoid real or imagined abandonment (Do not include suicidal or self-mutilating behavior covered in [5].)

Table from DSM-III-R, *Diagnostic and Statistical Manual of Mental Disorders,* ed 3, revised. Copyright American Psychiatric Association, Washington, 1987. Used with permission.

the context of the patient's ongoing treatment. Try to avoid hospitalization unless that is the therapist's plan (Table B.29–2). Patients may present in an emergency as a result of some conflict encountered in the ongoing psychotherapy.

5. Unless there is an indication for hospital admission, attempt to resolve the crisis without hospitalization. Manipulate the environment to reduce the stress, perhaps by recruiting the assistance of friends and relatives. Give the patient the opportunity to ventilate and discharge some hostile affect. Consider a family session for crisis intervention. Try to develop some rapport with the patient. Reassure the patient, as reasonably as possible, that someone does care.

6. Consider a wide range of psychotherapeutic and psychopharmacological approaches, ranging from insight-oriented psychotherapy to antidepressants, antipsychotics, benzodiazepines, lithium (Eskalith), and other drugs. Behavior therapy, family therapy, and group therapy may also be useful.

DRUG TREATMENT

Agitation or anxiety may be reduced with benzodiazepines, although the risk of abuse and dependence is great. Initiating a benzodiazepine in the emergency room or your office should be considered only as part of a complete plan (for example, to avoid hospitalization) and should be continued only during an acute episode. Benzodiazepines may cause disinhibition. For nonpsychotic patients, the risks of benzodiazepines are usually less severe than the risks of antipsychotic side effects, especially tardive dyskinesia. Borderline patients are subject to psychotic symptoms in response to stress. Brief treatment with antipsychotics can be considered for

Table B.29-2
Use of Hospitalization for Patients with Borderline Personality Disorder or Other Severe Personality Disorders

Indications for admission
- The patient's ongoing therapist wants the patient admitted as part of an ongoing treatment plan or for reevaluation.
- Suicidal gestures are escalating.
- Secondary major depression or psychoactive substance abuse requires admission.
- Psychotic reaction that does not respond to emergency interventions (structured environment and/or antipsychotic medication) occurs.
- Severe losses or other stresses occur.

Contraindications to admission*
- Repeating a treatment that has already failed
- Using the hospital because nothing else works
- Attempting to make major characterologic change
- Attempting to try a new medication in the absence of any positive indication for its success
- Trying to convince patients to change their living situations
- Treating the patient's unwillingness to follow treatment plans
- Sheltering malingerers or patients facing legal charges

*Table adapted from I D Glick, H Klar, P Broff: When should chronic patients be hospitalized? Hosp Community Psychiatry *35*: 934, 1984. Table from J R Hillard: Personality disorders. In *Manual of Clinical Emergency Psychiatry,* J R Hillard, editor, p 268. American Psychiatric Press, Washington, 1990. Used with permission.

those minipsychotic episodes. If depression is also present, serotonergic agents, such as paroxetine (Paxil), fluoxetine (Prozac), and sertraline (Zoloft), may be helpful.

Cross-References:

Agitation, brief reactive psychosis, homicidal and assaultive behavior, hospitalization, separation anxiety, suicide, violence.

30 / Brief Reactive Psychosis

The term *brief reactive psychosis* is used to describe patients who experience psychotic symptoms lasting for less than one month in response to some identifiable stressor.

CLINICAL FEATURES AND DIAGNOSIS

The psychotic symptoms may include disorganization, incoherence, loosening of associations, hallucinations, delusions, and catatonic behavior. Affective symptoms may be more common than the classic schizophrenic symptoms. The mental status of the patient may be indistinguishable from that of a patient with schizophrenia or a psychotic mood disorder, but the diagnosis is made on the basis of a history of brief duration and an identifiable stressor (Table B.30–1).

Features suggestive of a good prognosis are similar to those for schizophrenia and include a severe stressor, a sudden onset, prominent mood

Table B.30–1
Diagnostic Criteria for Brief Reactive Psychosis

A. Presence of at least one of the following symptoms indicating impaired reality testing (not culturally sanctioned):
   (1) incoherence or marked loosening of associations
   (2) delusions
   (3) hallucinations
   (4) catatonic or disorganized behavior

B. Emotional turmoil (i.e., rapid shifts from one intense affect to another, or overwhelming perplexity or confusion).

C. Appearance of the symptoms in A and B shortly after, and apparently in response to, one or more events that, singly or together, would be markedly stressful to almost anyone in similar circumstances in the person's culture.

D. Absence of the prodromal symptoms of schizophrenia, and failure to meet the criteria for schizotypal personality disorder before onset of the disturbance.

E. Duration of an episode of the disturbance of from a few hours to one month, with eventual full return to premorbid level of functioning. (When the diagnosis must be made without waiting for the expected recovery, it should be qualified as "provisional.")

F. Not due to a psychotic mood disorder (i.e., no full mood syndrome is present), and it cannot be established that an organic factor initiated and maintained the disturbance.

Table from DSM-III-R, *Diagnostic and Statistical Manual of Mental Disorders,* ed 3, revised. Copyright American Psychiatric Association, Washington, 1987. Used with permission.

symptoms, good premorbid functioning, the absence of schizoid traits, the absence of a family history of schizophrenia, subjective distress caused by the symptoms, and little blunting of affect.

INTERVIEWING AND PSYCHOTHERAPEUTIC GUIDELINES

Take a structured empathic approach. Keep the questions simple but, initially, open-ended. Thought-disordered patients may need gentle redirection and structuring. Explore the patient's experience of the psychotic symptoms without confronting the unreality of the symptoms. Use a flexible approach. Essential data can usually be obtained without adhering to a rigid interview structure, since the psychotic patient cannot accommodate such a structure. When offering medication to patients with limited insight, indicate that the medication can help them feel calm and think clearly.

EVALUATION AND MANAGEMENT

1. Rule out any possible organic causes. A rapid change in the patient's mental status suggests a possible organic cause. Obtain the patient's vital signs, a detailed history of alcohol and drug abuse, and a history of prescribed and over-the-counter drugs. Is there a history of the abuse of hallucinogenic drugs, especially phencyclidine (PCP) or lysergic acid diethylamide (LSD)? Psychosis can also be caused by steroids, antidepressants, and a wide variety of prescribed medications, including most psychotropic drugs. Evaluate the patient's thyroid function; both hyperthyroidism and hypothyroidism can cause psychosis. Complete a workup for delirium or dementia as indicated.

2. Hospitalization is usually indicated. Even if the symptoms can be controlled with medication in the emergency room or your office, a thorough evaluation can seldom be completed without hospitalization.

3. Determine the patient's premorbid personality traits. Brief reactive psychoses often occur in patients with borderline, schizotypal, narcissistic, histrionic, and paranoid personality disorders. Borderline, narcissistic, or histrionic personality disorder traits indicate that the possibility of depression should be considered thoroughly.

4. Refer the patient for psychotherapy. The approach depends on the needs of the patient and often focuses on recovery in the postpsychotic period. Patients who are very upset by the psychotic episode and have lost self-confidence may benefit from supportive, cognitive, family, or group therapy.

DRUG TREATMENT

Acute agitation can usually be controlled with benzodiazepines (oxazepam [Serax] 10 to 30 mg by mouth, estazolam [ProSom] 0.5 to 1 mg by mouth, alprazolam [Xanax] 0.5 to 1 mg by mouth, or lorazepam [Ativan] 1 to 2 mg by mouth or intramuscularly (IM)—all repeated as needed). Benzodiazepines should be tried first but should be abandoned rapidly if they are ineffective and then replaced by antipsychotics, such as haloperidol (Haldol) 2 to 5 mg by mouth or IM, fluphenazine (Prolixin) 2 to 5 mg by mouth or 1M, or thiothixene (Navane) 2 to 5 mg by mouth or IM repeated as needed. All medications should be given in the context of a brief (several weeks) treatment.

Cross-References:

Agitation, delirium, delusional disorder, hallucinations, hospitalization, ideas of reference.

---

31 / Bromide Intoxication

Bromide intoxication is an organic mental syndrome that follows the ingestion of bromides. Bromides are drugs with a long onset of action that were once used as anticonvulsants but are now largely obsolete. They are found in some over-the-counter preparations, such as Bromo-Seltzer. Their elimination half-life is more than one week; thus, the drugs tend to accumulate in the body. Bromide intoxication is thought to be uncommon. However, since most clinicians do not routinely consider the disorder in the differential diagnosis, it is likely to be missed. The patient's history is always one of long-term abuse of the drugs, since bromides accumulate slowly and cannot be taken in large doses because of gastric irritation.

CLINICAL FEATURES AND DIAGNOSIS

The patient's symptoms may be similar to those of a wide range of functional and organic disorders, including schizophrenia, mania, delirium, and depression. Bromide intoxication can present with almost any clinical picture and was once called the great masquerader. The differential diagnosis should include syphilis, alcoholism, encephalitis, multiple sclerosis, uremia, brain tumor, schizophrenia, mania, and depression. The symptoms may include labile affect, cognitive deficits, irritability, confusion, delusions, and hallucinations. The abuse of other sedative-hypnotics, such as benzodiazepines and barbiturates, may exist, further complicating the evaluation. The symptoms may persist for two to three weeks, since the half-life of bromide is about 12 days.

Associated symptoms include an acneform rash, primarily on the face and the scalp, nodular lesions on the legs, incoordination, tremor, ataxia, hyperreflexia, weakness, Babinski's sign, loss of gag and corneal reflexes (present in barbiturate intoxication), absence of nystagmus (present in barbiturate intoxication), and presence of delirium during intoxication (occurs during withdrawal from barbiturates). Additional signs include slurred speech, halitosis, cyanosis, papilledema, mydriasis, and furred tongue.

INTERVIEWING AND PSYCHOTHERAPEUTIC GUIDELINES

Reassure the patient that the condition is reversible. Educate the patient that symptoms can be controlled and that they are the result of bromide intoxication.

EVALUATION AND MANAGEMENT

1. Obtain the history of the long-term abuse of over-the-counter sedatives, and, if possible, obtain a sample of the drug.

2. Obtain the history of the abuse of other drugs, especially sedative-hypnotics. Determine whether withdrawal from sedative-hypnotics is likely.

3. If the serum bromide level is >50 mg/dL, the patient is bromide-intoxicated; however, the clinical symptoms are not directly related to blood levels.

4. Correct the patient's nutritional deficiencies.

DRUG TREATMENT

Stop all bromide-containing medications, and give large doses of saline (6 to 12 g a day) either orally or intravenously (IV). Hemodialysis may be needed in severe cases.

Avoid tranquilizers if possible, although concomitant sedative-hypnotic withdrawal may require treatment. Severe agitation may be treated with a high-potency antipsychotic—for example, thiothixene (Navane), trifluoperazine (Stelazine), fluphenazine (Prolixin), or haloperidol (Haldol)—all given at 2 to 5 mg orally or intramuscularly (IM).

Cross-References:

Confusion, delirium, delusional disorder, depression, hallucinations, intoxication, mania.

---

32 / Bulimia Nervosa

Bulimia nervosa is an eating disorder characterized by episodic uncontrolled binge eating followed by self-induced vomiting or other purgative maneuvers designed to prevent weight gain (for example, the use of laxatives).

CLINICAL FEATURES AND DIAGNOSIS

The diagnostic criteria for bulimia nervosa are listed in Table B.32–1. The disorder is much more common in women than in men. It usually begins in adolescence or early adulthood. The patient may engage in compulsive exercise and laxative abuse. Vomiting is a common feature and is usually induced by sticking a finger down the throat. Vomiting relieves postbinge bloating and allows the patient to binge without fear of gaining weight. The patient generally binges on sweet, soft, high-calorie foods, such as pastry and cakes. Binging may be planned, although it may be done impulsively when the person is angry. Substance abuse, suicide attempts, shoplifting, depression, and emotional lability may be present.

Most bulimic patients are concerned about their sexual attractiveness, body image, and appearance to others. Unlike patients with anorexia nervosa, most bulimic patients are of normal weight. In contrast to patients with anorexia nervosa, most bulimic patients are sexually active and rarely amenorrheic or incapacitated. They are more disturbed by their eating disorder than are anorexics and are, therefore, more likely to seek help.

The prognosis for bulimia nervosa is better than for anorexia nervosa; however, bulimia can be chronic, with resulting medical complications, including dehydration, electrolyte imbalances leading to arrythmias and sudden death, metabolic alkalosis, salivary gland enlargement, dental caries, esophagitis, esophageal tears, and gastric rupture.

The differential diagnosis includes seizure disorders, central nervous system (CNS) tumors, Kleine-Levin syndrome, and syndromes similar to Klüver-Bucy syndrome. Coexisting borderline personality disorder should be considered when assessing bulimic patients.

INTERVIEWING AND PSYCHOTHERAPEUTIC GUIDELINES

Assess the nature and the frequency of the binge-purge behavior in a way that does not come across as judgmental or punitive. Patients may already feel guilty and ashamed. Encourage the patients to describe their behavior and associated feelings of anger, dysphoria, and loss of control.

Table B.32–1
Diagnostic Criteria for Bulimia Nervosa

A. Recurrent episodes of binge eating (rapid consumption of a large amount of food in a discrete period of time).

B. A feeling of lack of control over eating behavior during the eating binges.

C. The person regularly engages in either self-induced vomiting, use of laxatives or diuretics, strict dieting or fasting, or vigorous exercise in order to prevent weight gain.

D. A minimum average of two binge eating episodes a week for at least three months.

E. Persistent overconcern with body shape and weight.

Table from DSM-III-R, *Diagnostic and Statistical Manual of Mental Disorders,* ed 3, revised. Copyright American Psychiatric Association, Washington, 1987. Used with permission.

Try to interest them in ongoing treatment, so that an effective referral can be made. In addition, educate them about the medical consequences of binge-purge behavior while showing concern about their physical health.

EVALUATION AND MANAGEMENT

1. A complete medical evaluation is needed to detect possible electrolyte imbalances (particularly hypokalemia and hypochloremia), dehydration, and gastrointestinal damage. Screen for laxative abuse. Rule out organic causes of bulimia.

2. Perform a complete psychiatric evaluation with attention to diagnosing comorbid depression, anorexia nervosa, substance abuse (for example, cocaine, alcohol, amphetamines, sedatives, and diet pills), and personality disorders.

3. Evaluate the patient for impulsivity and suicidality.

4. Consider hospitalizing patients with particularly poor impulse control, suicidality, or medical complications secondary to their eating disorders.

5. Refer the patient for cognitive-behavioral therapy, insight-oriented psychotherapy, or pharmacotherapy.

6. Consider admitting the patient to a specialized eating disorders unit if necessary.

DRUG TREATMENT

Antidepressants, including tetracyclics (imipramine [Tofranil]), serotonin-specific reuptake inhibitors (fluoxetine [Prozac]), and monoamine oxidase inhibitors (MAOIs) (phenelzine [Nardil]) are useful in treating bulimia. Those medications are used as part of a comprehensive treatment program and are ordinarily not initiated in the emergency room. Particularly anxious or agitated patients can be given lorazepam (Ativan) 1 to 2 mg by mouth or intramuscularly.

Cross-References:

Anorexia nervosa, borderline personality disorder, depression.

33 / Caffeine Intoxication

Caffeine is an alkaloid that acts as a psychomotor stimulant. It is present in many foods, beverages, and both over-the-counter drugs and prescribed drugs. *Caffeine intoxication* (also known as caffeinism) results from the excessive ingestion of caffeine.

CLINICAL FEATURES AND DIAGNOSIS

Caffeine is the most commonly used psychoactive drug. An estimated 20 to 30 percent of all adult Americans consume more than 500 mg of caffeine a day. Tolerance and dependence occur. The most common sources of caffeine are coffee, tea, and soft drinks (Table B.33–1).

The daily consumption of at least 250 mg of caffeine is needed to produce intoxication. Caffeine intoxication can exacerbate or cause the symptoms of a variety of psychiatric disorders, including anxiety disorders (especially panic disorder), depression, mania, and schizophrenia. The symptoms of caffeine intoxication include restlessness, nervousness, excitement, insomnia, flushed facies, diuresis, gastrointestinal disturbances, muscle twitching, rambling thoughts and speech, tachycardia or cardiac arrhythmia, periods of inexhaustibility, and psychomotor agitation (Table B.33–2). The effects of caffeine intoxication last only several hours and can usually be managed supportively. Assess caffeine intake in patients with anxiety or insomnia.

People show a wide range of variability in susceptibility to caffeine intoxication and dependence. Dependence is usually not a clinically important condition, but withdrawal from caffeine can be an unrecognized cause of such symptoms as headache, fatigue, decreased alertness, and social withdrawal. Headaches may persist for days.

INTERVIEWING AND PSYCHOTHERAPEUTIC GUIDELINES

Focus on the assessment of caffeine intake. Reassure and educate the patient regarding the effects of caffeine on mentation and physical signs and symptoms.

EVALUATION AND MANAGEMENT

1. Perform a complete psychiatric evaluation; focus on the amount of caffeine intake. Ask about sources other than coffee (for example, soft drinks and chocolate).

2. Rule out other psychopathology that may be exacerbated by caffeine (for example, bipolar disorder). Is the patient is self-medicating with caffeine to relieve depression with anergy?

3. Determine if the patient is taking medications that have significant interactions with caffeine. For example, caffeine lowers lithium (Eskalith) levels.

Table B.33–1
Some Common Sources of Caffeine and Representative Decaffeinated Products

Source	Approximate Amounts of Caffeine per Unit
Beverages and foods (5–6 oz)	
Fresh drip coffee, brewed coffee	90–140 mg
Instant coffee	66–100 mg
Tea (leaf or bagged)	30–100 mg
Cocoa	5–50 mg
Decaffeinated coffee	2–4 mg
Chocolate bar or ounce of baking chocolate	25–35 mg
Selected soft drinks (8–12 oz)	
Pepsi, Coke, Tab, Royal Crown, Pepsi Light, Dr. Pepper, Mountain Dew	25–50 mg
Canada Dry Ginger Ale, Caffeine-Free Coke, Pepsi Free, 7-Up, Sprite, Squirt, Caffeine-Free Tab	0 mg
Prescription medications (1 tablet)	
Cafergot, Migralam	100 mg
Anoquan, Aspir-code, BAC, Darvon, Fiorinal	32–50 mg
Over-the counter analgesics and cold preparations	
Excedrin	60
Aspirin compound, Anacin, B-C powder, Capron, Cope, Dolor, Midol, Nilain, Norgesic, PAC, Trigesic, Vanquish,	30–32.5 mg
Advil, aspirin, Empirin, Midol 200, Nuprin, Pamprin	0 mg
Over-the-counter stimulants and appetite suppressants	
Caffin-TD, Caffedrine	250 mg
Vivarin, Ver capsules	200 mg
Quick-Pep	140–150 mg
Amostat, Anorexin, Appedrine, Nodoz, Wakoz	100 mg

Table from J Jaffe: Drug dependence: Opioids, nonnarcotics, nicotine (tobacco), and caffeine. In *Comprehensive Textbook of Psychiatry,* ed 5, H I Kaplan, B J Sadock, editors, p 683. Williams & Wilkins, Baltimore, 1989. Used with permission.

Table B.33–2
Diagnostic Criteria for Caffeine Intoxication

A. Recent consumption of caffeine, usually in excess of 250 mg

B. At least five of the following signs:
    (1) restlessness
    (2) nervousness
    (3) excitement
    (4) insomnia
    (5) flushed face
    (6) diuresis
    (7) gastrointestinal disturbance
    (8) muscle twitching
    (9) rambling flow of thought and speech
    (10) tachycardia or cardiac arrhythmia
    (11) periods of inexhaustibility
    (12) psychomotor agitation

C. Not due to any physical or other mental disorder, such as an anxiety disorder

Table from DSM-III-R, *Diagnostic and Statistical Manual of Mental Disorders,* ed 3, revised. Copyright American Psychiatric Association, Washington, 1987. Used with permission.

4. Assess the patient for caffeine-related medical problems. Excessive intake can cause cardiac arrhythmias, hypertension, gastrointestinal upset, and, rarely, peptic ulcers.

5. Advise the patient to restrict caffeine intake or to taper and then discontinue caffeine intake.

6. Educate the patient about the effects of caffeine and the symptoms of withdrawal.

DRUG TREATMENT

Generally, no drug treatment is indicated. If the patient presents with severe anxiety, benzodiazepines such as oxazepam (Serax) 10 to 30 mg by mouth, diazepam (Valium) 5 to 10 mg by mouth, chlordiazepoxide (Librium) 10 to 25 mg by mouth, alprazolam (Xanax) 0.5 to 1 mg by mouth, or lorazepam (Ativan) 1 to 2 mg by mouth can be given. In cases of severe withdrawal, low-dose benzodiazepines can be given for several days.

Cross-References:

Anxiety, depression, intoxication, panic disorder, schizophrenia.

---

34 / Cannabis Intoxication (Marijuana)

Cannabis intoxication is an organic mental syndrome that follows the ingestion of cannabis. Cannabis (also known as marijuana, pot, grass, weed, hemp, Mary Jane, hashish, and many other names) is the most commonly abused illicit drug in the United States. It is a drug found in the resin of the plant *Cannabis sativa* that induces psychic or somatic changes when smoked or ingested in sufficient quantity.

CLINICAL FEATURES AND DIAGNOSIS

Although cannabis use has been decreasing, almost one third of all adult Americans have tried marijuana. Cannabis intoxication is caused most commonly by smoking marijuana in cigarettes (joints). Other forms include hashish, hash oil, and Δ-9-tetrahydrocannabinol (THC) (the active ingredient). All of those forms may be smoked or ingested. The onset of action after smoking is immediate. Oral ingestion produces a gradual onset of effects that may last for many hours. Advanced growing techniques developed in the United States have produced a potent type of marijuana called sinsemilla (without seeds).

The symptoms of cannabis intoxication are given in Table B.34–1. Additional symptoms include dose-dependent hypothermia and mild sedation. Urine toxicology testing results can remain positive for weeks.

Cannabis use usually occurs in the context of polysubstance abuse—most commonly with cigarettes, alcohol, and cocaine. Acute intoxication usually

Table B.34–1
Diagnostic Criteria for Cannabis Intoxication

A. Recent use of cannabis.

B. Maladaptive behavioral changes (e.g., euphoria, anxiety, suspiciousness or paranoid ideation, sensation of slowed time, impaired judgment, social withdrawal)

C. At least two of the following signs developing within two hours of cannabis use:
  (1) conjunctival injection
  (2) increased appetite
  (3) dry mouth
  (4) tachycardia

D. Not due to any physical or other mental disorder

Table from DSM-III-R, *Diagnostic and Statistical Manual of Mental Disorders,* ed 3, revised. Copyright American Psychiatric Association, Washington, 1987. Used with permission.

does not require any treatment, but a mild delusional disorder, usually persecutory, can occur with a brief acute state of panic. Less common symptoms are depersonalization and (rarely) hallucinations. Naive users are prone to cannabis-induced panic. Toxic delirium, usually self-limited, can occur after large doses are ingested or inhaled (Table B.34–2).

Although some long-term users are psychologically dependent, the diagnosis of cannabis dependence is controversial; dosage escalation (tolerance) and a withdrawal syndrome—consisting of insomnia, irritability, nausea, vomiting, and diaphoresis—can occur. Long-term use may lead to syndromes of amotivation and depression. Flashbacks may occur for several months after the last drug use. Some religions (for example, Rastafarianism) consider smoking cannabis a part of a religious practice.

Cannabis use can exacerbate schizophrenia in previously stable patients. Cannabis increases lithium (Eskalith) levels and the half-life of barbiturates. It has added physiological effects with amphetamines. Cannabis-opioid and cannabis-alcohol combinations can produce tachycardia.

INTERVIEWING AND PSYCHOTHERAPEUTIC GUIDELINES

Reassure the patient that the syndrome is drug-induced and will stop in several hours. Engage the patient in conversation and, if possible, have a trusted friend or a family member stay with the patient and provide reassurance. Provide a nonstimulating environment.

EVALUATION AND MANAGEMENT

1. Determine the route of administration. Oral ingestion produces effects lasting up to 12 hours or longer.

2. Evaluate the patient for the abuse of alcohol, cocaine, other stimulants, sedative-hypnotics, and other drugs. Obtain a urine toxicology screen.

3. Evaluate the patient for underlying psychotic, mood, and personality disorders.

4. Refer the patient for appropriate outpatient treatment when indicated.

Table B.34–2
Adverse Reactions to Marijuana

Type	Predisposing factors	Symptoms	Treatment
Acute panic	Inexperienced users, hysterical or obsessional characters, oral administration	Anxiety, depression, no psychotic symptoms	Reassurance; occasionally anxiolytics; episode usually short-lived
Toxic delirium	Large dose, oral use	Confusion, disorientation, hallucinations, depersonalization, delusions	Most remit in 12 to 48 hours; antipsychotics if necessary
Flashbacks	Days or weeks after last dose, prior history of hallucinogenic use	Like hallucinogenic experience except brief	Reassurance; anxiolytics if necessary
Chronic psychosis	Prolonged heavy use of very potent marijuana or hashish; rare in U.S.	Paranoia, delusions, hallucinations, panic, bizarre behavior, occasionally violence	Antipsychotics
Amotivational syndrome	Prolonged heavy use; existence of syndrome is controversial	Apathy, decreased attention span, poor judgment, poor interpersonal relations	No known treatment

Table from S M Mirin, R D Weiss: Drug use and abuse. In *Emergency Psychiatry*, E L Bassuk, A W Birk, editors, p 170. Plenum, New York, 1984. Used with permission.

DRUG TREATMENT

Medications are usually not required, but severe anxiety may be relieved with a benzodiazepine—for example, lorazepam (Ativan) 1 to 2 mg by mouth, alprazolam (Xanax) 0.5 to 1 mg by mouth, clonazepam (Klonopin) 0.25 to 0.5 mg by mouth, or oxazepam (Serax) 10 to 30 mg by mouth—which often leads to sleep. If psychotic symptoms predominate, use haloperidol (Haldol) 1 to 2 mg by mouth or intramuscularly (IM). Repeat in 20 to 30 minutes as needed.

Cross-References:

Anxiety, delusional disorder, depersonalization, intoxication, panic disorder.

---

35 / Cardiac Arrhythmia

Cardiac arrhythmia is a disorder characterized by irregular heartbeats, which the patient usually describes as a pounding heartbeat or a fluttering sensation. The disorder occurs as a symptom of anxiety or panic, as a side effect of cocaine or other psychostimulant drug, or as a toxic effect of psychotropic drugs, such as tricyclic antidepressants and antipsychotics. Cardiac arrhythmia may also be a sign of cardiac disease.

CLINICAL FEATURES AND DIAGNOSIS

Arrhythmia can be brought on by anxiety. Death as a result of overwhelming shock may be due to cardiac arrhythmia. Anxiety-related arrhythmia may be worsened by withdrawal from alcohol or sedative-hypnotics. Tachycardia is common in anxiety, but arrhythmia is uncommon and typically occurs only during the acute episode of anxiety.

INTERVIEWING AND PSYCHOTHERAPEUTIC GUIDELINES

Provide a nonstimulating environment and reassure the patient, who is likely to be anxious. Explain all medical procedures concisely and clearly, and tell the patient that all efforts are being made to make an accurate diagnosis and to initiate appropriate treatment.

EVALUATION AND MANAGEMENT

1. Obtain a full medical and psychiatric history from any patient with complaints that may indicate arrhythmia, such as dizziness, syncope, blackouts, light-headedness, and palpitations.
2. Obtain an electrocardiogram (ECG), thyroid function tests, toxicology screen, and other tests as indicated.

3. Find out if the patient has a history of substance abuse. Cocaine-induced and other stimulant-induced arrhythmias are potentially life-threatening. Tachycardia can be treated with β-blockers. Benzodiazepines are also helpful in relieving anxiety and reducing the patient's level of agitation, which may decrease the risk of arrhythmia. If arrhythmia persists, admission to an intensive care unit may be required.

4. Find out if the patient is taking psychotropic agents that may be arrhythmogenic. Tricyclic antidepressants at therapeutic blood levels have a quinidinelike antiarrhythmic effect. However, at toxic blood levels they are arrhythmogenic. Cardiac side effects that are more common than arrhythmia include conduction delays, tachycardia, and nonspecific ST changes. Patients taking tricyclic antidepressants who have arrhythmia should have the medication withheld until a blood level can be obtained; the antidepressant should be resumed only after a cardiology consultation.

5. The presence of arrhythmia should prompt an immediate medical consultation.

6. Arrhythmia induced by prescription medications mandates a discontinuation of those medications.

DRUG TREATMENT

Severe associated anxiety can be treated with a short-acting benzodiazepine—for example, estazolam (ProSom) 0.5 to 1 mg by mouth, lorazepam (Ativan) 1 to 2 mg by mouth, or oxazepam (Serax) 10 to 30 mg by mouth, all given every four to six hours—until the underlying problem is resolved. Associated diagnoses of substance abuse, anxiety disorders, and other disorders should be treated as needed.

Cross-References:

Anxiety, cocaine intoxication and withdrawal, impending death of a psychogenic origin, mitral valve prolapse, panic disorder.

---

36 / Cataplexy (Sudden Loss of Muscle Tone)

Cataplexy is the sudden temporary loss of voluntary muscle tone in response to emotional stimulation. Cataplexy is a symptom of narcolepsy, although it can also occur in neurological disorders.

CLINICAL FEATURES AND DIAGNOSIS

Typically, the patient's history includes uncontrollable daytime sleep attacks (from which the patient awakens refreshed), hypnagogic hallucinations (which occur while the patient is falling asleep), sleep paralysis (in which the patient feels unable to move while falling asleep), and restless sleep with vivid, terrifying dreams. Cataplectic attacks are typically brought on by laughter or elation, although other emotions may also trigger an attack. The patient is usually awake during the cataplectic attack and is aware of the surroundings, even though temporarily paralyzed. A sleep laboratory evaluation reveals that the electroencephalogram (EEG) during a cataplectic attack is that of rapid eye movement (REM) sleep, a sleep stage associated with decreased muscle tone (hence the paralysis). A polysomnogram reveals REM periods shortly after the onset of sleep (rather than the usual delay of at least 70 minutes) and an abnormal sleep architecture. Primary narcolepsy runs in families and is, at least in part, genetically based. Other causes of narcolepsy include brain tumors, encephalitis, head injury, and cerebrovascular diseases.

Cataplexy can be differentiated from petit mal seizures by the fact that the patient is awake during the attack and also by the characteristic precipitation of cataplexy by emotional stimuli. Hypoglycemia, multiple sclerosis, and myasthenia gravis must be differentiated from cataplexy.

INTERVIEWING AND PSYCHOTHERAPEUTIC GUIDELINES

Reassure the patient that treatment is available to ameliorate some symptoms. Explain that a thorough medical workup is necessary to rule out rare causes of the disorder, but that the condition is most likely a sleep disorder.

EVALUATION AND MANAGEMENT

1. Obtain a complete neurological examination and medical screening tests, including thyroid tests.

2. Refer the patient for an EEG, polysomnography, and daytime multiple sleep latency tests.

3. Advise patients to avoid emotionally provocative stimuli to prevent cataplectic attacks.

DRUG TREATMENT

Narcolepsy is usually treated with stimulants, such as amphetamines and methylphenidate (Ritalin), but those drugs usually do not help with the cataplectic attacks.

Tricyclic antidepressants, such as imipramine (Tofranil) and clomipramine (Anafranil), are often helpful. Monoamine oxidase inhibitors (MAOIs), such as phenelzine (Nardil), may also be useful if tricyclics are ineffective.

Cross-Reference:

Narcolepsy.

37 / Catatonia (Rigid Muscle Tone)

Catatonia is a condition characterized by alteration in muscle tone—for example, fixed posture or immobility, stupor, or rigidity. *Catalepsy* is a general term for a condition in which an immobile or awkward position is maintained for a prolonged period of time. A specific type of catalepsy is *waxy flexibility* (flexibilitas cerea), in which a part of the patient can be moved and, when the body part is released, it remains in the position in which it was left, as if it were made of wax.

CLINICAL FEATURES AND DIAGNOSIS

Symptoms associated with catatonia include mutism, echolalia, stupor, negativism, excitement, and repetitive motor behavior, as well as catalepsy. Catatonia is a syndrome that can be produced by organic disorders (for example, metabolic conditions and central nervous system [CNS] lesions), mood disorders, schizophrenia (for example, catatonic type), drug toxicity, and severe anxiety states (for example, posttraumatic stress disorder, dissociative disorders, and conversion disorder).

Lethal catatonia is a rare syndrome that occurs in patients receiving long-term treatment with antipsychotic medication. It is characterized by a prodrome of increasing mental and physical agitation that lasts for weeks to months. Lethal catatonia may culminate in stupor, coma, or death. It can resemble neuroleptic malignant syndrome. The two syndromes are compared in Table B.37–1.

INTERVIEWING AND PSYCHOTHERAPEUTIC GUIDELINES

Catatonic patients may be awake and aware, despite their appearance. Clinicians should identify themselves and explain their actions. Patients may remember events, especially conversations, occurring during their catatonic episodes.

EVALUATION AND MANAGEMENT

1. Perform a mental status examination if possible and check the patient's vital signs.
2. Complete a medical workup to rule out organicity.
3. Obtain a history of drug abuse and medications.
4. In the absence of a known organic condition, consider hypnosis for the relief of the catalepsy and related symptoms.
5. If the symptoms persist in spite of hypnosis or parenteral benzodiazepines, refer the patient for a full neurological workup, including brain imaging with computed tomography (CT) or magnetic resonance imaging (MRI).
6. Pursue treatments specific to the underlying diagnosis.

Table B.37–1
Clinical Differences Between Lethal Catatonia and Neuroleptic Malignant Syndrome

Stage	Lethal Catatonia	Neuroleptic Malignant Syndrome
	Prodrome lasting 2 weeks–2 months, consisting of behavioral and personality changes or frank schizophrenic symptoms Possible onset with no prodrome	Period of prior antipsychotic drug exposure can be hours to months Develops rapidly over a few hours to days No prodromal phase has been described
Initial symptoms	Excitement, intense anxiety, and restlessness lasting a few days Possible self-destructive or assaultive behavior Hallucinatory experiences and delusional thinking usually present Possible fever, tachycardia, and acrocyanosis Sudden death may occur	Tremors and dyskinesias are early signs Muscle hypertonicity described as lead-pipe or plastic rigidity Severe excitement and intense anxiety are not major features Autonomic instability with tachycardia, labile hypertension, and possible diaphoresis Fever may not be present initially Acrocyanosis has not been described May occur in nonpsychotic patients treated with antipsychotics No deaths reported during early phase
Full syndrome	Continued increasing excitement with wild agitation and violent, destructive behavior, lasting 3–15 days, and possible choreiform movements Mutism, rigidity, or stupor may alternate with excitement Refusal of food and fluids Increasing and fluctuating fever, rapid and weak pulse, profuse clammy perspiration, hypotension	Appearance of most major symptoms (severe muscle rigidity, persistent autonomic instability, fever) usually occurs after 2–9 days Possible agitation, confusion, and clouding of consciousness
Final stage	Cachexia, convulsions, delirium, coma, exhaustion Death may occur	Severe complications, e.g., rhabdomyolysis with elevated creatine phosphokinase, myoglobinuria, renal failure, and intravascular thrombosis with pulmonary embolism and respiratory failure Possible 20–30% mortality rate with full syndrome
Treatment	Antipsychotic drugs and other treatments to reduce severe psychotic symptoms	Immediate cessation of all dopamine-blocking antipsychotic drugs Dopamine agonists (to reduce central hypodopaminergic state), calcium channel blockers (to reduce muscle rigidity), β-adrenergic blockers (to reduce tachycardia), other supportive measures as needed Consider using electroconvulsive therapy (ECT)

Table adapted from E Castillo, R T Rubin, E Holsboer-Trachsler: Clinical differentiation between lethal catatonia and neuroleptic malignant syndrome. Am J Psychiatry *146*: 326, 1989. Used with permission.

DRUG TREATMENT

If the patient has a recent history of antipsychotic exposure, consider giving anticholinergic drugs—for example, benztropine (Cogentin) 2 mg by mouth or intramuscularly (IM)—to treat such extrapyramidal side effects as dystonia. However, if the patient has an underlying organic disorder, the anticholinergic drug could exacerbate the condition. Also consider the possibility of neuroleptic malignant syndrome (Table B.37-1).

Benzodiazepines—for example, lorazepam (Ativan) 1 to 2 mg IM or intravenously (IV)—may reduce the patient's anxiety and permit cooperation with the interview or relieve the symptoms altogether.

CROSS-REFERENCES:

Anxiety, catatonic schizophrenia, neuroleptic malignant syndrome, panic disorder.

---

38 / Catatonic Schizophrenia

Catatonic schizophrenia is a type of schizophrenia. It is characterized by muscular rigidity (catatonia), negativism, and stupor or excitement.

CLINICAL FEATURES AND DIAGNOSIS

The signs and the symptoms of catatonic schizophrenia include mutism, excitement, waxy flexibility, stupor, stupor alternating with excitement, negativism, mannerisms, and stereotypies (Table B.38-1). Mood disorders can present as catatonia. The differential diagnosis also includes organically caused coma, toxic psychosis, antipsychotic-induced rigidity and akinesia, conversion disorder, dissociative states, malingering, and factitious disorders.

INTERVIEWING AND PSYCHOTHERAPEUTIC GUIDELINES

Remember that unresponsive catatonic patients are awake and aware. Explain all actions and procedures to them. The patients often fully remember the events that occurred and the statements that were made during their stupor.

EVALUATION AND MANAGEMENT

1. Catatonic patients may need treatment for self-inflicted injuries, malnutrition, dehydration, exhaustion, or hyperpyrexia. Rule out any medical illness presenting as catatonic decompensation (for example, neuroleptic malignant syndrome).

Table B.38–1
Diagnostic Criteria for Catatonic Schizophrenia

A type of schizophrenia in which the clinical picture is dominated by any of the following:
(1) catatonic stupor (marked decrease in reactivity to the environment and/or reduction in spontaneous movements and activity) or mutism
(2) catatonic negativism (an apparently motiveless resistance to all instructions or attempts to be moved)
(3) catatonic rigidity (maintenance of a rigid posture against efforts to be moved)
(4) catatonic excitement (excited motor activity, apparently purposeless and not influenced by external stimuli)
(5) catatonic posturing (voluntary assumption of inappropriate or bizarre postures)

Table from DSM-III-R, *Diagnostic and Statistical Manual of Mental Disorders,* ed 3, revised. Copyright American Psychiatric Association, Washington, 1987. Used with permission.

2. Conduct a psychiatric evaluation to confirm the diagnosis and to assess the patient for an organic cause and for comorbid substance abuse. The patient's history obtained from collateral informants is particularly important.

3. Provide a safe environment for the patient and for staff members because catatonic patients can unpredictably erupt into an excited, violent state. Restraint and sedation may be needed.

4. Assess the patient for the side effects of medications, with particular attention to antipsychotic-induced akinesia, which can resemble catatonia.

5. Evaluate the patient for psychosocial stressors that may have led to an exacerbation. Has the patient's living situation changed? Was the patient traumatized?

6. Evaluate the patient for depression, which may be contributing to the catatonic decompensation.

7. Hospitalization may be needed. Catatonic patients are at serious risk for impulsive violence and are often unable to provide their own basic needs.

DRUG TREATMENT

Emergency treatment consists of an antipsychotic, such as fluphenazine (Prolixin) 2 to 5 mg intramuscularly (IM), haloperidol (Haldol) 2 to 5 mg IM, thiothixene (Navane) 5 mg IM, or trifluoperazine (Stelazine) 5 mg IM, all given every 30 minutes as needed. Lorazepam (Ativan) 1 to 2 mg IM every four to six hours may also be useful for treating the patient's catatonia.

Cross-References:

Agitation, akinesia, catatonia, chronic schizophrenia in acute exacerbation, delusional disorder, hallucinations, hospitalization, mutism, neuroleptic malignant syndrome, schizophrenia, violence.

39 / Chronic Schizophrenia in Acute Exacerbation

Schizophrenia in remission can unexpectedly erupt into an exacerbation characterized by delusions, hallucinations, incoherence, catatonic behavior, and grossly inappropriate affects. The symptoms cause functional impairment and are usually continuous. Chronic schizophrenia is diagnosed when the disorder has been present for more than two years.

CLINICAL FEATURES AND DIAGNOSIS

Early indications of schizophrenic exacerbation include increasing paranoia, grandiosity, or religiosity; ideas of reference; anger; anxiety; somatic symptoms; increased sleep disturbance; increased difficulty at work or in school; and increased social withdrawal. Patients often have their own characteristic patterns of signs and symptoms when they are decompensating.

INTERVIEWING AND PSYCHOTHERAPEUTIC GUIDELINES

The clinician should be supportive and empathic. The thought-disordered patient cannot accommodate a rigid interview schedule, but may need gentle redirection and structuring. Ask simple and direct questions. Flexibility is essential.

Explore the patient's experience of the psychotic symptoms without confronting the unreality of the symptoms. When offering medication to patients with no insight, indicate that the medication can help them feel calm, think more clearly, or make the voices they hear less disturbing.

EVALUATION AND MANAGEMENT

1. Evaluate the patient's medical needs. The patient may require medical attention for self-inflicted injuries, malnutrition, hyperpyrexia, or exhaustion. Medical illness may be masked by the schizophrenia or present as psychotic decompensation.

2. Differentiating an exacerbation of chronic schizophrenia from a psychotic mood disorder or an organic disorder is not possible if the only evidence is the clinical presentation. A definitive diagnosis can be made only on the basis of the patient's longitudinal history and after the needed laboratory tests have been performed. Contact the patient's regular physician, caseworker, and family for additional history. Such contacts also ensure good continuity of care.

3. Schizophrenic patients are at a high risk of drug abuse, most commonly alcohol and cocaine. Patients with schizophrenia may also consume large amounts of coffee and smoke incessantly; caffeine intoxication and with-

drawal may affect the patient's symptoms, and cigarettes may lower antipsychotic blood levels. In addition, schizophrenic patients may abuse the anticholinergic drugs—such as benztropine (Cogentin) and diphenhydramine (Benadryl)—that are prescribed for the extrapyramidal side effects of antipsychotics. If taken in sufficient doses, the anticholinergic drugs can produce a delirium with visual hallucinations. A thorough evaluation for substance abuse is indicated; if drugs are present, treatment may include a drug detoxification and rehabilitation program.

4. Antipsychotic side effects are common reasons for emergency presentation. The most dramatic side effect is acute dystonia. Other side effects include rigidity, cogwheel rigidity, bradykinesia, akinesia, akathisia, and tardive dyskinesia. Dystonia and rigidity are rapidly relieved by anticholinergic drugs—for example, benztropine 2 mg intramuscularly (IM). The drugs should be continued on a standing basis. The management of akathisia involves lowering the antipsychotic dosage (which is not helpful immediately), a trial of anticholinergic drugs (which are often ineffective), and trials of β-blockers—such as propranolol (Inderal)—or benzodiazepines. The treatment of tardive dyskinesia requires long-term planning and may include periodic adjustments of the antipsychotic dosage.

5. Evaluate the patient for traumatic events or stressful interpersonal situations that may have led to the exacerbation. Has the patient's living situation changed? Has a family member moved into or out of the household? Is the patient being scapegoated at home? Perhaps the situation is amenable to environmental manipulation and crisis intervention.

6. An exacerbation of chronic schizophrenia may be due to the development of a secondary depression, which occurs in up to 25 percent of all schizophrenic patients. Evaluate the patient for depressive symptoms, including suicidality.

7. Hospitalization is often indicated. The emergency reasons for hospitalization include the prevention of harm to the patients or others and the patients' inability to care for themselves. Patients with schizophrenia are more likely to commit suicide than are patients with any other diagnosis. Patients with fixed paranoid delusions are also at a high risk of homicide and other violence. After making a thorough diagnostic evaluation and stabilizing the patient on medication, refer the patient for rehabilitation and education. For patients who are receiving outpatient treatment and who present with acute symptoms, tranquilization with an antipsychotic (typically the antipsychotic already being prescribed) or a benzodiazepine—for example, oxazepam (Serax) 10 to 30 mg by mouth or lorazepam (Ativan) 1 to 2 mg by mouth or intramuscularly (IM)—and observation for several hours may stabilize the patient and avoid a hospital admission.

8. Behavior therapy, family therapy, group therapy, psychoeducation, and individual psychotherapy are all helpful in treating schizophrenia.

9. Use seclusion and restraint as necessary. Usually, try to provide chemical restraint with benzodiazepines or antipsychotics. If severe agitation or dangerousness persist after the IM administration of tranquilizers, seclusion and physical restraint may be necessary.

DRUG TREATMENT

Antipsychotics are the mainstay of the treatment of schizophrenia. They are helpful in relieving psychotic symptoms and agitation. Antipsychotics can be started in the emergency room or your office. They are rapidly effective in providing behavioral control. Low-potency antipsychotics, such as chlorpromazine (Thorazine) and thioridazine (Mellaril), are more sedating and less likely to cause extrapyramidal side effects than are high-potency antipsychotics, such as haloperidol (Haldol) and fluphenazine (Prolixin). Haloperidol and fluphenazine offer the advantage of being available in depot form for patients who, after being stabilized on an oral regimen, are likely to be noncompliant. The depot antipsychotics are administered by injection every two to four weeks.

Benzodiazepines (for example, lorazepam 1 to 2 mg IM) are also effective for acute agitation and may be used in addition to antipsychotics. However, benzodiazepines are not used as the primary antipsychotic treatment. Clozapine (Clozaril) is indicated in schizophrenic patients who have not responded to trials of other antipsychotics. Clozapine is reportedly most effective in treating negative symptoms, such as blunted affect and withdrawn behavior, but it is associated with agranulocytosis, which is potentially life-threatening.

Cross-References:

Agitation, catatonic schizophrenia, delusional disorder, hallucinations, homicidal and assaultive behavior, hospitalization, intoxication, mania, restraints, schizophrenia, seclusion, suicide, violence.

---

40 / Claustrophobia

Claustrophobia is a fear of enclosed places.

CLINICAL FEATURES AND DIAGNOSIS

For the claustrophic patient, exposure to enclosed spaces provokes immediate anxiety. Although the patient recognizes that the fear is unrealistic, the fear and the avoidance interferes with functioning. The symptoms of anxiety when in enclosed spaces include panic, tachycardia, sweating, palpitations, and dyspnea.

Claustrophobia is considered a simple phobia. Its onset is usually in the patient's 30s. It may be related to panic disorder and agoraphobia but should be differentiated from posttraumatic stress disorder and obsessive-compulsive disorder. Simple phobias are common (six-month prevalence is between 5 and 12 percent) and affect women more often than men. Although claustrophobic patients may be able to successfully avoid the phobic stimulus and function well, in adulthood the phobia seldom resolves without treatment.

Patients with simple phobias rarely present in the emergency psychiatry setting, although the psychiatrist may be called to see a claustrophobic patient who is unable to cooperate with such phobia-exacerbating procedures as computed tomography (CT) and magnetic resonance imaging (MRI) scans. Phobic patients may present in an acutely anxious state after a recent exposure to the phobic stimulus. They also come to emergency treatment when a change in their circumstances no longer accommodates the avoidance behavior.

INTERVIEWING AND PSYCHOTHERAPEUTIC GUIDELINES

Claustrophobic patients are often embarrassed about their irrational fears. Reassure them, and take their fears seriously. Allow the patients to express their fears while taking a history of the specific phobia-stimulating circumstances and a history of the illness. Explain to patients that phobias are treatable.

EVALUATION AND MANAGEMENT

1. Perform a complete psychiatric evaluation to rule out additional phobias and other psychiatric diagnoses that require treatment (for example, schizophrenia, personality disorders, and panic disorder).
2. Evaluate the patient for substance abuse; phobic patients may self-medicate to overcome their fears.
3. Assess the patient for any recent environmental change that no longer allows phobic avoidance (for example, the patient's workplace may have moved to a high floor in an office building that necessitates the use of an elevator).
4. Reassure the patient, and refer the patient for appropriate outpatient treatment, such as behavior therapy, hypnosis, relaxation techniques, and insight-oriented psychotherapy.

DRUG TREATMENT

If the patient is acutely anxious or must undergo an anxiety-provoking medical procedure, give a short-acting benzodiazepine, such as estazolam (ProSom) 0.5 to 1 mg by mouth, lorazepam (Ativan) 1 to 2 mg by mouth or intramuscularly (IM), or oxazepam (Serax) 10 to 30 mg by mouth, one hour before the procedure. Benzodiazepines should be given only as a single dose or a limited several-day prescription until the patient can be seen in outpatient treatment. Monoamine oxidase inhibitors (MAOIs) and β-blockers can also be of some help.

Cross-References:

Agoraphobia, anxiety, panic disorder, phobia, posttraumatic stress disorder.

41 / Clonidine Withdrawal

Clonidine (Catapres) is a centrally acting α_2-agonist that reduces peripheral adrenergic tone. It is often used to treat hypertension. Its psychiatric applications include mania, opioid withdrawal, cocaine intoxication, Tourette's disorder, posttraumatic stress disorder, and other conditions associated with autonomic arousal.

CLINICAL FEATURES AND DIAGNOSIS

Withdrawal from ongoing clonidine treatment can lead to anxiety, agitation, irritability, psychosis, violence, hypertension, and seizures.

INTERVIEWING AND PSYCHOTHERAPEUTIC GUIDELINES

Explain to the patient that withdrawal is a self-limiting process and that they will be given medication to deal with uncomfortable signs and symptoms. Determine the reason the patient was prescribed clonidine, the length of time prescribed the drug, the dose, and by whom.

EVALUATION AND MANAGEMENT

The elimination half-life of clonidine is about 13 hours, and a gradual reduction of the clonidine dosage may prevent withdrawal symptoms. Even untreated symptoms of clonidine withdrawal generally resolve after several days.

DRUG TREATMENT

Agitation and possible violence may require physical restraint or tranquilization with a benzodiazepine—for example, estazolam (ProSom) 0.5 to 1 mg by mouth, lorazepam (Ativan) 1 to 2 mg by mouth or intramuscularly (IM), or oxazepam (Serax) 10 to 30 mg by mouth. In psychotic or severely agitated patients, the short-term use of parenteral antipsychotics—for example, fluphenazine (Prolixin) 2 to 5 mg IM or haloperidol (Haldol) 2 to 5 mg IM—may be needed.

Cross-References:

Agitation, anxiety, cocaine intoxication and withdrawal, mania, opioid intoxication and withdrawal, posttraumatic stress disorder, psychotropic drug withdrawal, violence.

42 / Cocaine Intoxication and Withdrawal

I. COCAINE INTOXICATION

Cocaine intoxication is an organic mental syndrome that follows the ingestion of cocaine. It produces both physical and behavioral effects. Cocaine can be snorted, injected, smoked, or absorbed through the mucous membranes. The potential for dependence is related to the route of administration and is greatest when the drug is either injected or smoked in its pure (freebase) form. A purified form of freebase cocaine called crack is sold in small single doses and is smoked. The low cost of small doses of crack and its availability in ready-to-smoke form have led to the widespread use of cocaine in indigent urban areas. Increased urban crack use has clearly affected drug-related crimes and violence.

CLINICAL FEATURES AND DIAGNOSIS

The symptom onset is within minutes to one hour of administration (Table B.42–1). Since the duration of action of cocaine is short (the elimination half-life is one hour), except for cases of severe overdose, most of the drug is usually gone from the body by the time the patient presents to the emergency room or your office. Both the physical and behavioral sequelae of intoxication can produce emergencies.

The behavioral signs include agitation, aggressiveness or fighting, paranoid delusions or hallucinations, delirium, excitement, and poor judgment. The physical signs include tachycardia, hypertension, mydriasis, perspiration and chills, tremor, nausea and vomiting, fever, arrhythmia, syncope, chest pain, and, in overdoses, convulsions, respiratory depression, coma, and death.

INTERVIEWING AND PSYCHOTHERAPEUTIC GUIDELINES

Reassure the patient that the symptoms are of limited duration. Provide a quiet environment. Assess the patient for the quantity, the frequency, and the route of cocaine use. Explain all actions and procedures carefully. Approach the paranoid patient with caution. If possible, enlist the aid of family members who can reassure the patient.

EVALUATION AND MANAGEMENT

1. Take the patient's vital signs. If fever is present, treat it aggressively. Frequently monitor the patient's blood pressure and pulse.

2. Reassure the patient that the symptoms are self-limiting and will resolve soon.

Table B.42–1
Diagnostic Criteria for Cocaine Intoxication

A. Recent use of cocaine

B. Maladaptive behavioral changes (e.g., euphoria, fighting, grandiosity, hypervigilance, psychomotor agitation, impaired judgment, impaired social or occupational functioning)

C. At least two of the following signs within one hour of using cocaine:
   (1) tachycardia
   (2) pupillary dilation
   (3) elevated blood pressure
   (4) perspiration or chills
   (5) nausea or vomiting
   (6) visual or tactile hallucinations

D. Not due to any physical or other mental disorder

Table from DSM-III-R, *Diagnostic and Statistical Manual of Mental Disorders,* ed 3, revised. Copyright American Psychiatric Association, Washington, 1987. Used with permission.

3. Determine if the patient also took other drugs, especially opiates (for example, a speedball of intravenous [IV] heroin and cocaine), sedative-hypnotics, and alcohol.

4. Seclusion and restraint are a last resort and are seldom necessary.

5. The psychotic symptoms usually resolve after the acute episode but may persist in heavy abusers (cocaine delusional disorder), especially in vulnerable persons.

6. Consider admitting the patient to the hospital for cocaine detoxification if necessary. A cocaine intoxication visit to the emergency room is probably the best time to convince the patient to attend a drug rehabilitation program.

7. Educate the patient about cocaine withdrawal.

DRUG TREATMENT

Severe agitation, dangerousness, or delusions can be treated with benzodiazepines—for example, oxazepam (Serax) 10 to 30 mg by mouth or lorazepam (Ativan) 1 to 2 mg intramuscularly (IM) and repeat in one hour if needed. Benzodiazepines are usually effective and are preferable to antipsychotics, because benzodiazepines raise the seizure threshold and reduce central nervous system (CNS) irritability.

If agitation persists after several doses of benzodiazepines or if signs of benzodiazepine toxicity (ataxia, dysarthria, nystagmus) develop, give a high-potency antipsychotic—for example, fluphenazine (Prolixin) or haloperidol (Haldol), both given at 2 to 5 mg by mouth or IM. Antipsychotics should generally be avoided if possible, because they lower the seizure threshold and because the self-limited course of cocaine intoxication does not usually warrant the risks of antipsychotic side effects.

Tachycardia and hypertension, if severe or persistent, can be treated with β-blockers (propranolol [Inderal]) or clonidine (Catapres). Hemodynamic instability, seizures, respiratory depression, and other signs of an overdose are indications for admission to an intensive care unit (ICU).

II. COCAINE WITHDRAWAL

Cocaine withdrawal is characterized by a dysphoric mood persisting for more than 24 hours after a decrease in cocaine consumption and with at least one of the following: (1) fatigue, (2) insomnia or hypersomnia, and (3) psychomotor agitation. Patients may also have paranoid or suicidal ideation, irritability, and depressed mood.

CLINICAL FEATURES AND DIAGNOSIS

No well-defined physiological syndrome of cocaine withdrawal occurs after the discontinuation of heavy use, but the behavioral syndrome described above is common. Cocaine withdrawal implies cocaine dependence.

The most prominent symptom of cocaine withdrawal is a craving for cocaine. The severity of the withdrawal is related to the amount and the duration of use and to the route of administration. Snorting produces less dependence and withdrawal; intravenous abuse and smoking crack (freebase) produces more dependence and withdrawal (Table B.42–2).

The symptoms peak in several days but may last for up to several weeks. An underlying or secondary major depression may be diagnosed if the symptoms persist for more than several weeks. In addition, underlying personality disorders, dependence on alcohol, and dependence on sedative-hypnotics may be obscured by cocaine use.

INTERVIEWING AND PSYCHOTHERAPEUTIC GUIDELINES

Patients with cocaine withdrawal are dysphoric, and major depression is included in the differential diagnosis. But, since personality disorders (especially borderline and antisocial personality disorders) are often present, cocaine withdrawal patients are often perceived as manipulative. The patient will probably medicate the withdrawal symptoms by returning to cocaine use; the relapse rates, even after inpatient detoxification, are high.

Reassure the patient that the syndrome is likely to resolve in one to two weeks. Determine the route, the frequency, and the quantity of cocaine use and the time of the last use. Screen the patient for dependence on other drugs. Setting limits can help educate the patient about what behaviors are acceptable.

EVALUATION AND MANAGEMENT

1. Assess the suicide risk. Even though the syndrome will probably resolve in several days, suicidal patients may require psychiatric admission to the hospital.

2. Encourage the patient to attend a detoxification or rehabilitation program.

3. Refer the patient to a support group (for example, Narcotics Anonymous) or to family or group therapy.

4. Evaluate the patient for an underlying psychiatric disorder and the abuse of other drugs.

Table B.42-2
Diagnostic Criteria for Cocaine Withdrawal

A. Cessation of prolonged (several days or longer) heavy use of cocaine, or reduction in the amount of cocaine used, followed by dysphoric mood (e.g., depression, irritability, anxiety) and at least one of the following, persisting more than 24 hours after cessation of substance use:
(1) fatigue
(2) insomnia or hypersomnia
(3) psychomotor agitation

B. Not due to any physical or other mental disorder, such as cocaine delusional disorder.

Table from DSM-III-R, *Diagnostic and Statistical Manual of Mental Disorders,* ed 3, revised. Copyright American Psychiatric Association, Washington, 1987. Used with permission.

DRUG TREATMENT

Severe agitation and maladaptive behavior can be controlled with benzodiazepines (for example, estazolam [ProSom] 0.5 to 1 by mouth, oxazepam 10 to 30 mg by mouth, or lorazepam 1 to 2 mg by mouth or IM).

Antidepressants can be used for persistent symptoms of depression, but they are usually not started unless the patient has a full depressive syndrome two weeks after stopping the cocaine.

Cocaine dependence has been treated with desipramine (Norpramin), doxepin (Sinequan), and other antidepressants. Bromocriptine (Parlodel) has also been used. The goal of treatment of cocaine dependence is abstinence.

Cross-References:

Agitation, amphetamine or similarly acting sympathomimetic intoxication and withdrawal, anxiety, delusional disorder, depression, intoxication, mania, paranoia, phencyclidine or similarly acting arylcylohexylamine intoxication, psychotropic drug withdrawal, restraints, schizophrenia, seclusion, suicide, violence.

43 / Coma

Coma is a severe state of impaired consciousness that indicates depression of the central nervous system (CNS); the patient is unresponsive to the environment or to internal needs, shows no purposeful spontaneous movement, and shows no evidence of thinking.

CLINICAL FEATURES AND DIAGNOSIS

Coma is a neurological emergency that is often an end stage mental status; it indicates severe brain dysfunction. Coma may also be a sign of malingering. It can be distinguished from deep sleep in that the comatose patient cannot be awakened by any stimulus, and the patient's eyes never open (Table B.43-1).

Table B.43–1
Levels of Consciousness

Alert wakefulness—The patient responds immediately, fully, and appropriately to visual, auditory, or tactile stimulation.
Lethargy—The patient appears drowsy and inactive; responses are delayed or incomplete.
Obtundation—The patient seems indifferent and maintains wakefulness but little more.
Stupor—The patient can be aroused only by vigorous and continuous external stimulation.
Coma—The patient's responses to stimulation are either completely lost (deep coma) or reduced to only rudimentary reflex motor responses (moderately deep coma).

Table from F Plum, M Posner: *Diagnosis of Stupor and Coma,* p 2. Davis, Philadelphia, 1966. Used with permission.

Coma can be caused by a wide range of conditions. An acute onset suggests cerebrovascular disease, head trauma, toxic conditions, overdose, or heatstroke. A gradual onset suggests CNS infection, intracranial mass, or systemic disease. The clinical features of the various coma states are given in Table B.43–2.

INTERVIEWING AND PSYCHOTHERAPEUTIC GUIDELINES

Obtain the patient's history from the person accompanying the patient to the emergency room or your office. Some comatose patients are aware of their surroundings and remember events occurring during the coma. Patients with akinetic mutism and catatonia may erupt into explosive outbursts and should be approached with caution.

EVALUATION AND MANAGEMENT

1. Refer the patient for a complete neurological examination.
2. Differentiate true organic coma from psychogenic unresponsiveness. Normal muscle tone and reflexes, a normal electroencephalogram (EEG), forcible closing of the eyes, eyes kept open but interrupted by quick blinks, normally reactive pupils, and random or no eye movements in response to head turning (doll's-eye maneuver)—all suggest a psychogenic origin. Bárány's caloric test (putting 10 cc of ice water into the external ear and observing for the quick component of nystagmus) can be performed. The presence of the quick component of nystagmus during the caloric test suggests a state of alertness. In an organically comatose patient, the quick component is absent, and the eyes slowly deviate to the side of the cooled ear.
3. Determine the level of coma, using the Glasgow Coma Scale (Table B.43–3). Document any efforts to ward off painful stimuli. Document the specific stimuli used and the response, so that the tests may be repeated serially by other examiners to measure the patient's progress.
4. Obtain a full organic workup, including complete blood count (CBC) with differential, complete blood chemistries, Venereal Disease Research Laboratory (VDRL) test, thyroid profile, urine and blood toxicology screens, urinalysis, chest X-ray, computed tomography (CT) scan or magnetic res-

Table B.43–2
Coma States

Condition	Features
Akinetic mutism	Absence of muscle activity, lack of movement, mutism; alert-appearing eye movements; periods of sleep and decreased wakefulness in the lethargic form; midbrain lesion often present
Catatonic stupor	Perseveration, rigidity, waxy flexibility, mutism, negativism, tachycardia, low-grade fever, diaphoresis, mydriasis, tachypnea, choreiform movements, violent outbursts; possible multiple causes, including organicity, schizophrenia, and mood disorders
Coma vigil	Apparently asleep and ready to be aroused; similar to akinetic mutism
Locked-in syndrome	Total body paralysis secondary to brainstem damage, with preservation of eye movements and mentation; mute but alert with intact hemispheric function; communication by blinking
Persistent vegetative state	Rare random or absent motor responses; evidence of meaningful contact with the environment; blood pressure and respiratory control maintained, eye movements present, sleep-wake cycles present; usually caused by severe brain damage
Psychogenic coma	No signs of neurological disease or dysfunction or changes in respiratory function, pupils, or eye movements; sometimes apparently aware of surroundings; urinary or fecal incontinence, insensitivity to pain, and no swallowing of secretions or fluids placed in the mouth

Table B.43–3
Glasgow Coma Scale

Activity	Best Response	
Eye Opening	Spontaneous	4
	To speech	3
	To pain	2
	None	1
Verbal	Oriented	5
	Confused	4
	Inappropriate words	3
	Nonspecific sounds	2
	None	1
Motor	Follows commands	6
	Localizes pain	5
	Withdraws to pain	4
	Abnormal flexion	3
	Extend	2
	None	1

Table from Jennett B. Teasdale G. *Lancet*, 1977. Used with permission.

onance imaging (MRI) of the head, an EEG, a lumbar puncture, and other diagnostic tests as indicated.

5. Give supportive care and treat as indicated by the workup results.

DRUG TREATMENT

Medications are indicated only according to the definitive diagnosis. In general, CNS-depressant drugs should be avoided.

Cross-References:
Catatonic schizophrenia, confusion, delirium, malingering, opioid intoxication and withdrawal.

44 / Confusion

Confusion is a disturbance in the clarity and the coherence of thinking. Confusion is often considered a cardinal (although nonspecific) sign of organic disorders, but confusion can also occur in schizophrenia and psychotic mood disorders.

CLINICAL FEATURES AND DIAGNOSIS

Cognitive impairment is the major sign of confusion. Focus on cognition. Test the patient's orientation, concentration and attention, naming, reading, writing, verbal repetition, copying, and short-term, intermediate-term, and long-term memory. Consider administering the Mini-Mental State Examination (MMSE), which is a screening examination for a wide range of cognitive functions (Table B.44–1).

Although abnormal results on the MMSE do not provide information about organicity or cause, they do provide a reliable screening of cognitive functions that can be followed over time. Psychotic patients may have abnormal MMSE results because of poor cooperation or cognitive deficits.

Table B.44–2 lists several causes of acute confusional states requiring urgent attention.

INTERVIEWING AND PSYCHOTHERAPEUTIC GUIDELINES

The primary concern in interviewing a confused patient is the possible presence of organic disorders. Immediately assess the patient's condition; orient and reassure the patient. If the patient's behavior seems impulsive or unpredictable, providing enough staff members to ensure environmental control may help establish limits and prevent violent acts. Identify the rate of onset of the confusion and any physical or psychological stressors.

EVALUATION AND MANAGEMENT

1. Check the patient's vital and neurological signs. Abnormal findings suggest possible organic conditions. Is the patient epileptic? Is evidence of a cerebrovascular disease or a head injury present? Are risk factors for a cardiovascular disease, such as hypertension or heart disease, present?

2. Consider the patient's age. Is the patient elderly and likely to have an organic disorder? Is the patient a young person who may be abusing drugs?

3. Obtain the patient's past history of confused episodes and the rate of onset of the current episode.

Table B.44–1
Mini-Mental State Examination (MMSE) Questionnaire

Orientation (score 1 if correct)
  Name this hospital or building.
  What city are you in now?   _____
  What year is it?   _____
  What month is it?   _____
  What is the date today?   _____
  What state are you in?   _____
  What county is this?   _____
  What floor of the building are you on?   _____
  What day of the week is it?   _____
  What season of the year is it?   _____

Registration
  Name three objects, and have the patient repeat them. Score number _____
  repeated by the patient. Name the three objects several more times if
  needed for the patient to repeat correctly (record trials _____).

Attention and calculation
  Subtract 7 from 100 in serial fashion to 65. Maximum score = 5   _____

Recall
  Do you recall the three objects named before?   _____

Language tests
  Confrontation naming: watch, pen = 2
  Repetition: "No ifs, ands, or buts" = 1   _____
  Comprehension: Pick up the paper in your right hand, fold it in half, and set _____
    it on the floor = 3
  Read and perform the command "Close your eyes" = 1   _____
  Write any sentence (subject, object, verb) = 1   _____

Construction
  Copy the design below = 1   _____

Total MMSE questionnaire score (maximum = 30)   _____

Table adapted from M F Folstein, S Folstein, P R McHugh: Mini-mental state: A practical method for grading the cognitive state of patients for the clinician. J Psychiatr Res *12*: 189, 1975. Used with permission.

4. Perform a full mental status examination. Fluctuations in consciousness suggest delirium. Psychotic symptoms and blunted affect suggest schizophrenia. Prominent amnesia and global cognitive impairment suggest dementia. Prominent mood symptoms with psychosis suggest a mood disorder.

5. What are the patient's present medications and drugs of abuse? Could medications—prescribed, over-the-counter, or street drugs—be causing toxic side effects? Could delirium be caused by medications (for example, anticholinergic drugs, antipsychotics, or other psychotropic drugs)?

6. Obtain the patient's medical history. Are systemic diseases, liver disease, cancer, neurological disorders (especially epilepsy), or other diseases increasing the possibility of an organic disorder?

7. Obtain an organic workup, including a physical examination with neurological examination, complete blood count (CBC), chemistry profile,

Table B.44-2
Some Clues to Causes of Acute Confusional States Demanding Urgent Attention

Metabolic disorders
1. Hypoglycemia: history of diabetes or alcoholism; reduced level of consciousness, shaky, sweaty, perhaps combative
2. Hyperglycemia: history of diabetes; complaints of increased thirst, urination, or flulike symptoms
3. Hyponatremia: underlying illness like lung cancer, recent stroke, chronic pulmonary infections, heart failure, cirrhosis, diuretic use
4. Hypernatremia: dehydration from inadequate fluid intake or excessive fluid loss without replacement
5. Hypercalcemia: underlying disorder such as cancer metastatic to bone, sarcoidosis, lung and renal cell cancer, multiple myeloma, and/or prolonged immobilization
6. Hypoxia: inadequate oxygen supplied to the brain because of poor pulmonary or cardiac function or carbon monoxide poisoning
7. Hypercarbia: history of chronic lung disease characterized by carbon dioxide retention; may use oxygen at home
8. Hepatic encephalopathy: history of chronic liver disease or alcoholism; probably jaundiced; ascites
9. Uremia: history of kidney disease, enlarged prostate, recent inability to pass urine
10. Thiamine deficiency (Wernicke's encephalopathy): variable degrees of ophthalmoplegia, ataxia, and mental disturbance; history of nutritional deficiency secondary to alcoholism, particularly of thiamine; since remaining thiamine in the body is rapidly used when the patient is given intravenous glucose, any patient with alcoholism should immediately receive intramuscular thiamine before glucose infusion to prevent precipitating this encephalopathy; untreated, the disorder rapidly progresses to a permanent memory disorder (Korsakoff's syndrome) and, in some advanced cases, death
11. Hypothyroidism: history of progressive fatigue, constipation, sensitivity to cold, weight gain, coarsening of hair and skin, mental slowing; examination shows abnormally low temperature and enlarged heart and slow pulse; may be precipitated by the effects of lithium on thyroid function
12. Hyperthyroidism: patient may be either hyperactive or apathetic; history may reveal rapid weight loss, diarrhea, heat intolerance, and emotional instability; examination shows goiter, silky fine hair, warm moist skin, proptosis and wide-eyed stare, fine tremor, rapid or irregular pulse; in elderly patients muscle weakness and heart failure may be most apparent

Systemic illness
1. Decreased cardiac output from various causes, such as congestive heart failure, arrhythmia, pulmonary embolus, and myocardial infarction; acute myocardial infarction presents with confusion as the major symptom in 13% of elderly patients; aged patients do not complain of typical pain; often they complain of indigestion; vital signs may be abnormal, and patient may look ill (ashen coloring, weak, nauseated, sweaty) and be confused
2. Pneumonia: recent history of a cold, becoming bedridden and aspirating; fever may not be apparent, but tachycardia or hypotension are evident on vital signs
3. Urinary tract infection: especially in patients with indwelling urinary catheters, prostatic hypertrophy, diabetes, neurogenic bladder
4. Anemia: especially with acute blood loss (injury, intestinal bleeding), chronic illness, occult gastrointestinal malignancy
5. Acute surgical emergencies: infarction of the bowel, appendicitis, and volvulus are common and often present only with confusion and no other complaints
6. Hypertension: sustained or rapid increase in blood pressure may cause encephalopathy; often has history of elevated blood pressure; may occur in patient on MAO inhibitor antidepressants who has eaten food containing tyramine
7. Vasculitides: e.g., systemic lupus erythematosus; confusion arises from cerebral involvement or treatment with steroids
8. Any febrile illness and infection can cause confusion in the aged

Table B.44–2—*continued*

Central nervous system disorders
1. Subdural or epidural hematoma: may or may not have history of head trauma; fluctuating mental status often present; may have no focal neurological signs
2. Seizure: unwitnessed seizure may be suggested if patient was found on floor with evidence of incontinence or vomiting; history of seizure disorder or alcoholism
3. Stroke: history of transient ischemic attacks or strokes; may have no signs except confusion
4. Infection: meningitis (bacterial, fungal, or tuberculous), viral encephalitis
5. Tumor, primary or metastatic: with a growing mass, raised intracranial pressure may cause local compression of vital structures or herniation of the brain; in the elderly, brain atrophy allows for greater space inside the skull so that symptoms may not appear until the mass is quite large
6. Normal pressure hydrocephalus: presents with triad of gait disturbance, incontinence, dementia; surgery may be curative

Drugs and medication
1. Almost all drugs are capable of causing confusion in the elderly; the most commonly implicated drugs include those with strong anticholinergic effects (antidepressants, antipsychotics, and antiparkinsonian drugs, and many over-the-counter preparations), sedative-hypnotics (barbiturates, benzodiazepines), cardiac medications (digoxin, propranolol, lidocaine, quinidine), antihypertensives, anticonvulsants, cimetidene, nonnarcotic and narcotic analgesics, and corticosteroids
2. Alcohol: intoxication and withdrawal syndromes occur as in young patients, but poor health in the elderly may put geriatric patients at greater risk
3. Drug abuse: far less common in elderly persons, but chronic intoxication with bromides, minor tranquilizers (especially meprobamate, barbiturates) occurs

Table from S L Minden: Elderly psychiatric emergency patients. In *Emergency Psychiatry*, E L Bassuk, A W Birk, editors, p 360. Plenum, New York, 1984. Used with permission.

thyroid function tests, urinalysis, urine drug screen, blood levels of drugs being taken, Venereal Disease Research Laboratory (VDRL) test, and electrocardiogram (ECG). If an organic disorder is suspected, a computed tomography (CT) scan or a magnetic resonance imaging (MRI) of the head and an electroencephalogram (EEG) are indicated. Other tests, such as a lumbar puncture, may be ordered.

DRUG TREATMENT

Avoid medicating the patient until a definitive diagnosis is made. If severe agitation or potential violence is seen and tranquilization is necessary, a high-potency antipsychotic—for example, haloperidol (Haldol) 2 to 5 mg by mouth or intramuscularly (IM) or fluphenazine (Prolixin) 2 to 5 mg by mouth or IM—may be used, since benzodiazepines may worsen the confusion in organic patients.

Cross-References:

Agitation, delirium, dementia, sundowner syndrome.

45 / Delirium

Delirium is an acute organic mental syndrome involving global cognitive impairment.

CLINICAL FEATURES AND DIAGNOSIS

Delirium is often reversible; the course is usually brief and rapidly fluctuating. The symptoms of delirium are listed in Table B.45–1. The diagnostic criteria for delirium are given in Table B.45–2.

Delirium is considered a sign of acute brain dysfunction and is, therefore, a medical emergency. The immediate goals are to make a definitive diagnosis of the cause and to reverse the cause before further deterioration, permanent damage, or physical injury occurs. Delirium is common in the medically ill, inpatients on medical and surgical services, postburn patients, and patients in intensive care units. The very young and the elderly are most vulnerable. Brain damage, dementia, and a prior history of delirium are also risk factors.

INTERVIEWING AND PSYCHOTHERAPEUTIC GUIDELINES

Delirious patients may present a wide range of psychomotor activity, ranging from agitation with delirium tremens to apathy because of sensory deprivation. Try to use stimuli that balance the level of psychomotor activity—for example, minimally stimulate an agitated patient. The patient's behavior may change suddenly. Keep questions brief, since the patient's attention may be limited. Assess the patient's memory, orientation, and level of consciousness. Orient patients with repeated simple statements regarding their situation (for example, "You are in the hospital. Today is . . ."). Clinicians should give simple, repetitious explanations of who they are and what they are doing. A family member or any familiar face may help calm an agitated patient. The patient's mental status may change considerably within a period of hours. Physical restraints may be needed. Obtaining a history from collateral informants is important in establishing a diagnosis; for example, a relative may reveal that the patient is an insulin-dependent diabetic who has not been eating.

EVALUATION AND MANAGEMENT

1. Identify any likely causes from the patient's history; if any are identified, try to reverse them immediately. If untreated, delirium can lead to death. List all the patient's drugs—prescribed, over-the-counter, and drugs of abuse—especially anticholinergic drugs, antidepressants, antipsychotics, sedative-hypnotics, psychostimulants, hallucinogens, and alcohol.

Table B.45–1
Symptoms of Delirium in Approximate Order of Specificity

1. Instability of all mental status findings over time
2. Nonauditory hallucinations
3. Misperceptions and illusions
4. Impaired attention span
5. Disorientation
6. Impaired level of consciousness
7. Auditory hallucinations
8. Other cognitive impairment
9. Delusional ideation
10. Affective symptoms

Table from O Thienhaus: Delirium and dementia. In *Manual of Clinical Emergency Psychiatry*, J R Hillard, editor, p 164. American Psychiatric Press, Washington, 1990. Used with permission.

Table B.45–2
Diagnostic Criteria for Delirium

A. Reduced ability to maintain attention to external stimuli (e.g., questions must be repeated because attention wanders) and to appropriately shift attention to new external stimuli (e.g., perseverates answer to a previous question)

B. Disorganized thinking, as indicated by rambling, irrelevant, or incoherent speech

C. At least two of the following:
   (1) reduced level of consciousness (e.g., difficulty keeping awake during examination)
   (2) perceptual disturbances: misinterpretations, illusions, or hallucinations
   (3) disturbance of sleep-wake cycle with insomnia or daytime sleepiness
   (4) increased or decreased psychomotor activity
   (5) disorientation to time, place, or person
   (6) memory impairment (e.g., inability to learn new material, such as the names of several unrelated objects after five minutes, or to remember past events, such as history of current episode of illness)

D. Clinical features develop over a short period of time (usually hours to days) and tend to fluctuate over the course of a day.

E. Either (1) or (2):
   (1) evidence from the history, physical examination, or laboratory tests of a specific organic factor (or factors) judged to be etiologically related to the disturbance
   (2) in the absence of such evidence, an etiologic organic factor can be presumed if the disturbance cannot be accounted for by any nonorganic mental disorder (e.g., manic episode accounting for agitation and sleep disturbance)

Table from DSM-III-R, *Diagnostic and Statistical Manual of Mental Disorders,* ed 3, revised. Copyright American Psychiatric Association, Washington, 1987. Used with permission.

2. If the patient is agitated, physical restraint may be necessary, especially in medical and surgical inpatients. Restraint may be preferable to medication if a definitive diagnosis is not yet clear.

3. Check the patient's vital signs, and perform a complete physical examination. Fever suggests an infection; hypertension and tachycardia suggest withdrawal from alcohol or sedative-hypnotics. Examine the patient for focal neurological signs suggesting an acute central nervous system (CNS) event. Signs of cardiopulmonary instability require prompt treatment (Table B.45–3).

4. On the mental status examination, document the areas of cognitive impairment and the level of psychomotor activity. Test the patient's lan-

Physical Examination of the Delirious Patient

Parameter	Finding	Clinical Implications
Pulse	Bradycardia	Hypothyroidism Stokes-Adams syndrome Increased intracranial pressure
	Tachycardia	Hyperthyroidism Infection Heart failure
Temperature	Fever	Sepsis Thyroid storm Vasculitis
Blood pressure	Hypotension	Shock Hypothyroidism Addison's disease
	Hypertension	Encephalopathy Intracranial mass
Respiration	Tachypnea	Diabetes Pneumonia Cardiac failure Fever Acidosis (metabolic)
	Shallow	Drug or alcohol intoxication
Carotid vessels	Bruits or decreased pulse	Transient cerebral ischemia
Scalp and face	Evidence of trauma	
Neck	Evidence of nuchal rigidity	Meningitis Subarachnoid hemorrhage
Eyes	Papilledema	Tumor Hypertensive encephalopathy
	Pupillary dilatation	Anxiety Autonomic overactivity (e.g., delirium tremens)
Mouth	Tongue or cheek lacerations	Evidence of generalized tonic-clonic seizures
Thyroid	Enlarged	Hyperthyroidism
Heart	Arrhythmia	Inadequate cardiac output, possibility of emboli
	Cardiomegaly	Heart failure Hypertensive disease
Lungs	Congestion	Primary pulmonary failure Pulmonary edema Pneumonia
Breath	Alcohol Ketones	Diabetes
Liver	Enlargement	Cirrhosis Liver failure
Nervous system Reflexes-muscle stretch	Asymmetry with Babinski's signs	Mass lesion Cardiovascular disease Preexisting dementia
	Snout	Frontal mass Bilateral posterior cerebral artery occlusion
Abducent nerve (sixth cranial nerve)	Weakness in lateral gaze	Increased intracranial pressure
Limb strength	Asymmetrical	Mass lesion Cardiovascular disease
Autonomic	Hyperactivity	Anxiety Delirium

Table from R L Strub, F W Black: *Neurobehavioral Disorders: A Clinical Approach.* Davis, Philadelphia, 1981. Used with permission.

Table B.45–4
Causes of Delirium

Intracranial causes
  Epilepsy and postictal states
  Brain trauma (especially concussion)
  Infections
    Meningitis
    Encephalitis
  Neoplasms
  Vascular disorders

Extracranial causes
  Drugs (ingestion or withdrawal) and poisons
    Sedatives (including alcohol) and hypnotics
    Tranquilizers
    Other drugs
      Anticholinergic agents
      Anticonvulsants
      Antihypertensive agents
      Antiparkinsonian agents
      Cardiac glycosides
      Cimetidine
      Disulfiram
      Insulin
      Opiates
      Phencyclidine
      Salicylates
      Steroids
    Poisons
      Carbon monoxide
      Heavy metals and other industrial poisons
  Endocrine dysfunction (hypofunction or hyperfunction)
    Pituitary
    Pancreas
    Adrenal
    Parathyroid
    Thyroid
  Diseases of nonendocrine organs
    Liver
      Hepatic encephalopathy
    Kidney and urinary tract
      Uremic encephalopathy
    Lung
      Carbon dioxide narcosis
      Hypoxia
    Cardiovascular system
      Cardiac failure
      Arrhythmias
      Hypotension
  Deficiency diseases
    Thiamine deficiency
  Systemic infections with fever and sepsis
  Electrolyte imbalance of any cause
  Postoperative states

Table by Charles E. Wells, M.D.

guage functions. Administer the remainder of the Mini-Mental State Examination as the patient's cooperation permits.

5. Order laboratory tests, including a complete blood count (CBC) with differential, erythrocyte sedimentation rate (ESR), complete blood chemistries, liver and renal function tests, thyroid function tests, urinalysis, urine

toxicology screen, electrocardiogram (ECG), chest X-ray, computed tomography (CT) scan of the head, and a lumbar puncture if indicated.

6. Correct any metabolic, nutritional, electrolyte, or fluid abnormalities.

7. Obtain a neurological consultation.

8. Start the treatment when a definitive diagnosis has been made. Delirium may be due to multiple causes, so, even after one possible cause has been identified, continue to make a full evaluation (Table B.45–4).

DRUG TREATMENT

High-potency antipsychotics are usually the first-choice treatment. They have little anticholinergic effects and are less likely than are low-potency antipsychotics to lower the seizure threshold. Haloperidol (Haldol) 2 to 5 mg intramuscularly (IM) may be repeated after 30 minutes if the first dose is ineffective. Antipsychotics are less likely than benzodiazepines to worsen the patient's cognitive function. However, patients in alcohol or sedative-hypnotic withdrawal are best treated with a benzodiazepine.

Benzodiazepines—for example, lorazepam (Ativan) 1 to 2 mg by mouth, IM, or slow intravenous (IV) administration and repeated after one hour as needed—may also be used for agitation if antipsychotics are contraindicated. If several doses of an antipsychotic are ineffective, lorazepam may be added.

Cross-References:

Alcohol withdrawal; anticholinergic intoxication; barbiturate and similarly acting sedative, hypnotic, or anxiolytic intoxication and withdrawal; confusion; dementia; head trauma; intoxication, restraints.

46 / Delusional Disorder

Delusional (paranoid) disorder is characterized by false fixed beliefs not subject to reality testing.

CLINICAL FEATURES AND DIAGNOSIS

In delusional disorder, delusions are of at least one month's duration and are well systematized as opposed to bizarre or fragmented. The patient's emotional response to the delusional system is congruent with and appropriate to the content of the delusion. Their personality remains intact or deteriorates minimally. Patients often are hypersensitive and hypervigilant, which may lead, despite their high-functioning capacities, to a relatively socially isolated existence.

The patients are relatively free of psychopathology in areas other than the delusional system (Table B.46–1). The onset is often in middle adult or late adult life.

Table B.46–1
Diagnostic Criteria for Delusional Disorder

A. Nonbizarre delusion(s) (i.e., involving situations that occur in real life, such as being followed, poisoned, infected, loved at a distance, having a disease, being deceived by one's spouse or lover) of at least one month's duration

B. Auditory or visual hallucinations, if present, are not prominent

C. Apart from the delusion(s) or its ramifications, behavior is not obviously odd or bizarre

D. If a major depressive or manic syndrome has been present during the delusional disturbance, the total duration of all episodes of the mood syndrome has been brief relative to the total duration of the delusional disturbance

E. Has never met criterion A for schizophrenia, and it cannot be established that an organic factor initiated and maintained the disturbance

Specify type: The following types are based on the predominant delusional theme. If no single delusional theme predominates, specify as **Unspecified Type**

Erotomanic Type
Delusional disorder in which the predominant theme of the delusion(s) is that a person, usually of higher status, is in love with the subject

Grandiose Type
Delusional disorder in which the predominant theme of the delusion(s) is one of inflated worth, power, knowledge, identity, or special relationship to a deity or famous person

Jealous Type
Delusional disorder in which the predominant theme of the delusion(s) is that one's sexual partner is unfaithful

Persecutory Type
Delusional disorder in which the predominant theme of the delusion(s) is that one (or someone to whom one is close) is being malevolently treated in some way. People with this type of delusional disorder may repeatedly take their complaints of being mistreated to legal authorities.

Somatic Type
Delusional disorder in which the predominant theme of the delusion(s) is that the person has some physical defect, disorder, or disease

Unspecified Type
Delusional disorder that does not fit any of the previous categories, e.g., persecutory and grandiose themes without a predominance of either; delusions of reference without malevolent content

Table from DSM-III-R, *Diagnostic and Statistical Manual of Mental Disorders,* ed 3, revised. Copyright American Psychiatric Association, Washington, 1987. Used with permission.

INTERVIEWING AND PSYCHOTHERAPEUTIC GUIDELINES

Do not argue with or challenge the patient's delusions. A delusion may become even more entrenched if the patient feels it must be defended. Examine the stresses on life experiences that precipitated the patient requiring emergency treatment. If treatment is indicated, explain the rationale to the patient.

The main objectives in the initial interview are to gain the patient's trust, determine the patient's level of impairment, and evaluate the possibility of other diagnoses, such as depression, mania, schizophrenia, substance abuse (for example, cocaine), and organic conditions.

EVALUATION AND MANAGEMENT

1. A physical and neurological examination, and the patient's drug history can help identify the possible organic causes (for example, drugs and tumors).

2. Suicidal or homicidal ideation, if present, may require hospitalization.

3. Outpatient treatment is difficult because of poor patient cooperation. However, individual psychotherapy is indicated. An early goal is to enlist the patient's trust and then to focus on the impairments caused by the delusional system. Work toward eliminating the delusions.

DRUG TREATMENT

Acute agitation should be treated with benzodiazepines, such as lorazepam (Ativan) 1 to 2 mg by mouth or intramuscularly (IM), or antipsychotics, such as haloperidol (Haldol) 2 to 5 mg by mouth or IM.

Although antipsychotics are currently considered the drugs of choice for maintenance therapy, adequate proof of their efficacy is lacking. If a coexisting mood disorder exists, antidepressants, lithium (Estkalith), or carbamazepine (Tegretol) may be used. Pimozide (Orap) may also be of use.

Cross-References:

Depression, homicidal and assaultive behavior, mania, schizophrenia, suicide.

47 / Dementia

Dementia is a loss of cognitive and intellectual functions that is sufficiently severe to interfere with the patient's social or occupational functioning.

CLINICAL FEATURES AND DIAGNOSIS

The essential deficit is a loss of memory, both short-term and long-term. Abstract thinking and judgment are also frequently impaired, and there are often other signs of high cortical involvement as well as a marked change in personality (Table B.47–1).

Dementia must be differentiated from normal aging, delirium, and depression. In *normal aging* the patient may have some loss of cognitive function, but it is not progressive and does not cause impairments in social and occupational functioning. The differential diagnosis between dementia and delirium is summarized in Table B.47–2. The differential diagnosis between dementia and depression is summarized in Table B.47–3. Demented patients often have a superimposed delirium or depression.

Dementia, although possible at any age after which an intelligence quotient (I.Q.) can be determined, is primarily a syndrome of the elderly. In-

Table B.47–1
Diagnostic Criteria for Dementia

A. Demonstrable evidence of impairment in short- and long-term memory. Impairment in short-term memory (inability to learn new information) may be indicated by inability to remember three objects after five minutes. Long-term memory impairment (inability to remember information that was known in the past) may be indicated by inability to remember past personal information (e.g., what happened yesterday, birthplace, occupation) or facts of common knowledge (e.g., past Presidents, well-known dates).

B. At least one of the following:
   (1) impairment in abstract thinking, as indicated by inability to find similarities and differences between related words, difficulty in defining words and concepts, and other similar tasks
   (2) impaired judgment, as indicated by inability to make reasonable plans to deal with interpersonal, family, and job-related problems and issues
   (3) other disturbances of higher cortical function, such as aphasia (disorder of language), apraxia (inability to carry out motor activities despite intact comprehension and motor function), agnosia (failure to recognize or identify objects despite intact sensory function), and "constructional difficulty" (e.g., inability to copy three-dimensional figures, assemble blocks, or arrange sticks in specific designs)
   (4) personality change (i.e., alteration or accentuation of premorbid traits)

C. The disturbance in A and B significantly interferes with work or usual social activities or relationships with others.

D. Not occurring exclusively during the course of delirium.

E. Either (1) or (2):
   (1) there is evidence from the history, physical examination, or laboratory tests of a specific organic factor (or factors judged to be etiologically related to the disturbance)
   (2) in the absence of such evidence, an etiologic organic factor can be presumed if the disturbance cannot be accounted for by any nonorganic mental disorder (e.g., major depression accounting for cognitive impairment)

Criteria for severity of dementia:

Mild: Although work or social activities are significantly impaired, the capacity for independent living remains, with adequate personal hygiene and relatively intact judgment.

Moderate: Independent living is hazardous, and some degree of supervision is necessary.

Severe: Activities of daily living are so impaired that continual supervision is required (e.g., unable to maintain minimal personal hygiene; largely incoherent or mute).

Table from DSM-III-R, *Diagnostic and Statistical Manual of Mental Disorders,* ed 3, revised. Copyright American Psychiatric Association, Washington, 1987. Used with permission.

creasing age is the major risk factor for dementia. The primary short-term objectives in treating demented patients are identifying and reversing any reversible dementias, managing behavioral emergencies, and treating any other medical and psychiatric conditions.

The most common cause of dementia is Alzheimer's disease, followed by multi-infarct dementia. Mixed forms are also common. Acquired immune deficiency syndrome (AIDS) is a common cause in young patients. Other causes are listed in Table B.47–4.

Patients with dementia are typically brought in by their family, the police, or caretakers who complain of the patient's wandering, confusion, inappropriate behavior (for example, touching others in a sexually inappropriate way, walking out of the house partially clad), aggression, depression, anxiety, or delusionally driven behavior (for example, accusations of theft). Patients with a known diagnosis of dementia are frequently brought in because of a sudden change in their behavior.

Table B.47–2
Clinical Differentiation of Delirium and Dementia

Feature	Delirium	Dementia
History	Acute disease	Chronic disease
Onset	Rapid	Insidious (usually)
Duration	Days to weeks	Months to years
Course	Fluctuating	Chronically progressive
Level of consciousness	Fluctuating	Normal
Orientation	Impaired, at least periodically	Intact initially
Affect	Anxious, irritable	Labile but not usually anxious
Thinking	Often disordered	Decreased amount
Memory	Recent memory is markedly impaired	Both recent memory and remote memory are impaired
Perception	Hallucinations common (especially visual)	Hallucinations not common (except sundowning)
Psychomotor	Retarded, agitated, or mixed	Normal
Sleep	Disrupted sleep-wake cycle	Little disruption of sleep-wake cycle
Attention and awareness	Prominently impaired	Little impairment
Reversibility	Often reversible	Majority not reversible

Note: Demented patients are susceptible to delirium, and delirium superimposed on dementia is common.

Table B.47–3
Dementia versus Depression with Cognitive Changes (Pseudodementia)

Feature	Organic Dementia	Pseudodementia
Age	Usually elderly	Nonspecific
Onset	Vague	Days to weeks
Course	Slow, worse at night	Rapid, even through day
History	Systemic illness or drugs	Mood disorder
Awareness	Unaware, unconcerned	Aware, distressed
Organic signs	Often present	Absent
Cognition[1]	Prominent impairment	Personality changes
Mental status examination	Consistent, spotty deficits	Variable deficits in different modalities
	Approximates, confabulates, perseverates	Apathetic, "I don't know"
	Emphasizes trivial accomplishments	Emphasizes failures
	Shallow or labile mood	Depressed
Behavior	Appropriate to degree of cognitive impairment	Incongruent with degree of cognitive impairment
Cooperation	Cooperative but frustrated	Uncooperative with little effort
CT and EEG	Abnormal	Normal

[1]Benzodiazepines and barbiturates worsen cognitive impairments in the demented patient, whereas they help the depressed patient relax.

INTERVIEWING AND PSYCHOTHERAPEUTIC GUIDELINES

If patients are disoriented or confused, try to orient them and help them relax.

In evaluating the patient's mental status, focus on cognitive functions, and administer the Mini-Mental State Examination. If the patient seems

Table B.47–4
Diseases That Cause Dementia

Parenchymatous diseases of the central nervous system
  Alzheimer's disease (primary degenerative dementia)
  Pick's disease (primary degenerative dementia)
  Huntington's chorea
  Parkinson's disease*
  Multiple sclerosis
Systemic disorders
  Endocrine and metabolic disorders
    Thyroid disease*
    Parathyroid disease*
    Pituitary-adrenal disorders*
    Posthypoglycemic states
  Liver disease
    Chronic progressive hepatic encephalopathy*
  Urinary tract disease
    Chronic uremic encephalopathy*
    Progressive uremic encephalopathy (dialysis dementia)*
  Cardiovascular disease
    Cerebral hypoxia or anoxia*
    Multi-infarct dementia*
    Cardiac arrhythmias*
    Inflammatory diseases of blood vessels*
  Pulmonary disease
    Respiratory encephalopathy*
Deficiency states
  Cyanocobalamin deficiency*
  Folic acid deficiency*
Drugs and toxins*
Intracranial tumors* and brain trauma*
Infectious processes
  Creutzfeldt-Jakob disease*
  Cryptococcal meningitis*
  Neurosyphilis*
  Tuberculosis and fungal meningitis*
    Viral encephalitis
    Human immunodeficiency virus (HIV)-related disorders (e.g., AIDS and AIDS-related
      complex [ARC])
Miscellaneous disorders
  Hepatolenticular degeneration*
  Hydrocephalic dementia*
  Sarcoidosis*
  Normal pressure hydrocephalus*

Adapted from C E Wells: Organic syndromes: Dementia. In *Comprehensive Textbook of Psychiatry,* ed 4. H I Kaplan, B J Sadock, editors, p 855. Williams & Wilkins, Baltimore, 1985.
*Conditions calling for specific therapeutic intervention.

to be irritated or embarrassed by questions that reveal impaired cognition, change the subject, and return to examining the patient's cognition later. Try to determine the course of the impairment, whether it had a rapid onset or a slow onset and whether there were physical or psychological precipitants to the present episode.

Note the patient's affect, especially whether the patient is depressed or anxious. What is the patient's attitude toward the impairment? Does it bother the patient, or is the patient unconcerned? Determining the patient's attitude helps identify possible pseudodementia. Patients with dementia often minimize or deny their cognitive deficits; those with pseudodementia often have exaggerated complaints of memory loss (Table B.47–3).

EVALUATION AND MANAGEMENT

1. Obtain a full physical and neurological examination. The organic workup should include a complete blood count (CBC) with differential white blood count, liver function tests, the blood urea nitrogen (BUN) and creatinine test, thyroid function tests, a Venereal Disease Research Laboratory (VDRL) test, B_{12} and folate levels, a urinalysis, a urine toxicology screen, an electrocardiogram (ECG), a chest X-ray, and a computed tomography (CT) scan or magnetic resonance imaging (MRI) of the head. A lumbar puncture may also be indicated.

2. Interview collaborative sources, such as the family, for the patient's history.

3. The elderly take many more medications than do the young. Identify all the prescribed and over-the-counter drugs the patient takes. The patient may also take alcohol and drugs of abuse. Any drugs that could possibly cause dementia should be systematically discontinued if that is medically possible. Common candidates for discontinuation include antihypertensives, anticonvulsants, antipsychotics, sedative-hypnotics, steroids, antiarrhythmics, anticholinergics, methyldopa, and antidepressants.

4. Perform a mental status examination, including a detailed cognitive examination, and assess depressive or psychotic symptoms.

5. Identify and treat the patient's medical problems, and correct any nutritional and metabolic deficiencies. Assess any behavioral changes in a known dementia patient. Evaluate the patient for superimposed delirium, a brain injury (for example, a cerebral infarct or a subdural hematoma secondary to a fall), or an environmental change (for example, the recent replacement of a long-time home attendant or some other change in caretaking).

6. Decide whether admission to a hospital or a nursing home is needed. Unless the patient has an acute medical or behavioral emergency, try to avoid hospital admission, since disposition problems (for example, no nursing home beds) may produce a long, medically unnecessary hospitalization.

7. Counsel the patient's family regarding the prognosis; the possible need for placement in a nursing home, home care, or legal guardianship; the possible behaviors to expect from the patient; and the syndromes that may develop in the caretakers (for example, burnout, depression, and anxiety). When appropriate, refer the family to the Alzheimer's Disease and Related Disorders Association (ADRDA). The family can get information about local groups by writing to ADRDA, 70 East Lake Street, Chicago, IL 60601.

DRUG TREATMENT

Use low dosages of all psychotropic medications in the elderly. Adhere to the maxim, "start low, go slow."

Although antipsychotics such as haloperidol 0.5 to 5 mg a day are the primary psychotropic drugs for behavioral control in demented patients, the elderly clear many drugs more slowly than do young patients because of decreased hepatic and renal function. The primary problems with antipsychotics in the elderly are the acute side effects, including dystonia, parkinsonian side effects, anticholinergic side effects, and hypotension. High-potency antipsychotic agents, such as haloperidol, are preferable to low-potency agents, such as chlorpromazine (Thorazine), whose strong anticholinergic effects can further impair the patient's cognition.

Some clinicians recommend short-acting benzodiazepines for insomnia or anxiety in the elderly, but the risks of cognitive impairment and dependence must be considered. The use of conjugated benzodiazepines (oxazepam [Serax] 7.5 to 15 mg by mouth, lorazepam [Ativan] 0.5 to 1 mg by mouth, temazepam [Restoril] 7.5 to 15 mg by mouth) is recommended because the elimination half-life of those drugs is not increased in the elderly by their impaired liver function.

Antidepressants, lithium, and anticonvulsants may be used, but they should be started at low dosages, increased slowly, and monitored with frequent blood levels. Monoamine oxidase inhibitors (MAOIs) may be useful for depression associated with dementia.

Antihistamines may be used in low dosages for anxiety or insomnia, but they may cause anticholinergic side effects to which the demented are especially sensitive.

Cross-References:

Agitation, anxiety, confusion, delirium, delusional disorder, depression, hallucinations, insomnia, sundowner syndrome.

---

48 / Depersonalization

Depersonalization is a disturbance in perception that involves a sense that one is unreal or somehow changed and is strange to oneself. Depersonalization, like derealization, can occur briefly to normal people under stress (for example, during physical or psychological trauma). Mild symptoms may occur in normal people when they are exposed to an unfamiliar environment.

CLINICAL FEATURES AND DIAGNOSIS

Patients with depersonalization may describe feeling as though they were detached from their own bodies, viewing their lives as though they were spectators. They may also feel mechanical or robotlike. The patients are aware that the symptoms are not reality, and they find the experience unpleasant.

Depersonalization that is severe enough to cause impairment and that occurs repeatedly, without other prominent symptoms, may fulfill the diagnostic criteria for depersonalization disorder (Table B.48–1).

Depersonalization is also a symptom of a wide range of disorders—including other dissociative disorders, schizophrenia, anxiety disorders (es-

Table B.48–1
Diagnostic Criteria for Depersonalization Disorder

A. Persistent or recurrent experiences of depersonalization as indicated by either (1) or (2):
   (1) an experience of feeling detached from, and as if one is an outside observer of, one's mental processes or body
   (2) an experience of feeling like an automation or as if in a dream

B. During the depersonalization experience, reality testing remains intact.

C. The depersonalization is sufficiently severe and persistent to cause marked distress.

D. The depersonalization experience is the predominant disturbance and is not a symptom of another disorder, such as schizophrenia, panic disorder, or agoraphobia without history of panic disorder but with limited symptom attacks of depersonalization, or temporal lobe epilepsy.

Table from DSM-III-R, *Diagnostic and Statistical Manual of Mental Disorders,* ed 3, revised. Copyright American Psychiatric Association, Washington, 1987. Used with permission.

pecially posttraumatic stress disorder), depression, and organic disorders. Depersonalization can also be caused by intoxication with cocaine, hallucinogens, and cannabis and by withdrawal from alcohol and sedative-hypnotics. β-Blockers, anticholinergic drugs, and such medical conditions as epilepsy and endocrine disorders can also cause depersonalization.

INTERVIEWING AND PSYCHOTHERAPEUTIC GUIDELINES

The symptoms do not usually occur during the interview. But a patient who is depersonalizing during the interview may be in a dreamlike state and only partially responsive to the environment. Be directive and help the patient cooperate with the interview and the examination. With some reassurance the symptom may stop, especially if the depersonalization is in response to anxiety. The goal of the interview is a definitive diagnosis. Organic disorders, depression, personality disorders, schizophrenia, and anxiety disorders must be ruled out before a diagnosis of depersonalization disorder is made. As a rule, consider the most severe diagnoses first (for example, organic disorders), and rule them out before considering other diagnoses.

EVALUATION AND MANAGEMENT

1. Consider possible causes based on the patient's history. First consider a history of substance use or withdrawal, then organic mental syndromes. Schizophrenia usually presents with other associated symptoms, including thought disorder. A history of a recent severe trauma may indicate that the depersonalization is a normal reaction. A history of repeated episodes of depersonalization after a past trauma suggests posttraumatic stress disorder. A history of other dissociative symptoms suggests a dissociative disorder.

2. Prescribed medications, particularly steroids, can cause organic disorders of which depersonalization may be a symptom.

3. On the mental status examination, look for symptoms of mood disorders, anxiety disorders, psychosis, and dissociative disorders.

4. Conduct a physical examination. A neurological examination should also be performed. If the diagnosis still remains unclear, order an organic workup, including urine toxicology screening, an electroencephalogram (EEG), and a computed tomography (CT) scan of the head.

DRUG TREATMENT

Drug treatment depends on the definitive diagnosis. If the depersonalization is a symptom of severe anxiety, a short-acting benzodiazepine—for example, lorazepam (Ativan) 1 to 2 mg by mouth, oxazepam (Serax) 10 to 30 mg by mouth, estazolam (ProSom) 0.5 to 1 mg by mouth, or alprazolam (Xanax) 0.5 to 1 mg by mouth—may be used. In some cases a long-acting benzodiazepine—for example, clorazepate (Tranxene) 7.5 to 15 mg by mouth, clonazepam (Klonopin) 0.25 to 0.5 mg by mouth, diazepam (Valium) 5 to 10 mg by mouth, or chlordiazepoxide (Librium) 10 to 25 mg by mouth—may be used. The symptoms may resolve after benzodiazepines are given.

Cross-References:

Agitation, anxiety, cocaine intoxication and withdrawal, confusion, delusional disorder, depression, derealization, hallucinogen hallucinosis, posttraumatic stress disorder, schizophrenia.

---

49 / Depression

Depression is a period of impaired functioning associated with depressed mood and related symptoms, including sleep and appetite changes, psychomotor changes, impaired concentration, anhedonia, fatigue, feelings of hopelessness and helplessness, and thoughts of suicide.

CLINICAL FEATURES AND DIAGNOSIS

A depressive episode may be isolated or may occur in the course of either recurrent depression or bipolar disorder (Table B.49–1). Other diagnoses to consider are organic disorders; substance intoxication, dependence, and withdrawal; dysthymia; cyclothymia; personality disorders; bereavement (grief); and adjustment disorders. Bereavement is a normal, although painful, response to a major loss; it is responsive to support and empathy and improves over time. The important issue in bereaved patients is to look for major depression if the symptoms do not resolve with time.

Depressed patients do not always complain of sadness. They may be irritable or somatically preoccupied. Evaluate the patient for all associated signs and symptoms of depression, even in the absence of overt sadness. Any patient complaining of memory loss and depression must be evaluated for pseudodementia.

Table B.49–1
Diagnostic Criteria for Major Depressive Episode

Note: A major depressive syndrome is defined as criterion A below.

A. At least five of the following symptoms have been present during the same two-week period and represent a change from previous functioning; at least one of the symptoms is either (1) depressed mood or (2) loss of interest or pleasure. (Do not include symptoms that are clearly due to a physical condition, mood-incongruent delusions or hallucinations, incoherence, or marked loosening of associations.)

   (1) depressed mood (or can be irritable mood in children and adolescents) most of the day, nearly every day, as indicated either by subjective account or observation by others

   (2) markedly diminished interest or pleasure in all, or almost all, activities most of the day, nearly every day (as indicated either by subjective account or observation by others of apathy most of the time)

   (3) significant weight loss or weight gain when not dieting (e.g., more than 5 percent of body weight in a month), or decrease or increase in appetite nearly every day (in children, consider failure to make expected weight gains)

   (4) insomnia or hypersomnia nearly every day

   (5) psychomotor agitation or retardation nearly every day (observable by others, not merely subjective feelings of restlessness or being slowed down)

   (6) fatigue or loss of energy nearly every day

   (7) feelings of worthlessness or excessive or inappropriate guilt (which may be delusional) nearly every day (not merely self-reproach or guilt about being sick)

   (8) diminished ability to think or concentrate, or indecisiveness, nearly every day (either by subjective account or as observed by others)

   (9) recurrent thoughts of death (not just fear of dying), recurrent suicidal ideation without a specific plan, or a suicide attempt or a specific plan for committing suicide

B. (1) It cannot be established that an organic factor initiated and maintained the disturbance.

   (2) The disturbance is not a normal reaction to the death of a loved one (uncomplicated bereavement)

   Note: Morbid preoccupation with worthlessness, suicidal ideation, marked functional impairment or psychomotor retardation, or prolonged duration suggest bereavement complicated by major depression.

C. At no time during the disturbance have there been delusions or hallucinations for as long as two weeks in the absence of prominent mood symptoms (i.e., before the mood symptoms developed or after they have remitted).

D. Not superimposed on schizophrenia, schizophreniform disorder, delusional disorder, or psychotic disorder NOS.

Table from DSM-III-R, *Diagnostic and Statistical Manual of Mental Disorders,* ed 3, revised. Copyright American Psychiatric Association, Washington, 1987. Used with permission.

INTERVIEWING AND PSYCHOTHERAPEUTIC GUIDELINES

Engage the patients by being empathic and supportive. Many depressed patients feel isolated and hopeless. Be reassuring and inform them that they will be helped and that depression is readily treatable. Avoid glib, empty optimism ("Cheer up" or "It's not so bad"), which will be experienced as a lack of empathy. Address any ambivalence that the patients have about seeking treatment. Inform them that depression is common. Help identify specific stressors to make the patients feel less guilty and self-deprecating. Help reduce guilt by using a medical model, emphasizing that depression is an illness, like hypertension, that requires medical treatment. A collateral history from family members or friends is valuable in the assessment of depressed patients.

EVALUATION AND MANAGEMENT

1. Treat any acute medical problems that have resulted from suicide attempts or gestures. If the patient has taken a drug overdose, obtain emergency medical and toxicological evaluations immediately.

2. Evaluate and treat potential dangerousness and possible suicidal ideation.

3. Rule out the causes of depressive symptoms listed in Table B.49–2.

4. Probe for a history of manic or hypomanic episodes suggesting bipolar disorder. The diagnosis of bipolar disorder has implications for treatment and prognosis that are different from the implications for depression without mania.

5. Make a diagnosis, and document the severity of the depressive symptoms and the impairment to determine a disposition and treatment plan. Depression may be a life-threatening condition requiring involuntary hospitalization. If the patient is actively suicidal or has made a serious suicide attempt, hospitalization is indicated, and the patient may require constant one-to-one observation if still a suicide risk in the hospital. Although most suicidal patients are ambivalent about suicide, determinedly suicidal patients may not tell you about their suicidal intent for fear that you will intervene. The decision about whether to hospitalize mildly depressed patients may be difficult and should include a consideration of the patient's past history of depressive episodes, suicide attempts, response to treatment, identifiable stressors, support systems (family and friends), and likelihood of compliance with referral to outpatient treatment.

6. Engage the patient in the treatment process, and provide reassurance that the episode is treatable and will eventually be over. Most depressed patients never seek professional treatment.

DRUG TREATMENT

Definitive antidepressant treatment with medication or electroconvulsive therapy (ECT) takes several weeks or longer and is not done in an emergency setting. However, agitation, anxiety, and insomnia can be treated. The important information to determine is whether (1) the patient is psychotic, (2) the patient has taken drugs or alcohol, and (3) medical conditions are present. Unless the patient has an organic condition, the acute agitation, anxiety, or insomnia can be treated with a benzodiazepine such as lorazepam (Ativan) 1 to 2 mg by mouth or intramuscularly (IM), alprazolam (Xanax) 0.5 to 1 mg by mouth, or oxazepam (Serax) 10 to 30 mg by mouth, all given every four hours as needed. The dosage may be repeated or increased as needed unless signs of toxicity (for example, ataxia, dysarthria, and nystagmus) appear. Usually, sedation can be induced with benzodiazepines.

If psychotic symptoms are present, a benzodiazepine can still be used, but an antipsychotic may also be considered—for example, haloperidol (Haldol) 2 to 5 mg by mouth or IM, fluphenazine (Prolixin) 2 to 5 mg by mouth

Table B.49-2
Neurological, Medical, and Pharmacological Causes of Depressive Symptoms

Neurological
  Dementias (including Alzheimer's disease)
  Epilepsy*
  Fahr's disease*
  Huntington's chorea*
  Hydrocephalus
  Infections (including HIV and neurosyphilis)*
  Migraines*
  Multiple sclerosis*
  Narcolepsy
  Neoplasms*
  Parkinson's disease
  Progressive supranuclear palsy
  Sleep apnea
  Strokes*
  Trauma*
  Wilson's disease*

Endocrine
  Adrenal (Cushing's*, Addison's diseases)
  Hyperaldosteronism
  Menses-related*
  Parathyroid disorders (hyperparathyroidism and
    hypoparathyroidism)
  Postpartum*
  Thyroid disorders (hypothyroidism and apathetic
    hyperthyroidism)*

Infectious and inflammatory
  Acquired immune deficiency syndrome (AIDS)*
  Chronic fatigue syndrome
  Mononucleosis
  Pneumonia—viral and bacterial
  Rheumatoid arthritis
  Sjögren's arteritis
  Systemic lupus erythematosus*
  Temporal arteritis
  Tuberculosis

Miscellaneous medical
  Cancer (especially pancreatic and other GI)
  Cardiopulmonary disease
  Porphyria
  Uremia (and other renal diseases)*
  Vitamin deficiencies (B_{12}, C, folate, niacin, thiamine)*

Pharmacological (representative drugs)
  Analgesics and anti-inflammatory
    Ibuprofen
    Indomethacin
    Opiates
    Phenacetin

  Antibacterials and antifungals
    Ampicillin
    Clycloserine
    Ethionamide
    Griseofulvin
    Metronidazole
    Nalidixic acid
    Nitrofurantoin
    Streptomycin
    Sulfamethoxazole
    Sulfonamides
    Tetracycline

Antihypertensives and cardiac drugs
  Alphamethyldopa
  Bethtanidine
  β-Blockers (propranolol)
  Clonidine
  Digitalis
  Guanethidine
  Hydralazine
  Lidocaine
  Prazosin
  Procainanide
  Quanabenzacetate
  Rescinnamine*
  Reserpine
  Veratrum

Antineoplastics
  C-Asparaginase
  Azathioprine (AZT)
  6-Azauridine
  Bleomycin
  Trimethoprim
  Vincristine

Neurological and psychiatric
  Amantadine
  Antipsychotics (butyrophenones,
    phenothiazines, oxyindoles)
  Baclofen
  Bromocriptine
  Carbamazepine
  Levodopa
  Phenytoin
  Sedatives and hypnotics
    (barbiturates, benzodiazepines,
    chloral hydrate)
  Tetrabenazine

Steroids and hormones
  Corticosteroids (including ACTH)
  Danazol
  Oral contraceptives
  Prednisone
  Triamcinolone

Miscellaneous
  Acetazolamide
  Choline
  Cimetidine
  Cyproheptadine
  Diphenoxylate
  Disulfiram
  Methysergide
  Stimulants (amphetamines,
    fenfluramine)

*These conditions are also associated with manic symptoms.

or IM, or thiothixene (Navane) 2 to 5 mg by mouth or IM, all given every four hours as needed.

If an organic condition is present, the drug choice depends on the patient's condition. Antipsychotics lower the seizure threshold and should be used with caution in patients with epilepsy. Benzodiazepines raise the seizure threshold but are more likely to cause amnesia, other cognitive problems, or agitation in patients who are confused, delirious, or demented. Patients should be referred for psychiatric treatment that includes psychotherapy or pharmacotherapy or both.

Cross-References:

Agitation, alcohol intoxication, anxiety, cocaine intoxication and withdrawal, dementia, grief and bereavement, hospitalization, mania, suicide.

---

50 / Derealization

Derealization is a disturbance in perception that involves a sense that one's environment is unreal or somehow changed and strange.

CLINICAL FEATURES AND DIAGNOSIS

Patients may describe feeling as though they were actors on a stage. Derealization is often associated with depersonalization. Both derealization and depersonalization can occur in normal people under severe stress; the disorders are considered final defense mechanisms protecting against overwhelming distress.

Derealization is also a symptom of a wide range of disorders—including schizophrenia, dissociative disorders, anxiety disorders (especially posttraumatic stress disorder), borderline personality disorder, depression, and organic mental disorders. Derealization can be caused by intoxication with cocaine or other psychostimulants, hallucinogens, or cannabis or by withdrawal from alcohol or sedative-hypnotics. β-Blockers, anticholinergic drugs, epilepsy, and endocrine disorders can also produce derealization.

INTERVIEWING AND PSYCHOTHERAPEUTIC GUIDELINES

The patient may be in a dreamlike state and only partially responsive to the environment. Be directive and help the patient cooperate with the interview and the examination. With some reassurance to the patient, the derealization may stop, thus allowing a comprehensive evaluation. The goal of the interview is a definitive diagnosis. Derealization is a nonspecific symptom and seldom occurs alone, without other symptoms.

EVALUATION AND MANAGEMENT

1. Consider possible causes. A history of substance use and withdrawal should be considered first, then organic mental disorders. Schizophrenia usually presents with other associated symptoms, including psychosis and thought disorder. A history of recent severe trauma may indicate that the derealization is a normal reaction. A history of repeated episodes after a past trauma suggests posttraumatic stress disorder. A history of depersonalization or other dissociative symptoms suggests a dissociative disorder.

2. Prescribed medications, particularly steroids, can cause organic mental disorders, of which derealization may be a symptom.

3. Rule out organic conditions with an electroencephalogram (EEG), urine toxicology screen, full medical evaluation, and endocrine workup (thyroid, pancreas, adrenal).

4. Look for symptoms of mood disorders, anxiety disorders, psychosis, and dissociative disorders.

5. The patient's behavior is usually either withdrawn or anxious and agitated.

DRUG TREATMENT

Drug treatment depends on the definitive diagnosis. If derealization is a symptom of severe anxiety, benzodiazepines may be used for a short time. For schizophrenia and other psychotic conditions, antipsychotics may be indicated.

Cross-References:

Agitation, anxiety, cocaine intoxication and withdrawal, delusional disorder, depersonalization, depression, disaster survivors, epilepsy, hallucinogen hallucinosis, posttraumatic stress disorder, schizophrenia.

---

51 / Dermatitis, Self-Inflicted

Self-inflicted dermatitis (also called dermatitis artefacta and dermatitis factitia) is a disorder consisting of self-inflicted skin wounds.

CLINICAL FEATURES AND DIAGNOSIS

The patient may deny that the wounds are self-inflicted and complains of dermatological disease, but the pattern of the lesions (linear or in a geometric shape) is pathognomonic of a factitious disorder. Self-inflicted dermatitis is more common in women than in men and is associated with borderline personality disorder. It also occurs in anxiety disorders, depression, and other personality disorders. It is rarely a symptom of a psychotic disorder.

INTERVIEWING AND PSYCHOTHERAPEUTIC GUIDELINES

The patients with the disorder have a need to have a dermatological condition; they may be manipulating to achieve a secondary gain. After ruling out a true dermatological condition, try to identify the psychological needs that the symptom has been fabricated to satisfy. Do not lie or acknowledge that the injuries are from a genuine dermatological disorder. In addition, do not confront the patients directly and accuse them of malingering. Focus on the conflicts and the stresses that led to the behavior.

EVALUATION AND MANAGEMENT

1. Rule out genuine dermatological conditions; a dermatology consultation may be helpful.

2. Complete a psychiatric evaluation for personality disorders, anxiety disorders, depression, and psychotic disorders.

3. Focus on underlying conflicts and try to resolve the acute problems that led to the present episode.

4. Definitive treatment depends on the psychiatric diagnosis. Often, referral for psychotherapy is indicated.

DRUG TREATMENT

No specific drug treatment is required, although underlying depressive, anxiety, or psychotic disorders may warrant drug therapy.

Cross-References:

Anxiety, borderline personality disorder, depression, malingering, self-mutilation.

---

52 / Disaster Survivors

Disaster survivors are people who have survived a sudden, unexpected, overwhelming stress that is beyond a level normally expected in life. Typical stresses include earthquakes, floods, fires, plane crashes, mud slides, building collapses, concentration camp internment, famine, and radiation contamination.

CLINICAL FEATURES AND DIAGNOSIS

The common emotions in disasters include fear, panic, anger, frustration, numbness, confusion, helplessness, and guilt. The psychiatric syndromes that may be present in the patients include posttraumatic stress disorder, other anxiety disorders, and depression. Some victims experience brief depersonalization or derealization. Psychiatric syndromes may be identified in those who are physically injured, those who escaped physical injury, family members of the victims, and rescue workers.

INTERVIEWING AND PSYCHOTHERAPEUTIC GUIDELINES

Be empathic and supportive. Make the patients as comfortable as possible. Reassure them with whatever facts are available, and minimize the spread of rumors. If the facts may be overwhelming for a patient, delay telling the facts, but do not intentionally tell a patient something that is not true. Emotional reactions to the stress vary considerably, so be prepared to handle a wide range of emotional states. Work with the victims to mobilize supports and a plan of action. Remind the victims of their past successful coping skills.

Obtain a detailed account of the victims' experiences. Was the event unexpected, anticipated, or a repetition of a similar experience? Past histories can be useful in understanding the patients' present maladaptive reactions.

EVALUATION AND MANAGEMENT

1. Treat any acute medical problems.
2. Provide some psychological relief. Cognitive approaches may be useful. The survivors' feelings of guilt may respond to such interventions as, "What could anyone else have done in that situation?" Reassure the survivors that guilt, frustration, and hopelessness are normal reactions to the level of stress experienced and that those feelings will pass with time. Hopelessness may be relieved by recruiting survivors to help other victims.
3. Encourage the patients to talk about their feelings and how they experienced the disaster. Survivors who were not injured and family members of dead victims may feel guilty about not being hurt when their friends and family members have died. Rescue workers may have similar feelings, plus anger and frustration.
4. Group therapy with victims, families, and rescue workers may be helpful, especially in relieving the feelings of helplessness and of being alone.

DRUG TREATMENT

Medications are usually not needed, although severe anxiety may be relieved with a brief course of short-acting benzodiazepines—for example, oxazepam (Serax) 15 to 30 mg, alprazolam (Xanax) 0.5 to 1 mg, lorazepam (Ativan) 1 to 2 mg, or estazolam (ProSom) 0.5 to 1 mg, all given by mouth three times a day. In some cases a long-acting benzodiazepine—for example, diazepam (Valium) 5 to 10 mg by mouth two times a day, chlordiazepoxide (Librium) 10 to 25 mg by mouth three times a day, clorazepate (Tranxene) 2.5 to 5 mg by mouth three times a day, or clonazepam (Klonopin) 0.25 to 0.50 mg by mouth two times a day—may be used. Insomnia can be treated with flurazepam (Dalmane) 15 to 30 mg by mouth as needed, quazepam (Doral) 7.5 to 15 mg by mouth as needed, temazepam (Restoril) 15 to 30 mg by mouth as needed, or triazolam (Halcion) 0.125 to 0.25 mg by mouth as needed.

Cross-References:

Agitation, anxiety, depersonalization, depression, derealization, group hysteria, panic disorder, posttraumatic stress disorder.

---

53 / Disorientation

Disorientation is impaired awareness of time, place, or person. This symptom is often considered a hallmark of organic disorders that produce global cognitive impairment, particularly delirium and dementia.

CLINICAL FEATURES AND DIAGNOSIS

The primary objective is to determine whether an acute organic disorder is present and, if so, to reverse it. In general, assume that delirium is present, and proceed accordingly. Patients with psychiatric disorders who are severely psychotic may also be disoriented.

INTERVIEWING AND PSYCHOTHERAPEUTIC GUIDELINES

In testing the patient's orientation, do not give any information that reveals the correct answer. Test the patient's orientation in detail, and try to quantify the degree of disorientation. Ask for the patient's name and age. Testing for orientation to time initially includes questions about the day, date, month, and year. If the patient is not oriented to those facts, inquire about the season and whether it is day or night. Similarly, if the patient is not oriented to place (for example, does not know the name of the hospital), inquire whether the patient knows the function of the building ("Is this a police station? A train station?"). If the patient does not know the name or the function of the building, ask for the name of the town, the county, the state, and the country.

If a patient is disoriented, screen for other signs of cognitive impairment. Administer the Mini-Mental State Examination as a broad screening test.

EVALUATION AND MANAGEMENT

1. Obtain the patient's vital signs. If the signs are abnormal, suspect a central nervous system (CNS) infection, delirium from alcohol or sedative-hypnotic withdrawal, or delirium from other causes.

2. Ask about medications. Both psychotropic and medical drugs can cause delirium, of which disorientation may be a sign. Steroids, anticholinergic drugs, anticonvulsants, antiparkinsonian agents, antipsychotics, benzodiazepines, antihypertensives, cardiac glycosides, cimetidine (Taga-

met), and disulfiram (Antabuse) should be considered as possible causes of the cognitive impairment.

3. Consider drugs of abuse. Intoxication or withdrawal from alcohol or sedative-hypnotics and intoxication with hallucinogens or psychostimulants may disorient the patient.

4. Examine the patient for medical and neurological conditions. Consider such medical conditions as thyroid disease, cardiac failure, nutritional deficiencies, cancer, hepatic failure, renal failure, sepsis, and electrolyte imbalance. Consider such neurological conditions as head trauma, epilepsy, meningitis, encephalitis, CNS neoplasms, and vascular disorders.

5. Ask for the patient's history and the course of the disorientation. Is it a new condition? If so, the search for a reversible cause must be aggressive.

6. Consider the age of the patient. An adolescent is likely to be abusing street drugs, but an elderly person is likely to be demented or delirious from prescription drugs.

7. Perform a medical workup. The full workup consists of a detailed physical examination and laboratory tests, including a complete blood count with differential white cell count; a chemistry profile, including electrolytes, liver function tests, and blood urea nitrogen; thyroid function tests; tests for B_{12} and folate; Venereal Disease Research Laboratory (VDRL) test; a urinalysis; a urine toxicology screen; an electrocardiogram (ECG); and a chest X-ray. A computed tomographic (CT) scan of the head, an electroencephalogram (EEG), and a lumbar puncture may also be indicated. Neurological and medical consultations may be needed.

DRUG TREATMENT

Although medications should be avoided, pending the results of a definitive workup, severe agitation or uncooperativeness may require medication. High-potency antipsychotics—for example, haloperidol (Haldol), fluphenazine (Prolixin), thiothixene (Navane), and trifluoperazine (Stelazine), all given at 2 to 5 mg by mouth or intramuscularly (IM)—are the drugs of choice over benzodiazepines; antipsychotics are less likely than benzodiazepines to worsen the patient's cognition. However, benzodiazepines are indicated if withdrawal from alcohol or sedative-hypnotics is a possible diagnosis.

Cross-References:
Confusion, delirium, dementia.

---

54 / L-Dopa Intoxication

L-Dopa (levodopa [Larodopa, Dopar]) can cause intoxication. It is commonly used to treat Parkinson's disease and parkinsonian syndromes after a head injury, manganese intoxication, carbon monoxide poisoning, encephalitis, and cerebrovascular diseases. L-Dopa is also used for dystonia musculorum deformans.

CLINICAL FEATURES AND DIAGNOSIS

The psychiatric manifestations of *L-dopa intoxication* consist of psychotic symptoms (for example, hallucinations and delusions) and alterations of mood (for example, mania and depression). Additional reactions include anxiety, dyskinesias, dementia, and delirium. A common preparation is a combination of L-dopa and carbidopa (Sinemet). The medical complications of L-dopa intoxication include nausea, vomiting, urinary retention, hypotension, bradycardia, and toxicity in the gastrointestinal tract, liver, bone marrow, and blood.

INTERVIEWING AND PSYCHOTHERAPEUTIC GUIDELINES

The conduct of the interview depends on the symptoms present. Usually, L-dopa is prescribed by neurologists and internists, who should be contacted. Explain to the patient that symptoms are self-limited and will resolve.

EVALUATION AND MANAGEMENT

1. Determine the ingested amount of L-dopa or L-dopa-carbidopa.
2. Reduce the dosage of L-dopa or L-dopa-carbidopa if possible.
3. Consider alternatives to L-dopa, including anticholinergic drugs, amantadine (Symmetrel), and bromocriptine (Parlodel).
4. Depression is common in patients with Parkinson's disease and should be treated.

DRUG TREATMENT

Begin by reducing the dosage of L-dopa. Severe agitation or anxiety may be treated with short-acting benzodiazepines—for example, oxazepam (Serax) 10 to 30 mg by mouth, lorazepam (Ativan) 1 to 2 mg by mouth or intramuscularly (IM), or estazolam (ProSom) 0.5 to 1 mg by mouth. Avoid antipsychotics. Tricyclic antidepressants may improve the depressive symptoms of Parkinson's disease. Never give monoamine oxidase inhibitors (MAOIs) with L-dopa.

Cross-References:

Agitation, delusional disorder, depression, hallucinations, intoxication, paranoia, parkinsonism.

55 / Drug Flashback

A *drug flashback* (also called posthallucinogen perception disorder) is a recurrence of a drug-induced effect that occurs some time after the drug was last taken. Flashbacks are common after hallucinogen use (up to 25 percent of lysergic acid diethylamide [LSD] users experience flashbacks) and rare after cannabis use. Patients typically come to clinical attention when a flashback is distressing or dysphoric.

CLINICAL FEATURES AND DIAGNOSIS

Flashbacks cannot be easily explained by the pharmacokinetics of the drug, and they may occur years after the drug was used. They may be precipitated by stress, fatigue, illness, or even by walking into a brightly lit area. Visual hallucinations, distortions, and illusions are typical symptoms, but somatic and psychological symptoms may also occur. If the symptoms are associated with distress, a diagnosis of posthallucinogen perception disorder may be made.

Hallucinogen-induced flashbacks usually resolve in hours but may last up to two days and occasionally longer. Flashback complications include severe anxiety, panic, depression, suicidal ideation, and persistent psychosis. Recurrences of flashbacks may appear for months to years.

INTERVIEWING AND PSYCHOTHERAPEUTIC GUIDELINES

Usually, the patient is aware that the experience is a drug flashback, since the subjective experience is similar to what was experienced during active use of the drug. If the patients have had dysphoric or distressing trips before, they may be expecting distressing flashbacks. If the patients are not aware that they are experiencing flashbacks, they may believe that they are going insane. Reassure the patients that the symptoms will probably pass. That is referred to as "talking down" the patient.

EVALUATION AND MANAGEMENT

1. Obtain the patient's history of hallucinogen use, and rule out acute hallucinogen intoxication.

2. Rule out other possible causes, including physical or mental disorders.

3. Reassure the patient that the episode is temporary and due to previous drug use. Provide the companionship of a family member or a close friend if possible; otherwise, have a staff member stay with the patient.

DRUG TREATMENT

Drug treatment is usually not needed, but, in cases of severe anxiety or agitation, start with a benzodiazepine—for example, estazolam (ProSom)

0.5 to 1 mg by mouth, oxazepam (Serax) 10 to 30 mg by mouth, alprazolam (Xanax) 0.5 to 1 mg by mouth, or lorazepam (Ativan) 1 to 2 mg by mouth or intramuscularly (IM), all given every four hours as needed. If that medication is ineffective, consider an antipsychotic. The choice of antipsychotic depends on the desired side-effect profile. High-potency antipsychotics—for example, fluphenazine (Prolixin), thiothixene (Navane), and haloperidol (Haldol), all given at 2 to 5 mg by mouth or IM every four hours as needed— are usually used but often produce extrapyramidal side effects. If sedation is desired and if anticholinergic side effects and reducing the seizure threshold are not concerns, a low-potency antipsychotic—for example, thioridazine (Mellaril) or chlorpromazine (Thorazine), both given at 10 to 25 mg by mouth every four hours as needed—may also be considered. If acute hallucinogen intoxication is a possibility, low-potency antipsychotics should be avoided, because of their possible exacerbation of anticholinergic side effects and their lowering of the seizure threshold.

Cross-References:

Agitation, anxiety, delusional disorder, depression, hallucinations, hallucinogen hallucinosis, panic disorder.

56 / Dysarthria

Dysarthria is poor articulation (slurred speech), usually caused by neurological involvement of the motor systems controlling speech. Dysarthria is not necessarily associated with impaired word finding or grammar.

CLINICAL FEATURES AND DIAGNOSIS

Dysarthria can be caused by conditions affecting the lower motor neurons, cerebellum, extrapyramidal system, or brainstem. Intoxication with alcohol or sedative-hypnotics is a common cause of transient dysarthria through cerebellar involvement. Less commonly, dysarthria is a hysterical sign without any identifiable neurological basis. In children, dysarthria may be a sign of a developmental articulation disorder or a pervasive developmental disorder.

INTERVIEWING AND PSYCHOTHERAPEUTIC GUIDELINES

Ask the patient to speak slowly. If communication is still difficult, ask the patient to communicate by writing.

EVALUATION AND MANAGEMENT

1. Ask what medications or drugs the patient has taken. Look for obvious intoxication with alcohol or sedative-hypnotics. Anticonvulsants can also cause dysarthria. Urine and blood screens for drugs and blood drug levels may be helpful.

2. Look for associated neurological signs. The presence of other neurological signs and subtle differences in the quality of the dysarthria may indicate an involvement of specific neurological sites (for example, the lower motor neurons, cerebellum, extrapyramidal system, and brainstem). Unless the dysarthria can be easily explained (for example, by alcohol or sedative-hypnotic intoxication), a full neurological evaluation is indicated.

3. Dysarthria, unless it is a sign of an acute CNS event, is seldom an emergency. The patient can usually be referred for outpatient neurological evaluation.

4. If no definitive treatment is indicated after a neurological workup, refer the patient for speech therapy.

DRUG TREATMENT

No specific medications are indicated.

Cross-References:

Alcohol intoxication; barbiturate and similarly acting sedative, hypnotic, or anxiolytic intoxication and withdrawal; confusion; delirium; dementia; intoxication.

57 / Dyskinesia (Abnormal Movement)

Dyskinesia is any disturbance of movement.

CLINICAL FEATURES AND DIAGNOSIS

In psychiatry the most commonly seen dyskinesias are the acute and chronic movement disorders caused by antipsychotic drugs (for example, acute dystonia and tardive dyskinesia). Patients taking maintenance antipsychotic agents may experience withdrawal dyskinesia if the antipsychotic dosage is reduced. L-Dopa agonists and psychostimulants cause increased dopamine activity related to dyskinesia. 1-Methyl-4-phenyl-1,2,3,6-tetrahydropyridine (MPTP), a synthetic opioid drug of abuse, can destroy substantia nigra neurons and cause Parkinson's disease. In general, dyskinesias are not present during sleep.

A wide range of neurological conditions can also present with abnormal movements. The disorders with established genetic transmission include Huntington's chorea, Wilson's disease, Tourette's disorder, Lesch-Nyhan syndrome, and essential tremor; other disorders include Parkinson's disease, dystonia musculorum deformans, and many other syndromes related to either focal insults (for example, cerebrovascular diseases) or diffuse insults (for example, anoxia, hepatic failure, hypocalcemia, and hypothyroidism) to the basal ganglia. Connective tissue diseases, such as systemic lupus erythematosus, can cause dyskinesia. In women, dyskinesias may occur in pregnancy or as a side effect of oral contraceptives.

Dyskinesias in patients receiving antipsychotic medications are common. Acute extrapyramidal side effects—including parkinsonism, dystonia, and akathisia—can be caused by any antipsychotic, except perhaps clozapine (Clozaril), and are most common in patients receiving high-potency antipsychotics.

INTERVIEWING AND PSYCHOTHERAPEUTIC GUIDELINES

The interviewing style depends largely on the acuteness and the severity of the complaint. A patient with an acute antipsychotic-induced dystonia should be reassured that the condition can be treated. Less acute conditions should be carefully evaluated, looking for organic causes of a neurological condition.

EVALUATION AND MANAGEMENT

1. Determine whether antipsychotic medication is a possible cause of the dyskinesia. If the patient is taking an antipsychotic, consider acute extrapyramidal side effects, withdrawal dyskinesia, and tardive dyskinesia. If the patient has taken antipsychotics in the past, consider tardive dyskinesia. Dyskinesia may have multiple causes in one patient.

2. Consider other drugs—psychostimulants, L-dopa agonists, and oral contraceptives in particular. Also consider exposure to toxins (for example, MPTP and carbon monoxide) and head injury.

3. Consider the age of the patient. In the elderly, look for cerebrovascular diseases, Parkinson's disease, and tumors; in children, look for perinatal injury, kernicterus, juvenile Huntington's chorea, Sydenham's chorea (after rheumatic fever), Lesch-Nyhan syndrome, Tourette's disorder, athetosis, and myoclonus caused by subacute sclerosing panencephalitis.

4. Look for genetic disorders in the patient's family history.

5. Refer the patient for a neurological examination.

6. Conduct a full organic workup, including complete blood count (CBC), thyroid function tests, Venereal Disease Research Laboratory (VDRL) test, chemistry panel tests, erythrocyte sedimentation rate (ESR), urinalysis, urine toxicology screen, blood drug levels, electroencephalogram (EEG), and a computed tomographic (CT) scan or a magnetic resonance imaging (MRI) scan of the head. A lumbar puncture and further brain imaging may also be indicated.

DRUG TREATMENT

Treatment depends on making a definitive diagnosis. Some conditions are responsive to pharmacological manipulations of the cholinergic or dopaminergic systems. Tardive dyskinesia requires careful planning of any antipsychotic exposure. Although they cause the patient discomfort, dystonia and parkinsonism can usually be rapidly managed with anticholinergic agents, such as benztropine (Cogentin) 1 to 2 mg by mouth or intramuscularly. Akathisia is less responsive to anticholinergic medications, but other drugs, such as benzodiazepines and β-blockers, may be helpful.

Cross-References:

Akathisia; L-dopa intoxication; dystonia, acute; parkinsonism; tardive dyskinesia; tic.

58 / Dysprosody (Flat Speech)

Dysprosody is the loss of the normal ability to vary the intonation of speech to express emotions.

CLINICAL FEATURES AND DIAGNOSIS

Speech is flat, monotonous, and without inflection. Dysprosody is seldom a specific complaint. It is seen in cases of brain dysfunction, particularly in the elderly. Dysprosody may be similar to the monotonous speech of depressed patients and schizophrenic patients with negative symptoms.

INTERVIEWING AND PSYCHOTHERAPEUTIC GUIDELINES

Do not focus on the dysprosody. Attempt to determine the underlying cause of the disorder by conducting a psychiatric history and mental status. Pay particular attention to the presence of dementia by conducting a cognitive examination and performing a medical workup.

EVALUATION AND MANAGEMENT

1. In addition to dementia, depression and schizophrenia must be ruled out. Patients with substance use disorder—particularly sedatives or hypnotics—may also show dysprosody. Some persons with articulation or speech disorders may have a flat intonation of speech.

2. Treat the underlying disorder. Speech therapy is of value for articulation or speech disorders if present.

DRUG TREATMENT

Underlying psychiatric disorders are treated with the appropriate medication (for example, antipsychotic agents for schizophrenia). Depression will respond to standard antidepressants. As the underlying condition improves, dysprosody diminishes.

Cross References:

Delirium, dementia, depression, schizophrenia, stuttering.

---

59 / Dystonia, Acute (Muscle Contraction)

Acute dystonia is the slow, involuntary contraction of one or more muscle groups. It is a common complaint in the psychiatric emergency room, since up to 10 percent of patients taking antipsychotic medications experience an antipsychotic-induced dystonia. Dystonia causes the patient discomfort. It is frightening and a common reason for noncompliance with antipsychotic medications. Patients who refer to allergic reactions to past treatment with an antipsychotic are often referring to an acute dystonia.

Dystonia, an extrapyramidal side effect, is most common with high-potency antipsychotics, but it can be caused by all conventional dopamine receptor antagonist antipsychotics. Dystonia is most common in young men (under the age of 40), although children and brain-damaged patients of any age are also vulnerable. Dystonia typically occurs early in the course of treatment (50 percent of cases in the first two days) or after an intramuscular (IM) injection. Dystonia is a less common side effect than parkinsonism and akathisia. The mechanism is thought to be related to dopaminergic hyperactivity as the brain levels of the antipsychotic decrease.

Dystonia can usually be prevented by the prophylactic use of an anticholinergic medication, but that approach is controversial, since anticholinergic medications also have side effects. Prophylactic treatment may be indicated for several days when starting to give high-potency antipsychotics to patients at high risk for dystonia (for example, brain-damaged patients, young men, children).

CLINICAL FEATURES AND DIAGNOSIS

Antipsychotic-induced dystonia may involve the neck (torticollis), the jaw (forced opening or trismus), the tongue (protrusion or twisting), or the entire body (opisthotonos). Dystonia of the tongue may present as dysarthria (slurred speech). Involvement of the extraocular muscles can produce an oculogyric crisis in which the eyes deviate upward and laterally (it may also occur during the course of treatment). Blepharospasm, grimacing, dysphagia, and respiratory stridor may also occur. Laryngeal dystonia can be life-threatening. Writhing movements of the limbs or the trunk may be a form of dystonia.

The disorder must be differentiated from seizures, tetany, tetanus, tardive dyskinesia that does not involve spastic muscle contraction, encephalitis, metabolic illness, and hysterical or psychotic posturing. Some patients simulate dystonia to obtain antiparkinsonian agents, which can produce euphoria.

Other causes of dystonia include (1) dystonia musculorum deformans (torsion dystonia), a rare disorder in children marked by bizarre postures; (2) focal dystonia of a single muscle group, typically presenting in adulthood; (3) spastic torticollis, caused by dystonia of the sternocleidomastoid muscle; and (4) occupational spasms that result from the repeated use of a particular muscle group (for example, writer's cramp).

INTERVIEWING AND PSYCHOTHERAPEUTIC GUIDELINES

The patient with acute antipsychotic-induced dystonia should be treated immediately, since dystonia is frightening and uncomfortable and treatment is effective. Reassure the patient that the muscle contraction is a side effect of the antipsychotic drug that can be rapidly relieved. After the dystonia has been treated, discuss the importance of continued compliance with the medication, and tell the patient that, with anticholinergic medication, the dystonia is not likely to recur.

EVALUATION AND MANAGEMENT

1. Determine if the patient is taking any antipsychotic medication.

2. Examine the patient for involuntary prolonged muscle spasm of one or more muscle groups.

3. Document the type of dystonia as specifically as possible, since the location of the dystonia is often idiosyncratic for an individual patient. The information will be useful for the evaluation of similar complaints in the future.

DRUG TREATMENT

Treat antipsychotic-induced dystonia rapidly with benztropine (Cogentin) 1 to 2 mg IM or intravenously (IV); with other anticholinergic medications; or with antihistamines, such as diphenhydramine (Benadryl) 25 to 50 mg by mouth, IM, or IV. For the most rapid relief, an IM or an IV injection usually relieves the symptoms within several minutes. The dose can be repeated in 15 minutes. Suspect another diagnosis if three doses are ineffective. For dystonia that does not respond to anticholinergic drugs, give methylphenidate (Ritalin), caffeine sodium benzoate, a benzodiazepine, or a barbiturate.

Consider the prophylactic use of anticholinergic drugs, such as benztropine 2 to 6 mg a day in divided doses.

Laryngeal dystonias are medical emergencies that should be treated with benzotropine 2 mg IV at once, with a repeat dose in 5 to 10 minutes if the patient does not respond. If the patient still does not respond, try lorazepam (Ativan) 1 to 2 mg by slow IV. The patient rarely requires intubation.

Consider decreasing the antipsychotic dosage or changing to a lower-potency antipsychotic.

Cross-References:

Akathisia, parkinsonism, tardive dyskinesia.

60 / Epilepsy

Epilepsy is characterized by recurrent seizures caused by central nervous system (CNS) disease or dysfunction. The symptoms of a seizure can range from the tonic-clonic movements of a grand mal seizure to such subtle symptoms as akinesia, abnormal sensations and perceptions, disturbed behavior, automatisms, and impaired consciousness.

Epilepsy is the most common chronic neurological condition; it affects 1 percent of the population. Psychiatric problems are common; 30 to 50 percent of epileptic patients have a diagnosable mental disorder, and 7 to 10 percent have psychotic symptoms. Epilepsy is three to seven times more common in psychotic patients than in the general population.

Recurrent seizures are usually treated by a neurologist. Primary care physicians may be involved for many reasons, including the diagnosis of epilepsy when the symptoms are behavioral, perceptual, or affective; the differentiation of true seizures from pseudoseizures; the treatment of depression, personality changes, and psychotic symptoms; and the management of postictal and interictal behavioral problems.

CLINICAL FEATURES AND DIAGNOSIS

The definitive diagnosis of epilepsy relies on an electroencephalogram (EEG), although normal findings on an EEG do not exclude the diagnosis of epilepsy. Seizures can be broadly divided into generalized and focal (partial).

Generalized Seizures

In generalized seizures the EEG paroxysms are bilaterally symmetrical, synchronous, and present in all leads. Generalized seizures almost always involve altered or lost consciousness. The most common types are (1) generalized convulsive seizures (grand mal or tonic-clonic), which produce clinical convulsions and postictal confusion and are characterized by bilaterally synchronous polyspike and slow-wave bursts on the EEG, and (2) petit mal seizures, which usually begin between ages 5 and 10 years; are characterized by abrupt, brief (seconds), and frequent episodes of loss of consciousness (absences) associated with automatisms, akinetic episodes, and myoclonic jerks; and have a characteristic 3-cycles-per-second spike-and-slow-wave pattern on the EEG. (Table B.60–1 gives a classification of seizure types.)

Partial (Focal) Seizures

The type of seizure most likely seen by the physician in the emergency room or office is the partial (focal) seizure, which often mimics psychiatric disorders of various kinds.

Table B.60-1
Classification of Seizure Types

I. Generalized seizures

    A. Tonic-clonic (grand mal) seizures
        1. Primary—idiopathic or familial
        2. Secondary to a definable structural lesion (e.g., tumor, arteriovenous malformation, old infarct)
        3. Secondary to infection (e.g., meningoencephalitis, abscess)
        4. Secondary to drug intoxication (e.g., cocaine)
        5. Secondary to metabolic imbalance (e.g., hypoglycemia, hyponatremia)
        6. Grand mal status epilepticus

    B. Absence seizures
        1. Typical absence—electroencephalogram (EEG) with 3-per-second spike and wave, impairment of consciousness only
        2. Complex or variant absence—with one or more additional components of myoclonus, atonic episodes (drop attacks), automatisms, autonomic phenomena (e.g., enuresis), or tonic episodes

    C. Myoclonic seizures
        1. Infantile spasms (West's syndrome; myoclonic seizures in children, Lennox-Gastaut syndrome), EEG with hypsarrhythmia
        2. Adult generalized myoclonic seizures (following cerebral anoxia or familial)

    D. Atonic seizures—isolated or part of an absence seizure

    E. Tonic seizures—uncommon in adults

    F. Clonic seizures—uncommon in adults

II. Partial (focal) seizures

    A. Simple partial seizures—consciousness not impaired
        1. Motor: focal, jacksonian (focal, with a march), versive (usually contraversive), postural, phonatory (with vocalization or speech arrest)
        2. Sensory: somatosensory, visual, auditory, olfactory, gustatory, vertiginous
        3. Autonomic
        4. Psychic (e.g., *déjà vu, jamais vu*)

    B. Complex partial seizures—consciousness impaired; encompasses temporal lobe or psychomotor seizures
        1. Simple partial onset followed by impairment of consciousness
        2. Impairment of consciousness at onset, with or without automatisms

    C. Partial seizures evolving into secondarily generalized tonic-clonic seizures

Table from M E Ross: Seizures. In *Manual of Psychiatric Emergencies,* ed 2, S E Hyman, editor, p 209. Little, Brown, Boston, 1988. Used with permission.

Partial seizures show localized spike discharges on the EEG and are divided according to whether they show simple symptoms or complex symptoms. They may spread and develop into secondarily generalized seizures.

Partial simple seizures are usually motor seizures and involve clonic movements or the loss of muscle tone on the side of the body contralateral to the focus of the seizure discharge. Sensory symptoms—such as abdominal pain, pain localized elsewhere, paroxysmal autonomic discharges, and hallucinations (visual, auditory, olfactory, and gustatory)—are other presentations.

Partial complex seizures (psychomotor seizures) originating in the temporal lobe (temporal lobe epilepsy) produce many psychiatric symptoms. They are complex because they have autonomic, sensory, psychic, and motor manifestations. The varied and complex auras may include emotional symptoms, such as anxiety; a sensation of an intense emotional experience; depersonalization; derealization; *déjà vu;* and visual, olfactory, gustatory, and auditory hallucinations. Somatic sensations, such as discomfort in the abdomen and the head, are other symptoms of the aura.

INTERVIEWING AND PSYCHOTHERAPEUTIC GUIDELINES

In general, if epilepsy is a diagnostic consideration, assume first that the symptoms are related to an organic condition, rather than a psychiatric disorder. That approach leads to the full exploration of possible organic causes. All patients with seizure disorders should be asked about the frequency and the duration of the seizures; the events before, during, and after a seizure (is there an aura? loss of consciousness? postictal amnesia or fatigue?); the relation of the seizures to drug or alcohol use; and their treatment history. Do not overlook the many psychosocial factors that affect the patients. Work to identify the possible definitive organic causes, but also emphasize adaptation strategies for coping with any impairment. How have the symptoms affected the patient's work, family, sexual, and social functioning? Is the patient able to drive? Does driving affect the patient's ability to work? Might any personality changes benefit from psychotherapeutic interventions? What were the patient's premorbid psychological substrates and traits that may make adaptation easy or difficult?

EVALUATION AND MANAGEMENT

1. A full organic workup and a neurological evaluation are needed.
2. A thorough search for the cause is mandatory. The causes to rule out include anoxia, head trauma, cerebrovascular diseases, infections, intracranial bleeding, drug abuse and withdrawal, alcohol withdrawal, electrolyte imbalances, hypoglycemia, hyperglycemia, and CNS tremor. Start with a detailed clinical history, focusing on headache, head injury, childhood seizures, and febrile seizures. Order a complete neurological examination, EEG, computed tomography (CT) or magnetic resonance imaging (MRI) scan, and a full battery of blood tests and urine drug screens.
3. Epilepsy should be managed by a neurologist with appropriate anticonvulsant medication.
4. Psychotherapy and psychotropic medications may be indicated.

Depression

Depression is common in epilepsy. Among epileptic patients, those with partial complex seizures have the highest suicide rate. Treatment may include psychotherapy and antidepressants, such as serotonin-specific reuptake inhibitors, tricylics, or monoamine oxidase inhibitors (MAOIs). Electroconvulsive therapy is another option that itself has anticonvulsant effects.

Personality Changes

Personality changes are common, but their cause is controversial and may be related to the stress of coping with epilepsy, to anticonvulsant medications, or to a primary organic condition. Personality changes are more related to the duration of epilepsy than to the frequency of seizures.

Table B.60–2
Clinical Features Distinguishing Seizures and Pseudoseizures*

Feature	Organic Seizure	Pseudoseizure
Aura	Common stereotyped	Rare
Timing	Nocturnal common	Only when awake
Incontinence	Common	Rare
Cyanosis	Common	Rare
Postictal confusion	Yes	No
Body movement	Tonic-clonic	Nonstereotyped and asynchronous
Self-injury	Common	Rare
EEG	May be abnormal	Normal
Affected by suggestion	No	Yes
Secondary gain	No	Yes

*Some patients with organic seizure disorders may also have pseudoseizures.

Table B.60–3
Drugs of Choice for Various Types of Seizures

Generalized tonic-clonic (grand mal)
  seizures:
    Phenobarbital
    Phenytoin (Dilantin)
    Carbamazepine (Tegretol)

Absence (petit mal) seizures:
    Ethosuximide (Zarontin)
    Valproic acid (Depakene)
    Trimethadione (Tridione)

Simple partial (focal) seizures:
    Phenobarbital
    Phenytoin (Dilantin)

Complex partial (temporal lobe) seizures:
    Phenytoin (Dilantin)
    Carbamazepine (Tegretol)

Myoclonic, atonic, akinetic, and atypical
  absence seizures:
    Clonazepam (Klonopin)
    Diazepam (Valium)

Infantile spasms:
    Adrenocorticotropic hormone
    Corticosteroids

Status epilepticus:
    Diazepam (Valium)
    Phenobarbital
    Amobarbital (Amytal)
    Phenytoin (Dilatin)
    Paraldehyde
    Anesthetic agent

Psychosis

Psychosis of a schizophreniform type may develop in patients who have long-standing temporal lobe epilepsy. Usually, the psychosis is preceded by personality changes. Responses to treatment are unpredictable. Treatment may include antipsychotics and anticonvulsants; however, low-potency antipsychotics are likely to lower the seizure threshold and should be avoided.

Impaired Cognition

Impaired cognition is not common, although some patients clearly show a progressive deterioration in cognition. The possible causes include anticonvulsant drugs, a CNS lesion (often the same one causing the seizures), and repeated prolonged seizures. Consider whether the patient can be treated with a lower dosage of an anticonvulsant or a different anticonvulsant.

Status Epilepticus

In status epilepticus, seizures follow one another with no intervening periods of consciousness; the seizures may be fatal. Partial continuous epilepsy is a rare type of sensory or motor seizure that may last for days to weeks. These conditions are considered neurological emergencies.

Pseudoseizures

The identification of pseudoseizures is a frequent reason for a psychiatric consultation. Some cases of pseudoseizures are obvious; for difficult cases, the distinctions in Table B.60–2 may help.

Violence

Violence rarely occurs during a seizure, but it may be a problem in some epileptic patients as an interictal or postictal phenomenon, particularly in patients with temporal lobe epilepsy. Carbamazepine (Tegretol), other anticonvulsants, antipsychotics, or β-blockers may help.

DRUG TREATMENT

In general, use a single anticonvulsant drug, and increase the dosage until it is effective or not tolerated. Table B.60–3 lists the drugs of choice for various types of seizures. Polypharmacy should be avoided because of drug interactions and the compounding of side effects.

Cross-References:

Alcohol seizures, depersonalization, depression, derealization, fugue state, panic disorder, temporal lobe epilepsy, violence.

---

61 / Fugue State

Fugue state is a prolonged dissociative period during which the patient performs complex activities, including unexpected travel and the assumption of a new identity. The episode usually lasts for hours to days but occasionally lasts for years. The new identity is apparently normal, and there is no obvious indication of a mental disorder. During the episode the patient is amnestic for the previous identity; after recovery, the patient is amnestic for the episode. Usually, the patient makes a complete recovery, and recurrences are uncommon.

CLINICAL FEATURES AND DIAGNOSIS

In the majority of cases, the new identity is incomplete, and the activities during the episode are only semipurposeful. The patient may avoid complex social interactions during the episode. In a minority of cases, a completely new personality is assumed. The new personality is usually more outgoing and friendly than the original personality.

Fugue states typically occur after a severe stress (such as a natural disaster), during wartime, or after a significant personal failure. Alcohol use may precipitate a fugue state. Patients with mood disorders and certain personality disorders (such as borderline, histrionic, and schizoid) are predisposed to psychogenic fugue.

Table B.61-1
Using Amobarbital During a Patient Interview

1. Have the patient recline.

2. Explain that the medication should make the patient relax and feel like talking.

3. Insert a narrow-bore scalp-vein needle into the forearm or hand.

4. Begin injecting a 5% solution of amobarbital (Amytal)—500 mg dissolved in 10 mL of sterile water—at a rate no faster than 1 mL/minute (50 mg/minute) to prevent sleep or sudden respiratory depression.

5. Interview:
   a. With a verbal patient, begin with neutral topics, gradually approaching areas of trauma, guilt, and possible repression.
   b. With a mute patient, continue to suggest that soon the patient will feel like talking. Prompting with known facts about the patient's life may also help.

6. Continue the infusion until the patient shows sustained rapid lateral nystagmus or drowsiness. Slight slurring of speech is common; the sedation threshold is usually reached at a dose between 150 mg (3 mL) and 350 mg (7 mL) but can be as little as 75 mg (1.5 mL) in an elderly patient or one with organic illness. Prompts to talk should have their strongest effect at this point.

7. To maintain the level of narcosis, continue the infusion at the rate of 0.5 to 1.0 mL every 5 minutes.

8. Conduct the interview as you would any other psychiatric interview, but with several caveats:
   a. Approach affect-laden or traumatic material gradually, and then work over it again and again to recover forgotten details, attendant feelings, and the patient's current reactions to them.
   b. In the mute or verbally inhibited patient, do not concentrate on traumatic topics (such as murderous rage toward someone) to prevent the development of panic after the interview.

9. Terminate the interview when enough material has been produced (about 30 minutes for a mute patient) or when the therapeutic goals have been reached (sometimes an hour or more). Have the patient recline for an additional 15 minutes until able to walk with close supervision.

Table from W R Dubin, K J Weiss: *Handbook of Psychiatric Emergencies,* p 100. Springhouse, Springhouse, Penn, 1991. Adapted from J C Perry, D L Jacobs: Overview: Clinical applications of the Amytal interview in psychiatric emergency settings. Am J Psychiatry *139:* 552, 1982. Used with permission.

INTERVIEWING AND PSYCHOTHERAPEUTIC GUIDELINES

In general, the patient comes to clinical attention either when the episode is over and the patient has a memory gap or when someone who knew the patient previously brings the patient to clinical attention. Under either of those conditions, the patient is perplexed and bewildered by the situation and requires reassurance.

In the initial evaluation the objective is to engage the patient in an ongoing treatment plan. The goals are to explore the conflicts that led to the episode, to eliminate any persistent amnestic barriers, and to prevent recurrences.

EVALUATION AND MANAGEMENT

1. The differential diagnosis includes intoxication, temporal lobe epilepsy, psychogenic amnesia, multiple personality disorder, factitious dis-

order, and malingering. Urine drug screening and an electroencephalogram (EEG) help in the evaluation of possible drug intoxication or temporal lobe epilepsy. Psychogenic amnesia seldom involves travel or the assumption of a new identity. In multiple personality disorder, the old (also known as host) and new identities fluctuate. Malingerers may avoid probing, detailed questions; may refuse to undergo laboratory tests; and are often difficult to identify. In general, do not assume that a patient is malingering unless strong evidence suggests it.

2. Identify the conflicts that led to the dissociation. Relaxation, hypnosis, and an interview facilitated by sedative-hypnotics—usually intravenous (IV) diazepam (Valium) or amobarbital (Amytal)—may help reduce the amnestic barriers (Table B.61-1).

3. Evaluate the extent of the lost memory. The most important objective of treatment is to break down the amnestic barriers and to restore the lost memory. Persistent lost memories can form the nidus for further amnesia and possible recurrence. Evaluate the patient for suicidality; some patients enter a fugue state when suicidal and again become suicidal when emerging from the fugue.

4. Refer the patient for psychotherapy to explore and to resolve the conflicts that led to the dissociation.

DRUG TREATMENT

Drug treatment is usually not needed, but severe anxiety may be treated with benzodiazepines.

Cross-References:

Amnesia, blackouts, borderline personality disorder, epilepsy, intoxication, malingering, temporal lobe epilepsy.

---

62 / Grandiosity

Grandiosity is an exaggerated feeling of one's importance, power, knowledge, or identity. The degree of grandiosity can range from a mild exaggeration of a true characteristic to psychotic delusions of grandeur. The content of the delusion may be that the patient has made some important discovery or possesses some unrecognized talent or great wealth. Sometimes grandiose delusions are religious and involve beliefs that the patient has a special relationship with God or is on an important religious mission (for example, to convert the psychiatric patients in hospitals).

CLINICAL FEATURES AND DIAGNOSIS

Persistent grandiosity is often a sign of a personality disorder. Grandiose delusions indicate a psychotic disorder, commonly mania, schizophrenia, or organic delusional disorder (for example, intoxication with cocaine, amphetamine, or hallucinogens). The most important goals of evaluating grandiosity are determining the severity, the duration, and the cause.

INTERVIEWING AND PSYCHOTHERAPEUTIC GUIDELINES

Grandiose patients are often easily engaged in an interview if you allow them to discuss the content of their grandiose beliefs, although some manic patients may be irritable and uncooperative. Do not challenge the patient's grandiose beliefs, even if they are obviously false. However, do not agree that they are true. If the patient asks you directly, "Don't you believe I can fly?" the best response is that you do not know, that you understand the patient believes it, and that the belief will be investigated further.

During the interview try to determine the severity and the duration of the grandiose ideas. Is the patient grandiose about other areas? Explore for paranoid thoughts. Some paranoid ideas have a grandiose core—that is, paranoid patients believe that they are important enough for others to be against them. Try to assess the degree of impairment caused by the grandiose ideas.

EVALUATION AND MANAGEMENT

1. Determine if the patient is psychotic, and evaluate the degree of impairment in judgment. Delusional patients may have such impaired judgment that they are dangerous to self or others and require hospitalization, involuntarily if necessary. Does the patient plan to act on the gradiose beliefs? Has the patient fought with people who challenge the grandiose convictions? Are there homicidal plans? Is the patient at risk of self-harm because of the nature of the grandiose delusions?

2. Rule out organic causes, especially if the patient is psychotic or if the symptoms are new in a patient without a previous history of similar symptoms. The patient's drug history, a urine drug screening, and a complete list of the medications taken are mandatory. Prescribed drugs (for example, steroids, tricyclic antidepressants, monoamine oxidase inhibitors [MAOIs], L-dopa, and phenylephrine) can cause grandiose delusions. Metabolic and endocrine disorders, withdrawal from alcohol or sedative-hypnotics, and organic conditions should be considered. Are the patient's vital signs normal?

3. Make a definitive diagnosis. Focus on the severity, the duration, and the related symptoms. Mildly grandiose patients who have been that way for many years may fulfill the diagnostic criteria for narcissistic, borderline, histrionic, or paranoid personality disorder. Determine whether other long-standing maladaptive patterns are present. Patients who have a persistent and well-circumscribed grandiose delusional system, who are not depressed or manic, and who do not have either prominent hallucinations or bizarre delusions may receive a diagnosis of delusional disorder, grandiose type.

4. Disposition depends on the diagnosis, the severity of the symptoms, and the availability of treatment options. If the grandiosity is not psychotic,

refer the patient for outpatient treatment. If the patient has a possible organic disorder, hospitalization may be needed for a complete workup. If the patient is psychotic, determine the likelihood that the patient will go to outpatient appointments and receive adequate evaluation and treatment. Find out if family members can supervise the patient and bring the patient to outpatient appointments.

DRUG TREATMENT

Drug treatment depends on a definitive diagnosis. Acute agitation may require tranquilization with a benzodiazepine (for example, oxazepam [Serax] 10 to 30 mg by mouth, estazolam [ProSom] 0.5 to 1 mg by mouth, lorazepam [Ativan] 1 to 2 mg by mouth or intramuscularly [IM]) or an antipsychotic (for example, trifluoperazine [Stelazine], thiothixene [Navane], fluphenazine [Prolixin], or haloperidol [Haldol], all given at 2 to 5 mg by mouth or IM) if the patient is psychotic. The drug treatment of patients with personality disorders should be focused on specific symptoms. Delusional disorders are generally treated with antipsychotics, although their effectiveness is questionable. Mania and schizophrenia require a psychopharmacological treatment plan.

Cross-References:

Agitation; alcohol withdrawal; amphetamine or similarly acting sympathomimetic intoxication and withdrawal; anxiety; barbiturate and similarly acting sedative, hypnotic, or anxiolytic intoxication and withdrawal; borderline personality disorder; delusional disorder; mania; paranoia.

---

63 / Grief and Bereavement

Grief is the characteristic feeling precipitated by the death of a loved one or by some other significant loss. *Bereavement* is the state of being deprived of a loved one by death and implies a state of mourning through which grief may be relieved.

CLINICAL FEATURES AND DIAGNOSIS

Grief is seen most frequently in doctor's offices and may be present in either identified patients or their family members or friends. Usually, grief is a normal, self-limiting process that can be managed with supportive, common-sense measures. The course of grief is affected by the patient's preparation for the loss, the abruptness of the loss, and its significance to the patient.

The clinician must look for signs of complications, including major depression, psychotic features, agitation, suicidality, alcohol abuse, and drug abuse. Persistent visual hallucinations or dreams that beckon the patient to reunite with the deceased are particularly ominous.

Although symptoms of grief and depression overlap, the symptoms of the grieving patient are generally considered to be appropriate for the circumstances. The depressed patient has inappropriate symptoms, such as prolonged functional impairment, morbid preoccupation with feeling worthless, and marked psychomotor retardation (Table B.63–1).

Although grief is generally described as occurring after the death of a loved one, other major losses—such as divorce, the death of a pet, the loss of a job, the loss of a body part, and the loss of status—can also precipitate grief. The clinical presentation of grief varies with cultural background. The clinician must determine what is considered an appropriate response in the patient's culture.

The clinical symptoms of normal grief include depressed mood, insomnia, anxiety, poor appetite, loss of interest, guilt feelings about what could have been done to prevent the loss (survivor guilt), dreams about the deceased, irritability, anger at medical professionals who were treating the deceased, poor concentration, focus on objects or activities that are reminiscent of the deceased (linkage objects), sensations that the deceased is still present (identification phenomena) such as hearing the deceased call out, shortness of breath, difficulty in talking, and other somatic symptoms. Psychological states encountered in grieving patients include shock, denial, yearning and searching for the deceased, depression, and reorganization. The active symptoms generally last from three to six months, followed by several months in which normal functioning and behavior are restored.

The stages of grief and bereavement are given in Table B.63–2.

INTERVIEWING AND PSYCHOTHERAPEUTIC GUIDELINES

The amount of effort expended in managing grieving patients should not be diminished because grief is considered a normal reaction. Clinicians can assist patients through the painful process. Treating a patient with an acute grief reaction may prevent the development of major depression.

Encourage grieving patients to express their feelings about the deceased and to review the relationship, describing its positive and negative aspects. Many patients are angry at the deceased for dying and should be encouraged to express that anger, even though they feel guilty about it.

Reassure patients that the symptoms are normal and will pass and that they are not psychiatrically ill. But avoid simplistic reassurances that suppress patients' abilities to express their feelings, such as, "It's destiny." Some patients with unresolved grief present with repeated somatic complaints and should be encouraged to talk about their losses. Providing a quiet place may make grieving patients comfortable.

EVALUATION AND MANAGEMENT

1. The goals of treatment are to facilitate a normal grieving process and to identify and treat a pathological process.

2. Determine the details of the loss. What was the importance of the relationship? How sudden or unpredicted was the loss? What is the signif-

Table B.63–1
Grief Versus Depression

Grief	Depression
Normal identification with deceased. Little ambivalence toward deceased	Abnormal overidentification with deceased. Increased ambivalence and unconscious anger toward deceased
Crying, weight loss, decreased libido, withdrawal, insomnia, irritability, decreased concentration and attention	Similar to grief
Suicidal ideas rare	Suicidal ideas common
Self-blame relates to how deceased was treated	Self-blame is global.
No global feelings of worthlessness	Person thinks he or she is generally bad or worthless
Evokes empathy and sympathy	Usually evokes interpersonal annoyance or irritation
With time, symptoms abate; self-limited; usually clears within six months	Symptoms do not abate and may worsen; may still be present after years
Vulnerable to physical illness	Vulnerable to physical illness
Responds to reassurance, social contacts	Does not respond to reassurance, pushes away social contacts
Not helped by antidepressant medication	Helped by antidepressant medication

Table B.63–2
Stages of Grief and Bereavement

Stage	John Bowlby	Stage	C. M. Parkes
1	**Numbness or protest.** Characterized by distress, fear, and anger. Shock may last moments, days, weeks, or months	1	**Alarm.** A stressful state characterized by physiological changes, e.g., rise in blood pressure and heart rate; similar to Bowlby's first stage
2	**Yearning and searching for the lost figure.** World seems empty and meaningless, but self-esteem remains intact. Characterized by preoccupation with lost person, physical restlessness, weeping, and anger. May last several months or even years	2	**Numbness.** Person appears superficially affected by loss but is actually protecting himself or herself from acute distress
3	**Disorganization and despair.** Restlessness and aimlessness. Increase in somatic preoccupation, withdrawal, introversion, and irritability. Repeated reliving of memories	3	**Pining (searching).** Person looks for or is reminded of the lost person. Similar to Bowlby's second stage
		4	**Depression.** Person feels hopeless about future, cannot go on living, and withdraws from family and friends
4	**Reorganization.** With establishment of new patterns, objects, and goals, grief recedes and is replaced by cherished memories. Healthy identification with deceased occurs	5	**Recovery and reorganization.** Person realizes that his or her life will continue with new adjustment and different goals

icance of the loss to the patient? Does the patient feel responsible for causing the death?

3. Does the patient have a history of major depression? If so, the risk of depression as a complication of grief is increased. How has the patient dealt with losses in the past?

4. Evaluate the patient for psychotic symptoms, agitation, increased activity, alcohol abuse, drug abuse, and suicidality. Look for severe depression, insomnia, appetite changes, and somatic symptoms. Has the patient done anything destructive or shown uncharacteristic poor judgment? Does the patient have the symptoms of the illness that the deceased had? The presence of such symptoms indicates complicated or unresolved grief and requires appropriate intervention.

5. Do not overlook patients who do not express significant grief in the context of a major loss. Those patients may have an increased risk of subsequent complicated or unresolved grief. The patients may be in shock or may have cultural or personality features that cause limited emotional expression. Encourage patients to express their emotions, and explore why it is difficult for them to do so. Delayed grief reactions may occur, typically, on the anniversary of the death.

6. Encourage patients to spend time with their families and friends; that will help fill the space vacated by the deceased. Returning to work or school may help the patients' sense of self-esteem. Group therapy and self-help groups are also beneficial for the grieving. Give patients simple structured tasks, such as getting up and dressing before noon every day, writing down feelings for a specified period of time each day, and scheduling daily chores and free time.

7. Complicated grief reactions require significant interventions. Suicidal or severely depressed patients may require hospitalization. Patients with unresolved grief may be referred to supportive outpatient psychotherapy. Those patients may come to the emergency room or doctor's office with somatic or depressive complaints while denying the significance of their losses. Unresolved grief may result from family conflicts, ambivalent feelings toward the deceased, or traumatic loss. The presence of psychosis, severe agitation, or alcohol or substance abuse requires appropriate intervention. Allow patients to see the deceased to say good-bye.

DRUG TREATMENT

Most grieving patients should not be medicated, especially since they may later feel that medications interfered with the mourning process. Severe insomnia or anxiety may be treated with benzodiazepines—for example, estazolam (ProSom) or lorazepam (Ativan), both given at 0.5 to 1 mg by mouth every four hours as needed for anxiety or flurazepam (Dalmane) or temazepam (Restoril), both given at 15 to 30 mg by mouth at bedtime as needed for insomnia. Patients with major depression may require a course of antidepressants. Patients dependent on alcohol or drugs may require detoxification. Antipsychotics are not required unless the patient has an underlying psychotic disorder or the grief reaction is complicated by psychotic depression.

Cross-References:

Anger, anniversary reaction, depression, disaster survivors, suicide.

---

64 / Group Hysteria

Group hysteria is seen in a group of people who have experienced a significant stress, such as a personal or collective tragedy, and who present with various psychiatric symptoms of a similar nature.

CLINICAL FEATURES AND DIAGNOSIS

The common characteristics of the group suggest that the individual members have experienced a stress in a common way. They may be a family, the residents of a single building, coworkers, or the victims of a disaster. Usually, the cultural background of the group is uniform.

Usually, a few members of the group manifest symptoms, and the rest of the group follow; as the leaders' symptoms escalate, so do those of the rest of the group. The symptoms may include screaming, panic, fainting, agitation, and other symptoms of hysteria.

INTERVIEWING AND PSYCHOTHERAPEUTIC GUIDELINES

The group must be dispersed before an intervention can begin. Start with the persons who are leading in the manifestation of symptoms. Provide a reassuring environment that emphasizes that the situation is under control. Give each patient an opportunity to ventilate. Point out potential resources, such as families and social networks.

EVALUATION AND MANAGEMENT

1. To whatever extent is possible, isolate the individual members whose symptom manifestations are leading the group; encourage less emotional family members and paraprofessional staff members to calm the others.

2. Consider the culture of the group. Emotional reactions are encouraged in some cultures (for example, Latin American cultures) and discouraged in others (for example, Asian cultures). Devise a culturally appropriate plan.

3. Enlist the help of important people in the culture (for example, priests, neighborhood leaders) who may be the best equipped to dissipate the crisis in an appropriate fashion.

4. Reassure the patients by providing an environment that shows that the situation is under control with the presence of enough staff members, rapid attention, and minimal unnecessary traffic in and out of the emergency area.

5. Give each patient a chance to discuss the stressful experience, to ventilate, and to describe the emotional process leading to the symptoms.

6. Encourage the patients to stay with extended-family members who are not involved in the hysteria. Close friends and other social networks can also be used. Try to avoid immediately reassembling the group, since doing so may lead to a recurrence of the group hysteria.

DRUG TREATMENT

Treat the severe agitation or anxiety with a brief course of short-acting benzodiazepines—for example, alprazolam (Xanax) 0.5 to 1 mg, lorazepam (Ativan) 1 to 2 mg, or oxazepam (Serax) 10 to 30 mg, all given by mouth every four hours as needed.

Cross-References:

Depression, disaster survivors, grief and bereavement, panic disorder.

---

65 / Hallucinations

Hallucinations are false sensory perceptions occurring in the absence of any external stimulus. They are distinguished from distortions and illusions, which involve misperceptions of real stimuli. The patient perceives the hallucination, at least temporarily, as real.

CLINICAL FEATURES AND DIAGNOSIS

Hallucinations are related to specific sensory modalities (for example, auditory, visual, tactile, olfactory, and gustatory), which should be clearly identified. The duration, the circumstances, and the interpretation of the significance of the hallucination are important. Past hallucinatory experiences and delusional interpretations (fixed false beliefs) of hallucinations should be identified. Hallucinations often occur in multiple sensory modalities and are usually associated with delusions—that is, false beliefs or judgments.

Hallucinations are psychotic symptoms; their presence requires a diagnosis before treatment is initiated. Visual, olfactory, and gustatory hallucinations are most common in organic disorders (for example, in temporal lobe epilepsy). Tactile hallucinations of bugs crawling on or under the skin (formications) are common in cocaine intoxication and in withdrawal from alcohol and sedative-hypnotics. Hallucinations that occur only when the patient is falling asleep (hypnagogic) or waking up (hypnopompic) are generally considered nonpathological.

Intoxication with hallucinogens, cocaine, amphetamines, or other stimulants can cause hallucinations, as can withdrawal from alcohol and sedative-hypnotics. Many medications can cause hallucinations as a side effect.

Such organic conditions as epilepsy are commonly associated with hallucinations. Delirium may have hallucinations as a feature. Drugs used to treat Parkinson's disease (for example, L-dopa [Larodopa, Dopar]) can cause hallucinations.

Hallucinations are also symptoms of several psychiatric disorders, such as schizophrenia, schizophreniform disorder, schizoaffective disorder, mania, depression with psychotic features, borderline personality disorder, brief reactive psychosis, and induced psychotic disorder. In unusual circumstances and in some cultures, certain hallucinations are normal—for example, hearing the voice or seeing an image of a deceased loved one during grief and bereavement. Typically, though, the patient recognizes that those hallucinations are not real. Patients may pretend to have hallucinations in certain situations (for example, to escape prosecution).

INTERVIEWING AND PSYCHOTHERAPEUTIC GUIDELINES

As with any psychotic patient, do not directly challenge the symptom, even if the patient seems uncertain about whether it is real. Do not say, for example, "You know those voices aren't real, don't you?" Observe whether the patient is distressed by the hallucination. Is it an extremely foreign experience, or is it something that the patient seems familiar with? If the patient seems to be responding to internal stimuli during the interview, ask what the patient is seeing or hearing. Is the content of the hallucination congruent with the patient's mood? Focus on obtaining a history that provides most of the information necessary for a diagnosis. Ask about command hallucinations—whether auditory hallucinations come from inside or outside the patient's head—since true auditory hallucinations are usually perceived as coming from outside one's head. Ask how the patient copes with the hallucinations.

EVALUATION AND MANAGEMENT

1. Obtain the patient's vital signs and a urine toxicology screen, which may suggest possible organic causes.

2. Review all the patient's medications—including prescribed, over-the-counter, and drugs of abuse—and consider whether drug intoxication or withdrawal is the cause or whether the hallucination is a drug side effect.

3. Evaluate the patient for possible medical and neurological conditions. Is delirium present? Is the patient hyperthyroid or hypothyroid? Does the patient have epilepsy or a central nervous system (CNS) infection?

4. Does the patient have a history of a primary psychiatric condition of which the hallucinations are a symptom? If so, what has been the course of the disorder? Have previous episodes been characterized by similar hallucinations? Is the patient coming to treatment attention because the hallucinations have increased in frequency or intensity?

5. Is the patient contemplating a dangerous act in response to the hallucinations (for example, committing suicide to obey the voices)?

6. Treatment depends on the diagnosis. Identified organic disorders should be reversed or treated accordingly. For psychiatric conditions the two main clinical questions concern hospitalization and medication.

7. Dangerous patients require hospitalization, involuntarily if necessary. Severely psychotic patients and those who are unable to care for themselves may also require hospitalization. Consider whether the patient is participating in and compliant with outpatient treatment, whether such resources as family and friends and a place to live are available, and whether other aspects of the case (for example, withdrawal from alcohol or drugs, medical complications, and neurological conditions) warrant hospital admission.

8. Patients who are not dangerous or severely disorganized can be referred for outpatient treatment.

DRUG TREATMENT

Hallucinations that are expected to resolve rapidly (for example, hallucinogen hallucinosis and hallucinations during grief and bereavement) may be treated with benzodiazepines. The tranquilization of agitated patients can be achieved with benzodiazepines or antipsychotics, both of which produce rapid behavioral control.

Antidepressants, lithium (Eskalith), and anticonvulsants are usually not initiated in the emergency setting and should, instead, be started when the patient is engaged in ongoing treatment, since the effective use of those drugs requires time and compliance.

Cross-References:

Agitation, alcohol withdrawal, amphetamine or similarly acting sympathomimetic intoxication and withdrawal, borderline personality disorder, cocaine intoxication and withdrawal, delirium, depression, epilepsy, hallucinogen hallucinosis, intoxication, malingering, mania, psychotropic drug withdrawal, schizophrenia, suicide, sundowner syndrome.

---

66 / Hallucinogen Hallucinosis

Hallucinogen hallucinosis (intoxication) is characterized by impaired perception and maladaptive behavior in an alert patient, with related physical signs after the use of a hallucinogen.

CLINICAL FEATURES AND DIAGNOSIS

Usually, the history of hallucinogen use is available, and the patient associates the symptoms with the drug use (Table B.66–1). Common hallucinogens include lysergic acid diethylamide (LSD), dimethoxymethylamphetamine (DOM, STP), a 4-bromo homologue of dimethoxymethylamphetamine (DOB), dimethyltryptamine (DMT), trimethoxyamphetamine

Table B.66–1
Diagnostic Criteria for Hallucinogen Hallucinosis

A. Recent use of a hallucinogen

B. Maladaptive behavioral changes (e.g., marked anxiety or depression, ideas of reference, fear of losing one's mind, paranoid ideation, impaired judgment, impaired social or occupational functioning)

C. Perceptual changes occurring in a state of full wakefulness and alertness (e.g., subjective intensification of perceptions, depersonalization, derealization, illusions, hallucinations, synesthesias)

D. At least two of the following signs:
   (1) pupillary dilation
   (2) tachycardia
   (3) sweating
   (4) palpitations
   (5) blurring of vision
   (6) tremors
   (7) incoordination

E. Not due to any physical or other mental disorder

Table from DSM-III-R, *Diagnostic and Statistical Manual of Mental Disorders,* ed 3, revised. Copyright American Psychiatric Association, Washington 1987. Used with permission.

(TMA), psilocybin, mescaline (peyote, tops, cactus), methylenedioxyamphetamine (MDA), methylenedioxymethamphetamine (MDMA, ecstasy), and phencyclidine (PCP) (Table B.66–2). Often, contaminants—such as anticholinergic drugs, cocaine and other stimulants, and strychnine—have been added to the hallucinogen.

The symptoms usually begin one hour after ingestion and generally last 8 to 12 hours. The typical clinical presentation is a panic reaction (bad trip). After taking a hallucinogen, the patients have trouble in distinguishing drug-induced symptoms from reality and believe that they have gone mad. Associated fears are that the patients have done permanent damage to their brains or chromosomes and will never recover. Bad trips most often occur in first-time users and in those who are anxious or isolated.

Most hallucinogenic drugs have stimulant effects and produce increased activity, insomnia, and elevated vital signs. Other symptoms include suspiciousness, synesthesias (stimulation of one sensory modality is perceived in another sensory modality), intense anxiety, visual hallucinations, fear of losing control, and depression. Hepatotoxicity and death have been attributed to MDMA.

The patients can usually be stabilized in one to two days. Severe agitation, dangerousness, or persistent psychotic symptoms may warrant hospitalization.

INTERVIEWING AND PSYCHOTHERAPEUTIC GUIDELINES

Reassure the patient that the symptoms are drug-induced and will resolve with time. Encourage the patient with constant reassurance and orientation (for example, "You're OK; you're in the hospital; you're going to be all right; it's now Monday afternoon").

Table B.66–2
Commonly Abused Hallucinogenic Drugs

Drug	Source	Psychedelic Dose	Peak Symptoms	Duration of Action	Prominent Somatic Effects	Prominent Psychological Effects
d-Lysergic acid diethylamide (LSD)	Synthetic (from fungi)	50 μg	2 to 3 hrs	8 to 12 hrs undulating activity as effect declines	Increased sympathetic nervous system activity: dilated pupils, increased BP, pulse, deep tendon reflexes, temperature, blood sugar, tremor	Hypervigilance, illusions, emotional lability, loss of body boundaries, time slowing, increased intensity of all sensations
Psilocybin	Mushroom	10 mg	90 mins	4 to 6 hrs	Like LSD but milder	Like LSD but less intense, more visual, more euphoria; paranoia
Dimethyl-tryptamine (DMT)	Synthetic	50 mg	5 to 20 mins	30 to 60 mins	Like LSD but with more intense sympathomimetic symptoms	Like LSD but usually more intense, in part because of sudden onset; must be smoked or injected; cannot be taken orally
Mescaline	Peyote cactus	200 mg	2 to 3 hrs	8 to 12 hrs	Nausea, vomiting; otherwise like LSD, perhaps more intense sympathomimetic effects	Like LSD but perhaps more sensory and perceptual changes; euphoria prominent
Dimethoxymethyl-amphetamine (DOM, STP)	Synthetic	5 mg	3 to 5 hrs	6 to 8 hrs at doses below 5 mg; 16 to 24 hrs at high doses (10 to 30 mg)	Minimal effects at low dose; autonomic effects prominent at doses above 5 mg	May resemble amphetamine combined with LSD but long-lasting; high incidence of flashbacks, psychosis; chlorpromazine may aggravate symptoms

Table from S M Mirin, R D Weiss: Drug use and abuse. In *Emergency Psychiatry*, E L Bassuk, A W Birk, editors, p 162. Plenum, New York, 1984. Used with permission.

EVALUATION AND MANAGEMENT

1. Place the patient in a nonstimulating environment.

2. Unless the patient seems violent, have a friend or a family member stay with the patient constantly.

3. Monitor the patient's vital signs, which may be elevated.

4. Urine toxicology screens and blood levels of the drug taken should be done if possible.

5. Consider intoxication with multiple drugs, particularly when the symptoms persist. The agents are frequently contaminated with other drugs, such as amphetamines and PCP.

6. If the patient is severely agitated and potentially dangerous, physical restraint may be needed. Avoid physical restraint, if possible, in PCP intoxication.

7. Organic delusional and mood disorders that last more than several days may develop in some patients.

8. Evaluate whether the psychotic symptoms preceded the use of the hallucinogen and whether other diagnoses should be considered (for example, schizophreniform disorder and mood disorder with psychotic features).

DRUG TREATMENT

If tranquilization is needed, benzodiazepines are preferred, since antipsychotics (especially low-potency antipsychotics) may produce anticholinergic effects, which can exacerbate the signs of hallucinogen intoxication. Start with oxazepam (Serax) 10 to 30 mg by mouth or lorazepam (Ativan) 1 to 2 mg by mouth or intravenously (IV), both given every four hours as needed. If that is ineffective after several doses or if the signs of benzodiazepine toxicity occur (ataxia, dysarthria), a high-potency antipsychotic may be added—for example, fluphenazine (Prolixin), thiothixene (Navane), or haloperidol (Haldol), all given at 2 to 5 mg by mouth or intramuscularly (IM) every four hours as needed.

Cross-References:

Amphetamine or similarly acting sympathomimetic intoxication and withdrawal, anticholinergic intoxication, cocaine intoxication and withdrawal, delusional disorder, drug flashback, hallucinations, intoxication, phencyclidine or similarly acting arylcyclohexylamine intoxication.

67 / Headache

Headache is a clinical complaint experienced by more than 75 percent of the population each year. Headaches have a wide range of causes, ranging from mild stress to life-threatening intracranial disease. The most important task in evaluating headaches is identifying the minority caused by serious organic disease.

CLINICAL FEATURES AND DIAGNOSIS

The differential diagnosis of headache includes chronic syndromes, such as migraine, tension, cluster, and postconcussive headaches (Table B.67–1). Trigeminal neuralgia (tic douloureux), other neuralgias, and temporomandibular joint syndrome are other causes of pain in the head area. Headaches, both acute and chronic, may also herald serious intracranial pathology, including subdural and subarachnoid hemorrhage, tumors, pseudotumor cerebri, meningitis, temporal arteritis, and uncontrolled hypertension.

Unless a headache is mild, transitory, and clearly in response to an identified stress, it warrants a workup. The patient's description of the headache does not usually lead to a definitive diagnosis. Laboratory tests and brain imaging are all part of the workup, which typically includes computed tomography (CT) or magnetic resonance imaging (MRI) of the brain, even though the results of the majority of brain-imaging studies are negative.

Migraine

Migraine is often (but not always) preceded by an aura, including visual abnormalities (scotoma, scintillating scotomata, tubular vision) and autonomic dysfunction.

The headache is described as throbbing, unilateral, often periorbital. It is precipitated by bright light, alcohol, certain foods (for example, chocolate), changes in sleep or eating habits, and medications (for example, oral contraceptives), and it may be associated with hypersensitivity to noise or light. The headache can occur when a person is asleep or awake. Migraine is thought to be related to cerebral vasoconstriction.

Tension Headache

Tension headache (muscle contraction headache) is caused by the contraction of muscles of the head and the neck. The onset is late in the day. The headache is exacerbated by fatigue, stress (the same as in migraine), and emotional factors. Combined migraine and tension headaches are common. In combined cases, the focus is on first treating the migraine.

Cluster Headaches

Several headaches daily that persist for days to weeks are known as cluster headaches. Each lasts several hours. The headache is typically periorbital and nonthrobbing but with sharp pain. It may be associated with local symptoms, such as Horner's syndrome, tearing, and nasal congestion. The headache is precipitated by alcohol and may occur during sleep.

INTERVIEWING AND PSYCHOTHERAPEUTIC GUIDELINES

Although headaches are often affected by psychological factors, the patient should be approached with the assumption that the headache is due to an organic condition until proved otherwise. However, the majority of headaches do not have an identifiable organic cause. Headaches often respond to medication and psychotherapeutic interventions.

Table B.67–1
Differentiating Features of Common Types of Headache

	Muscle Contraction (Tension) Headache	Vascular Headaches	
		Migraine	Cluster Headache
Sex	Male = female	Female > male	Male > female
Age of onset	Not specific	Puberty to menopause	20 to 50 years
Family history	Not specific	Often familial	Not familial
Quality of pain	Pressure, tightness, bandlike, or not specific	Throbbing	Excruciating, boring, piercing, burning
Location of pain	Bilateral, occipital > frontal	Unilateral, often temporal	Unilateral orbital or adjacent head or face or both
Time of onset	Afternoon or evening more than morning	Early morning, often on weekends	Soon after onset of sleep, and daytime
Mode of onset	Gradual	Abrupt or gradual, often prodromata	Abrupt
Duration	Hours, days, or weeks; often continuous	Hours, 1 to 2 days	20 minutes to 2 hours
Frequency	Not specific; chronic daily headache	Not specific	Cluster, such as one or more a day for 2 to 10 weeks
Precipitating aggravating factors	Emotional stress or not apparent	Emotional stress, menstruation, vasodilators; alcohol, certain foods; change in weather	Alcohol, lying down, REM sleep
Ameliorating factors	Nonspecific: relaxation, alcohol; Rx: analgesics, tricyclics	Rest, compression of scalp arteries; pregnancy; Rx: ergotamine, propranolol	Activity; Rx: oxygen, ergotamine, methysergide, lithium, steroids
Associated symptoms or signs	None or not specific symptoms—tenderness of scalp or neck muscles	Prodromata: scintillating scotomata, hemianopsia, other brain signs During attack: nausea, vomiting, photophobia, irritability; tender scalp	Ipsilateral redness and tearing of eye, stuffiness and discharge of nostril, ptosis and myosis
Personality traits	Competitive, sensitive, conscientious > perfectionistic	Perfectionistic, neat, efficient, restrained, ambitious > compulsive	Not specific > perfectionist

Table from S Solomon, J C Masdeu: Neuropsychiatry and behavioral neurology. In *Comprehensive Textbook of Psychiatry*, ed 5, H I Kaplan, B J Sadock, editors, p 217. Williams & Wilkins, Baltimore, 1989. Used with permission.

EVALUATION AND MANAGEMENT

1. The patient's history should include the headache's location, duration, quality (sharp, throbbing, tight), timing, rate of onset, frequency, and precipitating and ameliorating factors. Find out whether the headaches occur during sleep and whether associated symptoms and signs, such as hallucinations and gastrointestinal disturbances, are present. A family history of migraine headache is often found in migraine sufferers.

2. Document the pattern of the headaches in a written record of all the headaches, their circumstances, possible precipitants, and what relieved them.

3. Over-the-counter medications—such as acetaminophen, aspirin, nonsteroidal anti-inflammatory drugs, caffeine, and phenacetin—may have been taken. Prescription medications—such as barbiturates, opioids, benzodiazepines, anticholinergics, tricyclic antidepressants, β-blockers, ergot alkaloids, lithium (Eskalith), and steroids—may have been taken. The evaluation should include inquiring about which medications have helped and those still being taken that may produce side effects.

4. A thorough physical and neurological examination is mandatory. Intracranial masses may be stretching or irritating the meninges. Nuchal rigidity is a sign of meningeal irritation and may be caused by hemorrhage or infection. Headaches caused by a brain tumor progress in intensity and duration as the tumor grows but are usually constant in location. Such headaches may be worsened by coughing or changing positions.

5. Biofeedback may be useful in tension headache. Oxygen inhalation is useful in cluster headaches.

6. Although psychotherapy is not a definitive treatment of headache, psychological stressors can often exacerbate headaches, and the relief of stress may improve the symptoms. Chronic headache syndromes can lead to disability and depression and should be dealt with by using a rehabilitation model that emphasizes functioning.

DRUG TREATMENT

Medications are given either abortively (to be taken after the headache has started) or prophylactically.

Start with common analgesics, such as aspirin, acetaminophen, and nonsteroidal anti-inflammatory drugs.

If those drugs are ineffective, treat migraines with ergot alkaloids, tension headaches with benzodiazepines, and cluster headaches with steroids and lithium. Sumatriptan (Imitrex) is also used to treat migraines.

β-Blockers and methysergide (Sansert) have been used for the prophylaxis of migraine. Tricyclic antidepressants—for example, low to moderate doses of amitriptyline (Elavil)—are effective in the prophylaxis of both migraine and tension headache.

Trigeminal neuralgia is treated with carbamazepine (Tegretol), and temporal arteritis is treated with steroids.

Cross-References:

Hypertensive crisis, hypochondriasis, pain.

---

68 / Head Trauma

The most common causes of *head trauma* are motor vehicle accidents. Head trauma can produce a wide range of clinical syndromes, including depression, mania, psychosis, organic personality disorder, and (rarely) dementia.

CLINICAL FEATURES AND DIAGNOSIS

Patients with the postconcussive syndrome may experience episodic dizziness, anxiety, lability, headache, and personality change. The symptoms may be exacerbated by alcohol, exercise, or exposure to heat or sunlight. Those factors may help differentiate the syndrome from emotional responses to the trauma. The duration of disorientation is an approximate guide to the prognosis. The acute syndrome is typically amnesia, which may resolve abruptly. Computed tomography (CT) or magnetic resonance imaging (MRI) classically shows a contrecoup lesion, with atrophy in the frontal and occipital poles and widespread edema from an anteroposterior injury.

INTERVIEWING AND PSYCHOTHERAPEUTIC GUIDELINES

Try to obtain as much information as possible from anyone who has witnessed the trauma. The patient may be able to provide bits of information, but they may be unreliable.

EVALUATION AND MANAGEMENT

1. In the mental status examination, focus on cognition. In the physical and neurological examinations, check for signs of intracranial hemorrhage (for example, focal neurological signs, nuchal rigidity, headache, sudden mental status change, delirium), which warrant an immediate CT or MRI of the head.

2. Factors affecting the prognosis include the presence of epilepsy, litigation, the patient's premorbid personality and coping mechanisms, the emotional repercussions of the injury, and the severity and the location of the brain damage.

3. With time, an organic personality syndrome may develop (Table B.68–1).

Table B.68–1
Diagnostic Criteria for Organic Personality Syndrome

A. A persistent personality disturbance, either lifelong or representing a change or accentuation of a previously characteristic trait, involving at least one of the following:
   (1) affective instability (e.g., marked shifts from normal mood to depression, irritability, or anxiety)
   (2) recurrent outbursts of aggression or rage that are grossly out of proportion to any precipitating psychosocial stressors
   (3) markedly impaired social judgment (e.g., sexual indiscretions)
   (4) marked apathy and indifference
   (5) suspiciousness or paranoid ideation

B. There is evidence from the history, physical examination, or laboratory tests of a specific organic factor (or factors) judged to be etiologically related to the disturbance.

C. This diagnosis is not given to a child or adolescent if the clinical picture is limited to the features that characterize attention-deficit hyperactivity disorder.

D. Not occurring exclusively during the course of delirium, and does not meet the criteria for dementia.

Specify explosive type if outbursts of aggression or rage are the predominant feature.

Table from DSM-III-R, *Diagnostic and Statistical Manual of Mental Disorders,* ed 3, revised. Copyright American Psychiatric Association, Washington, 1987. Used with permission.

DRUG TREATMENT

Drug treatment depends on the specific syndromes present. Head trauma patients may be vulnerable to the side effects of psychotropic drugs, including amnesia from benzodiazepines, and to extrapyramidal side effects, including tardive dyskinesia caused by antipsychotics. Medication may also mask more severe pathology, such as impending subdural hematoma; therefore, it is rarely used.

Cross-References:

Confusion, dementia, depression, mania.

---

69 / Hemodialysis

Hemodialysis is a complex treatment process that can cause many maladaptive behaviors for which psychiatric consultation is requested. Most hemodialysis patients are coping with a chronic debilitating, lifelong disease; its treatment requires tedious and time-consuming attachment to a machine for up to six hours three or more times each week. Hemodialysis patients spend a major portion of their lives coping with the consequences of renal failure, and the process of dialysis itself severely disrupts their daily lives, depriving them of their autonomy. Although psychiatrists are often consulted for acute situations, they must evaluate the patients in terms of chronic symptoms and long-term plans.

CLINICAL FEATURES AND DIAGNOSIS

Depression is common in hemodialysis patients, and suicide is 300 times more common in hemodialysis patients than in otherwise comparable normal controls. The behavioral problems that can arise include acting out, noncompliance with the prescribed diet, missing dialysis sessions, anger toward staff members, regression, infantilization, bargaining, and pleading. The premorbid personalities of the patients are important determinants of how they will handle the process of hemodialysis.

INTERVIEWING AND PSYCHOTHERAPEUTIC GUIDELINES

Provide counseling routinely for all hemodialysis patients. Hemodialysis patients are confronted by disturbances of body image, by depression, and by fears of death. Counseling should start before dialysis has begun and should directly address the issues of denial and unrealistic expectations. Discuss the benefits of alternatives, such as home dialysis and renal transplants. Evaluate the family and how the hemodialysis will change the roles of the family members. How will dialysis affect the patient's financial situation and ability to work? During dialysis, make periodic evaluations of the patient's adaptation to the process.

EVALUATION AND MANAGEMENT

1. Hemodialysis patients are subject to frequent and rapid shifts in fluids, electrolytes, and nutrients. Those changes can produce vitamin deficiencies, electrolyte imbalances, and osmotic disequilibrium in the brain.

2. Some patients complain of headache during dialysis, probably because the rapid changes in osmolality cause edema and increased water in the brain. In severe cases, nausea, muscle cramps, short-term mental status changes, delirium, and seizures can occur.

3. Long-term hemodialysis (several years) can lead to dementia characterized by the associated symptoms of dyspraxia, myoclonus, asterixis, grimacing, and seizures. Organic mental syndromes may also result from hypercalcemia, anemia, nitrogen retention, and cerebral infections.

4. Subdural hematomas can be caused by the anticoagulants that are administered to keep the arteriovenous shunt open.

5. Patients should strive to achieve an adaptive acceptance of the situation. The new hemodialysis patient may start with a feeling of euphoria, which then progresses to a stage of depression before progressing to acceptance. A steady supportive family and treatment team are important in facilitating the process. Group therapy with other dialysis patients is often helpful.

DRUG TREATMENT

Any medications used must have their dosages adjusted according to their effects on the patient's renal function and should be prescribed in consultation with a nephrologist. Antidepressants are often indicated. Blood levels of drugs should be measured after each dialysis treatment.

Cross-Reference:

Depression.

70 / Homicidal and Assaultive Behavior

Threats of homicide or assaultive behavior are common in psychiatric settings. Since a statement of violent intent is a predictor of violence, determine which threatening patients are actually dangerous.

CLINICAL FEATURES AND DIAGNOSIS

Factors that increase the likelihood of an assault include agitation, psychosis (especially paranoid delusions and command hallucinations), previous violence, recent stressors, intoxication with drugs or alcohol, withdrawal from alcohol or sedative-hypnotics, and organic disorders.

Some threats of assault (typically from borderline, antisocial, or histrionic personality disorder patients) are manipulative and without true intent. The evaluation of those patients can be difficult, but always err on the side of caution. Assume, at least initially, that all threats are potentially genuine. Threatening manipulative patients, on perceiving that they are not being taken seriously, may commit violent acts simply to prove that the clinician should have believed them.

INTERVIEWING AND PSYCHOTHERAPEUTIC GUIDELINES

Interaction should be firm, and limits should be clear. The patient must realize that any threats of homicide or assault are taken seriously and will elicit predictable responses from the authorities. A thorough search for weapons may be indicated. Perform a complete psychiatric evaluation, with special emphasis on obtaining a history of previous episodes of assault.

EVALUATION AND MANAGEMENT

1. Is a psychiatric illness responsible for the patient's threatening behavior? How specific are the patient's plans for violence? Does the patient have a specific intended victim? Has the patient obtained the means (for example, a weapon)? Does the patient have a specific reason for committing the violent act (for example, a domestic dispute, revenge against a rival drug dealer, or a response to command hallucinations)?

2. Has the patient committed violent acts in the past?

3. Has the patient been using drugs or alcohol? When was the last alcohol or drug ingestion?

4. Does the patient have a criminal record? If so, what are the specifics (for example, arrests, convictions, the nature of the crimes).

5. Was the patient abused as a child? Did the patient have childhood conduct problems or the triad of bed-wetting, fire setting, and cruelty to animals?

6. The clinician has a duty to warn and protect the intended victim. If a specific intended victim is likely to be attacked, the clinician must notify that person, the police, or the family or friends of the intended victim who are likely to be able to intervene. In addition, the clinician must do anything reasonable to protect the intended victim. The duty to warn and to protect takes priority over the patient's confidentiality. Threats against the President of the United States must be reported to the Secret Service.

7. Hospitalization, medication, and restraint may be needed.

DRUG TREATMENT

Acutely agitated patients who are already being treated with antipsychotics or benzodiazepines should be given an additional dose of their medication. Violent, psychotic patients can be given haloperidol (Haldol) 2 to 5 mg by mouth or intramuscularly (IM), thiothixene (Navane) 2 to 5 mg by mouth or IM, fluphenazine (Prolixin) 2 to 5 mg by mouth or IM, or perphenazine (Trilafon) 8 mg by mouth or 5 mg IM. Patients who are intoxicated or in withdrawal from drugs or alcohol can be given lorazepam (Ativan) 1 to 2 mg by mouth or IM, estazolam (ProSom) 0.5 to 1 mg by mouth, or oxazepam (Serax) 10 to 30 mg by mouth. If the patient has delirium or dementia, give haloperidol 1 to 5 mg by mouth or IM.

Cross-References:

Agitation, borderline personality disorder, hospitalization, intermittent explosive disorder, intoxication, restraints, suicide, violence.

---

71 / Homosexual Panic

Homosexual panic does not occur in people who are comfortable with issues related to homosexuality. Rather, it typically occurs in patients with strong latent homosexual drives who deny being homosexual but who have had recent experiences that suggest someone of the same gender is sexually interested in them. The experience triggers unrecognized feelings of homosexuality, causing the patient to mount a massive defense, which produces a panic state characterized by anxiety, fear, agitation, and possibly violence and paranoid delusions.

CLINICAL FEATURES AND DIAGNOSIS

Homosexual panic is not specifically described in the revised third edition of *Diagnostic and Statistical Manual of Mental Disorders* (DSM-III-

R), but it is considered either an adjustment disorder or an anxiety disorder not otherwise specified. The population with the highest rate of homosexual panic are adolescent boys.

The precipitant of homosexual panic may be a sexual conversation with a friend or, more commonly, physical contact, such as bathing together, fondling, sleeping together, or wrestling. In those situations a patient's unacceptable homoerotic fantasies may be aroused and then projected onto the other person involved in the encounter, precipitating a strong reaction in the patient. Homosexual panic may occur when a patient is impotent during heterosexual sex. Less often, a sexual act to the point of orgasm, such as mutual masturbation or anal intercourse, triggers the panic. Often, the precipitant occurred while the patient was intoxicated with alcohol or some other drug. Common settings are military barracks and college dormitories.

Homosexual panic is not normal, and it may be related to a serious psychiatric condition, such as schizophrenia. In severe cases the patient can be violent. Patients may have ideas of reference or paranoid delusions in which they believe that others accuse them of homosexuality.

INTERVIEWING AND PSYCHOTHERAPEUTIC GUIDELINES

Be supportive and reassuring. Give the patient an opportunity to emotionally ventilate and process what has occurred. A clinician who is the same sex as the patient should not be overly friendly so as to avoid any possibility that the patient will misperceive it as sexual interest.

EVALUATION AND MANAGEMENT

1. Arrange for a clinician of the opposite sex to evaluate the patient if possible.

2. Evaluate the patient for possible paranoid delusions. Homosexual panic may represent the beginning of a paranoid disorder or schizophrenia.

3. Get the patient's drug history. Could the homosexual panic have been exacerbated by alcohol or sedative-hypnotic withdrawal or by cocaine or other stimulant intoxication?

4. Minimize the physical examination unless it is clinically necessary. The patient can easily misinterpret the physical examination as a sexual assault. Defer the rectal, pelvic, and genital examinations if possible. Hospitalization is usually indicated for patients who are violent or acutely psychotic.

5. Refer the patient for psychotherapy.

DRUG TREATMENT

For severe anxiety, a benzodiazepine may be needed (for example, alprazolam [Xanax] 0.5 to 1 mg by mouth or lorazepam [Ativan] 1 to 2 mg by mouth). If the patient is psychotic, antipsychotics may be indicated—for example, thiothixene (Navane), trifluoperazine (Stelazine), fluphenazine

(Prolixin), or haloperidol (Haldol), all given at 5 mg by mouth for a short term. If possible, avoid giving medication by injection, which can be perceived as a sexual assault.

Cross-References:

Anxiety, delusional disorder, hospitalization, ideas of reference, impotence, panic disorder, rape and sexual abuse.

---

72 / Hospitalization

The decision about whether a patient requires psychiatric *hospitalization* is one of the most important decisions made by physicians. As the gatekeepers for inpatient treatment, emergency psychiatrists are familiar with the indications for hospitalization in the community in which they are working. In addition, emergency psychiatrists should be familiar with the available alternatives to hospitalization, such as outpatient clinics, day programs, crisis-intervention programs, psychosocial manipulations of the patient's environment, and jail.

Patients may be hospitalized in several ways. Since state laws vary, psychiatrists should be familiar with their local regulations. In general, patients should be hospitalized under the least restrictive statute (that is, voluntary hospitalization, if possible). However, that sometimes presents a management problem; dangerous patients admitted on a voluntary status may, shortly after admission, request discharge and require conversion to involuntary status, a difficult process.

In adolescents, hospitalization is usually indicated for new-onset psychosis and cases in which the psychiatric symptoms seriously disrupt the patients' functioning in school and at home and sufficiently disturb them and their families.

Informal Hospitalization

Admission and discharge may be requested orally, and the patient may leave at any time, even against medical advice. Most medical and surgical patients are admitted informally.

Voluntary Hospitalization

Voluntary hospitalization requires a written application for both admission and discharge. After the patient requests a discharge, the physician may convert a voluntary hospitalization to involuntary hospitalization.

Involuntary Hospitalization

Involuntary hospitalization severely limits the patient's autonomy and rights. It does not require the patient's consent and is often used for patients who are dangerous to themselves or others. Involuntary hospitalization requires certification by two physicians; the certificate may last up to 60 days and can be renewed. It may be ordered by a court in response to a petition by a hospital or the patient's family.

Emergency Hospitalization

Emergency hospitalization (temporary or one-physician commitment) is a convenient form of involuntary commitment that requires certification by only one physician; the certificate lasts up to 15 days. The patient must be examined by a second physician within 48 hours to confirm the need for emergency admission. After 15 days, the patient must be discharged, converted to involuntary status, or converted to voluntary status.

Short-Term Involuntary Protective Order

Patients with life-threatening medical illnesses who refuse treatment and who have mental disorders that prevent them from making decisions about their medical care can be involuntarily hospitalized for medical care by order of a judge. Patients who are dangerous to themselves or others must always be hospitalized or otherwise detained to prevent the occurrence of a dangerous act. Other indications for hospitalization include the presence of a mental illness, a need for treatment that is not available in other settings, and a lack of ability to care for oneself.

INTERVIEWING AND PSYCHOTHERAPEUTIC GUIDELINES

If patients are expected to be uncooperative with hospitalization, have sufficient staff members present before informing them. Explain to patients clearly what their rights are and what the procedures are for being discharged. Voluntary patients and parents requesting voluntary admission of a minor may incorrectly believe that they must be discharged immediately after they request it. Explain that they must request discharge in writing and that the physician has an option to convert them to involuntary status.

EVALUATION AND MANAGEMENT

1. Is the patient dangerous (for example, suicidal or homicidal)? Suicidal patients must be admitted to prevent a suicide attempt if outpatient care is not feasible. Some suicidal patients may continue to be actively suicidal even in the hospital and may require constant observation or one-to-one observation. Homicidal patients may also be admitted, but there should be an indication for treatment. Some homicidal persons are appropriately referred to the police if no treatable mental illness is detected. If a homicidal patient is not admitted or otherwise detained, the clinician has a duty to warn and protect the intended victim.

2. Does the patient have a mental illness? Make a diagnosis before deciding on the disposition. Does the mental illness warrant inpatient treatment? Would manipulation of the environment, referral to outpatient treatment, medication, crisis intervention, or family therapy reduce the need for hospitalization?

3. Does the patient have a new-onset psychosis? New-onset psychoses generally require inpatient evaluation and treatment.

4. Is hospitalization the appropriate treatment? Some patients, including those with borderline personality disorder, may become dependent on the hospital and regress when admitted. During crises they may require admission, but hospitalization should be avoided if possible, and a long-term treatment plan should be devised, usually in cooperation with the outpatient therapist.

5. Does the patient have sufficient supports if not hospitalized? The supports may include family, friends, the community, a church, and mental health providers.

6. How will the patient perceive not being hospitalized? If a patient has requested hospitalization, will not admitting the patient cause the patient to feel neglected and abandoned? Will a minor suicide gesture escalate to a dangerous attempt?

7. How will hospitalization affect the patient's work or school functioning? Hospitalization that creates absence from work or school may cause more problems.

8. Are family, friends, and hospital records available as sources of history? Clinicians are often faced with the difficult decision of whether to hospitalize with only limited data. Collateral sources of history can provide information crucial to making the most appropriate decision.

9. Is the patient medically ill? Emergency psychiatrists must be careful not to hospitalize patients on a psychiatry unit if they have medical problems that cannot be managed adequately. In some cases the medical or surgical problem may be responsible for the psychiatric presentation. For some patients, admission to a medical or surgical unit, with follow-up by the psychiatric consultation service, may be indicated.

DRUG TREATMENT

If the patient is violent an antipsychotic or antianxiety agent may be used in the emergency room. In most situations medication can be withheld until the patient has gone through the admission process and has been more thoroughly evaluated as an inpatient.

Cross-References:

Agitation, anxiety, homicidal and assaultive behavior, suicide, violence.

---

73 / Hypersexuality

Social evaluation of what is considered appropriate sexual behavior is highly dependent on culture. Although the symptom of hypersexuality has been poorly studied, the vast majority of hypersexual patients suffer from psychological conditions, rather than organic conditions. Hypersexuality must be defined in a social context; it is not based strictly on the quantity of sexual activity. A wide range of quantity of sexual activity can be considered normal.

Hypersexuality is usually used for repeated sexual activity with different partners in the absence of ongoing relationships. In homosexual patients it is more difficult to determine when a patient is hypersexual, since the range of socially acceptable sexual behavior may be wider in the gay community than among heterosexuals.

CLINICAL FEATURES AND DIAGNOSIS

Mental disorders that may present with hypersexuality include personality disorders (such as borderline and histrionic personality disorders), mania, intoxication with such stimulant drugs as amphetamine and cocaine, and, less commonly, schizophrenia.

The terms "nymphomaniac" for women and "satyr" and "Don Juan" for men are commonly used for heterosexuals who repeatedly have sex with multiple partners, often compulsively. The theories about Don Juanism include unconscious homosexual desires that are defended against by repeated heterosexual contacts. Hypersexual women (nymphomaniacs) are often highly dependent and may have anorgasmia. They engage in sexual activities repeatedly out of a fear of loss of love.

Hypersexuality is rarely a symptom of an organic disorder, such as epilepsy, especially temporal lobe epilepsy. Frontal lobe disease may present with hypersexuality as a form of disinhibited behavior.

INTERVIEWING AND PSYCHOTHERAPEUTIC GUIDELINES

Be nonjudgmental in interviewing the patient. In addition to a sexual history, the evaluation should include a full psychiatric history and a mental status examination.

EVALUATION AND MANAGEMENT

1. Perform a complete psychiatric evaluation and make a diagnosis.

2. Complete a sexual history, with detail about possible sexual disorders.

3. Evaluate the patient for possible exposure to human immunodeficiency virus (HIV) and other sexually transmitted diseases. Refer the patient for medical treatment if appropriate.

4. Consider giving a female patient a pregnancy test.

5. Is the hypersexual behavior placing the patient in potentially dangerous situations, especially if the patient is psychotic? Consider hospitalization in those cases.

6. When hospitalizing a hypersexual patient, consider a one-to-one watch to prevent destructive sexual interactions with other patients.

DRUG TREATMENT

No specific medication is used on an emergency basis for this condition. If the behavioral pattern is a manifestation of an underlying disorder pharmacotherapy can be considered.

Cross-References:

Incest, mania, obsessions and compulsions, pregnancy, rape and sexual abuse, temporal lobe epilepsy.

---

74 / Hypertensive Crisis

Hypertensive crisis is a potentially life-threatening emergency that occurs when patients taking monoamine oxidase inhibitors (MAOIs) eat food containing tyramine or take contraindicated drugs, such as sympathomimetic agents.

CLINICAL FEATURES AND DIAGNOSIS

The symptoms of hypertensive crisis include severe occipital headache, stiff neck, sweating, nausea, and vomiting.

Interactions of MAOIs with sympathomimetic agents and other specific drugs are potentially fatal (Table B.74–1). MAOIs combined with meperidine (Demerol) or dextromethorphan (Dexedrine and many over-the-counter cough medications) can produce restlessness, dizziness, tremor, sweating, muscle twitching, seizures, and severe hyperpyrexia—in some cases eventually leading to shock and death. The concomitant use of serotonin-specific reuptake inhibitors (SSRIs) (for example, fluoxetine [Prozac], paroxetine [Paxil], and sertraline [Zoloft]) and MAOIs can produce rigidity, fever, confusion, and death. MAOIs cannot be used until the SSRIs has been discontinued for five weeks.

Tricyclic antidepressants have been safely and effectively combined with MAOIs in closely monitored patients. The best rule is to use low dosages of both drugs, increase them slowly, and monitor the patients closely.

Patients should continue a tyramine-free diet for at least two weeks after the MAOI has been discontinued (Table B.74–2).

The most common side effects of MAOIs are unrelated to diet and drug interactions; the side effects include orthostatic hypotension, weight gain, edema, insomnia, and sexual dysfunction. Both orthostatic hypotension and hypertensive crisis can present with symptoms of fainting.

INTERVIEWING AND PSYCHOTHERAPEUTIC GUIDELINES

Keep the interview brief, and focus on identifying the type and the amount of any tyramine-containing food eaten and contraindicated medications taken. Patients with potentially dangerous conditions should be referred for possible intensive care unit (ICU) admission. Medications taken in an overdose attempt present a much greater risk than do inadvertent toxic combinations.

Table B.74-1
Drugs to Be Avoided during MAOI Treatment

Never use:

Anesthetic—never spinal anesthetic or local anesthetic containing epinephrine (lidocaine and
procaine are safe)
Antiasthmatic medications
Antihypertensives (α-methyldopa, guanethidine, reserpine, pargyline)
L-Dopa, L-tryptophan
Narcotics (especially meperidine [Demerol]; morphine or codeine may be less dangerous)
Over-the-counter cold, hay fever, and sinus medications, especially those containing
dextromethorphan (aspirin, acetaminophen, and menthol lozenges are safe)
Sympathomimetics (amphetamine, cocaine, methylphenidate, dopamine, metaraminol,
epinephrine, norepinephrine, isoproterenol)

Use carefully:

Antihistamines
Hydralazine (Apresoline)
Propranolol (Inderal)
Terpin hydrate with codeine

Table B.74-2
Tyramine-Rich Foods to Be Avoided while Taking MAOIs

Very high tyramine content:

Alcohol (particularly beer and wines, especially Chianti; a small amount of scotch, gin, vodka,
or sherry is permissible)
Fava or broad beans
Aged cheese (e.g., Camembert, Liederkranz, Edam, and cheddar; cream cheese and cottage
cheeses are permitted)
Beef or chicken liver
Orange pulp
Pickled or smoked fish, poultry, or meats
Soups (packaged)
Yeast vitamin supplements
Meat extracts (e.g., Marmite, Bovril)
Summer (dry) sausage

Moderately high tyramine content (no more than one or two servings a day):

Soy sauce
Sour cream
Bananas
Avocados
Eggplant
Plums
Raisins
Spinach
Tomatoes
Yogurt

EVALUATION AND MANAGEMENT

1. Check the patient's vital signs. Rule out orthostatic hypotension
caused by the MAOI itself. Hypotension may also be related to the rate of
the MAOI dosage increase. Headaches may have many different causes, so
do not assume that a patient taking an MAOI is in a hypertensive crisis

until the patient's blood pressure has been taken, even if the headache is severe.

2. Identify the quantity of the tyramine-containing food or contraindicated medication taken.

3. Obtain a medical consultation.

4. Provide ICU monitoring and supportive treatment of the patient's vital functions as needed.

5. Evaluate the patient for suicidality.

DRUG TREATMENT

Give phentolamine (Regitine) 5 mg intravenously (IV) repeated as needed or phenoxybenzamine (Dibenzyline) 100 mg IV drip over an hour (both are α-adrenergic receptor blockers). Another alternative drug is diazoxide (Hyperstat) 300 mg IV, which relaxes the arteriolar smooth muscles. Nifedipine (Procardia) can be used by having the patient bite into a 10 mg capsule before swallowing its contents with water. Chlorpromazine (Thorazine) 50 to 100 mg by mouth also has prominent hypotensive effects and can be used to lower the patient's blood pressure. Some psychiatrists prescribe chlorpromazine to their patients taking MAOIs and advise them to carry the pills with them in case they experience a hypertensive crisis.

Cross-References:

Headache, neuroleptic malignant syndrome, serotonin syndrome.

---

75 / Hyperthermia

Hyperthermia is a heat illness associated with an elevated body temperature. The general categories of heat illness include heat cramps, heat exhaustion, and heatstroke. Children, the elderly, and the medically ill are the most susceptible.

CLINICAL FEATURES AND DIAGNOSIS

All antipsychotics can induce hyperthermia, particularly low-potency antipsychotics, which have prominent anticholinergic effects. Typically, the patient has also been exposed to heat or has engaged in physical activity. Men and women are equally susceptible.

Symptoms of hyperthermia begin with sweating, thirst, fatigue, giddiness, ataxia, and hysteria. As the condition progresses, the body's temperature rises, eventually leading to delirium. The patient may be hypoactive or hyperactive. If the patient becomes dehydrated, sweating may stop, and symptoms of profound central nervous system (CNS) disturbance may develop, including restlessness, rigidity, seizures, coma, and death.

Antipsychotic drugs can decrease the body's central thermoregulation. In addition, sweating is impaired, further reducing the patient's ability to dissipate heat. Hyperthermia is most likely to develop shortly after the patient starts taking an antipsychotic or after the dosage is changed.

Hyperthermia may also accompany substance abuse withdrawal (for example, withdrawal from alcohol or opioids).

INTERVIEWING AND PSYCHOTHERAPEUTIC GUIDELINES

Reassure the patient that the condition can be treated. Explain that it is a reaction to drugs. Evaluate the patient's recent level of exertion and heat exposure. Ask about antipsychotic drug exposure. Also ask about possible signs of infection, which can cause fever. Is the patient taking any other drugs that can cause a drug fever, such as antibiotics?

EVALUATION AND MANAGEMENT

1. Obtain the patient's history of antipsychotic exposure, heat exposure, and exertion. Is the patient taking anticholinergic drugs or an antipsychotic with prominent anticholinergic side effects?

2. Measure the patient's temperature, and examine the patient for rigidity. Is the patient sweating? Is the patient's pulse elevated? Is the patient hypotensive? Rigidity may suggest neuroleptic malignant syndrome. Anhidrosis, tachycardia, and hypotension are signs of dehydration.

3. Order blood tests, including those for blood urea nitrogen (BUN), creatinine, electrolytes, and complete blood count (CBC). If the patient is dehydrated, provide intravenous (IV) hydration, and correct any electrolyte abnormalities.

4. Is it a drug fever? Does the patient have a skin rash? An uncommon side effect of antipsychotics, drug fever is commonly caused by antibiotics, antihistamines, barbiturates and other anticonvulsants, and antiarrhythmics. Discontinue any drugs that could be causing drug fever.

5. Does the fever have a medical cause? Perform a full fever workup. Also perform a full battery of laboratory screening tests, including creatine phosphokinase (CPK), erythrocyte sedimentation rate (ESR), CBC, chemistry panel, electrolytes, glutamic acid (Glu), BUN, creatinine, hepatic enzymes, and blood and urine cultures.

6. Place the patient in an air-conditioned environment. In severe cases, consider either an ice bath or evaporative cooling by spraying the patient with lukewarm water and then blowing with a fan. Evaporative cooling may be more effective, since it produces less peripheral vasoconstriction than do ice packs or ice baths.

7. If the fever is mild, follow the temperature closely, consider discontinuation of the antipsychotic, and encourage the patient to drink liberal amounts of fluids.

DRUG TREATMENT

If neuroleptic malignant syndrome is diagnosed, treat that disorder immediately. Supportive measures, such as cooling, monitoring in an intensive care unit, and the maintenance of vital functions, are necessary. Antipyretics (for example, acetaminophen and aspirin) may be helpful, but they are of little use in treating heat exhaustion and heatstroke. Moreover, those drugs do not reduce the patient's elevated temperature when the hyperthermia involves an antipsychotic medication.

Cross-Reference:

Neuroleptic malignant syndrome.

76 / Hyperventilation

Hyperventilation occurs when a person breathes rapidly and deeply for several minutes, producing hypocapnia and respiratory alkalosis. When the voluntary hyperventilation stops, the hypocapnia reduces the normal drive to breathe, which leads to a mild hypoxia.

CLINICAL FEATURES AND DIAGNOSIS

The symptoms of hyperventilation include dizziness, light-headedness, fainting, paresthesias, and carpopedal spasm. The differential diagnosis includes seizures, hysteria, hypoglycemia, vasovagal attacks, myocardial ischemia, asthma, porphyria, pheochromocytoma, and Ménière's disease. The psychiatric conditions associated with hyperventilation include panic disorder, phobia, obsessive-compulsive disorder, histrionic and borderline personality disorders, schizophrenia, and other syndromes in which anxiety is prominent.

INTERVIEWING AND PSYCHOTHERAPEUTIC GUIDELINES

Help the patient relax. Inform the patient that the symptoms are due to hyperventilation and will pass. Show them that they can hold their breath during an attack, despite their complaints of suffocation.

EVALUATION AND MANAGEMENT

1. If the patient is still hyperventilating, have the patient blow into a paper bag and rebreathe the air from the bag. That counters the hypocapnia.

2. Rule out possible medical causes.

3. Perform a full psychiatric evaluation. If the problem is chronic, evaluate the patient for personality and anxiety disorders. Refer the patient to appropriate outpatient treatment.

DRUG TREATMENT

Drug treatment is usually not necessary, but, if the patient is severely anxious, a single dose of a benzodiazepine—for example, lorazepam (Ativan) 1 mg by mouth or intramuscularly or alprazolam (Xanax) 0.5 to 1 mg by mouth—usually relieves the symptoms.

Cross-References:

Alcohol withdrawal, anxiety, borderline personality disorder, cocaine intoxication and withdrawal, panic disorder.

77 / Hypochondriasis

Hypochondriasis is characterized by an unreasonable concern about one's health and an unrealistic conviction that physical signs or symptoms are indicative of serious medical disease, despite reasonable assurance that such a disease is not present.

CLINICAL FEATURES AND DIAGNOSIS

The fear of disease is persistent, and itself leads to functional impairment. Several organ systems may be the focus of concern, or one system may predominate (Table B.77–1).

About 10 to 15 percent of all patients seen in general medical practice have hypochondriasis. The peak incidence is in the fourth or fifth decade. Hypochondriasis may be more common in the relatives of patients with hypochondriasis than in the general population.

Hypochondriasis may be common in cultures that encourage somatization as an expression of psychic distress. Psychodynamically, hypochondriasis offers the patient a way to assume the sick role in avoidance of insurmountable problems or some overwhelming stress. The possible origins include (1) aggression toward others that is repressed and displaced into physical symptoms and (2) defense against guilt in which the physical symptoms are a deserved punishment for some sin. Psychosocially, the onset of symptoms often follows a major stressor.

The clinical features that indicate a good prognosis include the presence of depression or anxiety, a sudden onset, young age, a high socioeconomic status, the absence of organic disease, and the absence of a personality disorder. Hypochondriacal patients are often resistant to psychiatric treatment; offering them treatment in a medical setting that emphasizes coping with chronic medical illnesses may improve their cooperation. The outcome is poor in about 25 percent of patients, and another two thirds run a long-term fluctuating course.

INTERVIEWING AND PSYCHOTHERAPEUTIC GUIDELINES

Hypochondriacal patients may also have genuine medical conditions. Begin by assuming that all somatic complaints are due to medical conditions, and proceed with an appropriate medical evaluation, including con-

Table B.77–1
Diagnostic Criteria for Hypochondriasis

A. Preoccupation with the fear of having, or the belief that one has, a serious disease, based on the person's interpretation of physical signs or sensations as evidence of physical illness.

B. Appropriate physical evaluation does not support the diagnosis of any physical disorder that can account for the physical signs or sensations or the person's unwarranted interpretation of them, **and** the symptoms in A are not just symptoms of panic attacks.

C. The fear of having, or belief that one has, a disease persists despite medical reassurance.

D. Duration of the disturbance is at least six months.

E. The belief in A is not of delusional intensity, as in delusional disorder, somatic type (i.e., the person can acknowledge the possibility that his or her fear of having, or belief that he or she has, a serious disease is unfounded).

Table from DSM-III-R, *Diagnostic and Statistical Manual of Mental Disorders,* ed 3, revised. Copyright American Psychiatric Association, Washington, 1987. Used with permission.

sultations if appropriate. Medical conditions with symptoms in multiple systems—such as acquired immune deficiency syndrome (AIDS), systemic lupus erythematosus, endocrinopathies, multiple sclerosis, myasthenia gravis, central nervous system (CNS) diseases, cancer, and syphilis—can be missed in a patient who appears to be hypochondriacal. Regular physical examinations and other noninvasive tests help reassure patients that their somatic complaints are not being ignored by the doctor. Maintain an understanding attitude without reinforcing the patient's behavior.

Identify pervasive psychiatric disorders, such as depression and anxiety disorders, since the presence of such disorders suggests definitive treatments that can improve the prognosis.

EVALUATION AND MANAGEMENT

1. Rule out genuine medical conditions; even a known hypochondriac can get sick. However, avoid repetitive unnecessary medical testing.

2. Evaluate the patient for depressive and anxiety disorders, especially panic disorder. Also examine the patient for somatic delusions, obsessions, and compulsions.

3. Group therapy may be the treatment of choice, especially in medical settings that emphasize coping skills. Groups also provide social contacts and support. Individual insight-oriented psychotherapy may also be effective.

DRUG TREATMENT

No specific drug treatment is indicated in cases of hypochondriasis. In the hypochondriacal anxious state the patient may benefit from an anxiolytic—for example, alprazolam (Xanax) 0.5 to 1 mg by mouth, oxazepam (Serax) 10 to 30 mg by mouth, or lorazepam (Ativan) 1 mg by mouth or intramuscularly (IM). If the course is episodic and similar to that of a depressive disorder, diagnose depression. A new onset of hypochondriasis in an elderly patient also suggests depression. Treatment with an antidepressant medication may relieve both the underlying depression and the hypochondriasis. In panic disorder, hypochondriasis may respond to benzodiazepines or antidepressants. If psychotic symptoms suggest a delusional disorder or schizophrenia, consider antipsychotics.

Cross-References:

Anxiety, borderline personality disorder, depression, headache, malingering, panic disorder.

---

78 / Hypothermia

Hypothermia is a medical emergency that is usually caused by prolonged exposure to cold temperatures.

CLINICAL FEATURES AND DIAGNOSIS

The behavioral symptoms include confusion, lethargy, combativeness, low body temperature and shivering, and a paradoxical feeling of warmth. The typical patient with hypothermia has been exposed for a prolonged period to cold external temperature after the heavy use of alcohol or other central nervous system (CNS) depressants. Medically ill patients may have hypothermia even without prolonged exposure to the cold.

The presence of hypoglycemia or hypothyroidism predisposes the patient to hypothermia. Antipsychotic medications can decrease the central thermoregulation, causing patients to be susceptible to hypothermia when exposed to the cold. Other medical conditions that increase the patient's susceptibility to the cold include pituitary insufficiency, Addison's disease, cerebrovascular disease, Wernicke's encephalopathy, myocardial infarction, cirrhosis, and pancreatitis. The most common clinical feature is alcohol intoxication.

INTERVIEWING AND PSYCHOTHERAPEUTIC GUIDELINES

Focus on the medical emergency and its potential sequelae. Inquire about the duration of exposure to the cold, the medications taken (especially antipsychotics), and the use of alcohol and drugs of abuse. If the patient is confused or delirious, focus on maintaining a safe, controlled environment and initiating immediate emergency medical treatment.

EVALUATION AND MANAGEMENT

1. Obtain a medical consultation immediately.
2. Monitor the patient's temperature frequently, and institute cardiac monitoring. Order blood tests (including a complete blood count), thyroid function tests, blood urea nitrogen (BUN) and creatinine tests, electrolytes,

liver function tests, amylase tests, blood alcohol level, and other screening tests for possible medical problems.

3. Warm the patient. Mild hypothermia can be treated by wrapping the patient in blankets in a warm room, but moderate hypothermia may require warm baths. In severely hypothermic patients, external warming can cause vasodilation that diverts blood from the viscera and can lead to rewarming shock. Patients with severe hypothermia require core warming with hemodialysis or peritoneal dialysis with warmed blood or dialysate.

4. Do not give the patient alcohol, which causes vasodilation and increases heat loss in spite of producing a subjective feeling of warmth.

5. If frostbite is present, warm the affected area gradually (starting with water at 50°F) after raising the patient's core temperature.

DRUG TREATMENT

Provide intravenous (IV) fluids, and carefully monitor the patient's pH and potassium. Treat acidosis with IV bicarbonate, and treat hypokalemia to reduce the risk of cardiac arrhythmias. No specific drugs are used for this condition.

Cross-References:

Alcohol intoxication, delirium.

---

79 / Ideas of Reference

Ideas of reference are misinterpretations of external events, thinking that they directly relate to oneself.

CLINICAL FEATURES AND DIAGNOSIS

Although ideas of reference may occur occasionally in anyone, they are common in paranoid patients and may be the initial nidus for a paranoid delusional system. If the ideas of reference are severe or persistent or become organized into a well-formed system, they become delusions of reference. Typical ideas of reference include "People are talking about me" and "The news on television is about me."

Ideas of reference often occur in schizophrenia, delusional disorder, and paranoid personality disorder. They may also occur in other disorders, including mania, psychotic depression, and substance-induced psychoses.

INTERVIEWING AND PSYCHOTHERAPEUTIC GUIDELINES

Do not challenge ideas of reference directly. Explore the degree to which the referential thinking is fixed. Evaluate the patient for delusions, particularly paranoid thoughts, thought control, thought insertion, thought broadcasting, and mind reading. How do people around the patient react to the referential ideas? Does the patient avoid talking about those ideas with others? Does the patient firmly believe something that is not possible? Does the patient plan to take action against the objects of the referential thinking?

Reassure the patient that the material can be discussed with you in confidence. Do not do anything that may make the patient more suspicious, lest you become incorporated into a paranoid delusional system.

EVALUATION AND MANAGEMENT

1. Make a definitive diagnosis. Consider schizophrenia, delusional disorder, and paranoid personality disorder in the differential diagnosis. Rule out psychotic mood disorders.

2. Drugs, especially such hallucinogens as lysergic acid diethylamide (LSD) and phencyclidine (PCP) and such psychostimulants as cocaine and amphetamine, can cause psychotic symptoms, including ideas of reference. The patient's vital signs and the results of a urine toxicology screen may help with the diagnosis.

3. Assess the degree to which the patient responds to referential thinking. Hospitalize dangerous patients.

DRUG TREATMENT

Drug treatment depends on the diagnosis and the severity of the impairment. Depression, schizophrenia, and mania—all require different approaches to drug treatment, so the proper diagnosis is critical.

If well-formed, systematized referential delusions are present in the context of a delusional disorder, antipsychotic medications may be only minimally helpful. Patients with delusional disorder often refuse treatment, and their delusions are often refractory to antipsychotic medications.

Cross-References:

Agitation, anxiety, chronic schizophrenia in acute exacerbation, delusional disorder, depression, hallucinations, mania, paranoia, schizoaffective disorder.

---

80 / Illusions

Illusions are perceptual misinterpretations of real external stimuli. By contrast, hallucinations are not related to any real external stimuli.

CLINICAL FEATURES AND DIAGNOSIS

Illusions are much less significant symptoms than are hallucinations. Illusions often occur in normal people, especially when they are falling asleep, tired, or overstimulated. The important clinical task is to determine when illusions are symptoms of psychotic disorders, such as schizophrenia.

In psychotic patients, distinguishing illusions from hallucinations may be difficult. The clinician must also determine whether the illusions are secondary to delirium, intoxication, or withdrawal.

In normal people, sensory deprivation can produce illusions, particularly in the elderly who have decreased sensory acuity. Physical and psychological stress can also precipitate illusions.

INTERVIEWING AND PSYCHOTHERAPEUTIC GUIDELINES

If hallucinations are also present, the interview should include a full evaluation for psychotic disorders. If the illusions are mild, reassure the patient that illusions are often normal and do not necessarily indicate a major psychiatric problem, especially when the illusions occur only after sensory deprivation or when the patient is under stress.

EVALUATION AND MANAGEMENT

1. Focus initially on whether such frank psychotic symptoms as hallucinations and delusions are present.

2. Perform a complete mental status examination, and obtain the patient's history. The cognitive examination should evaluate the patient for such disorders as schizophrenia, depression, mania, anxiety disorders, psychoactive substance abuse, and organic mental disorders. Assess the patient medically, since illusions may be related to underlying medical illnesses.

3. Identify the course of the illusions and what impairment, if any, is present. Illusions are usually transitory. The presence of persistent illusions and of any impairment caused by the illusions suggests serious psychopathology.

4. In the elderly who experience illusions after sensory deprivation, the restoration of an appropriately stimulating environment usually resolves the symptoms.

DRUG TREATMENT

No specific drug treatment is indicated. If the patient is extremely upset by the symptom, such benzodiazepines as diazepam (Valium) 5 to 10 mg by mouth one or two times a day, clonazepam (Klonopin) 0.25 to 0.5 mg by mouth one or two times a day, or lorazepam (Ativan) 1 to 2 mg by mouth one or two times a day may be helpful for short-term use. If the illusion is a symptom of another disorder, such as psychosis, antipsychotics may be indicated.

Cross-References:

Anxiety, confusion, hallucinations, intoxication, schizophrenia.

81 / Impending Death Associated with Antipsychotic Medication

The introduction of antipsychotic medications has not increased the rate of sudden death in psychiatric patients. Patients with acute psychoses may die as a result of stresses related to the acute psychosis, rather than to the treatment. Nonetheless, antipsychotic medications do have potentially dangerous side effects, especially for the medically ill. Life-threatening complications are not more commonly associated with either high-potency or low-potency antipsychotics.

CLINICAL FEATURES AND DIAGNOSIS

The side effects of antipsychotics that may possibly contribute to sudden death include (1) ventricular fibrillation (antipsychotics are not arrhythmogenic); (2) depressed gag reflex, leading to asphyxia from the aspiration of regurgitated food; (3) lowering of the seizure threshold, causing seizures; (4) dystonia of the larynx and pharynx, leading to asphyxiation; (5) orthostatic hypotension, leading to a cerebrovascular event or myocardial infarction; (6) neuroleptic malignant syndrome; (7) anticholinergic effects, reducing gastrointestinal (GI) motility and leading to shock in patients with acquired megacolon; (8) endobronchial mucous plugs in asthmatic patients; and (9) clozapine (Clozaril)-induced agranulocytosis, leading to opportunistic infection.

INTERVIEWING AND PSYCHOTHERAPEUTIC GUIDELINES

No evidence indicates that the use of antipsychotic medications increases the likelihood of sudden death. Carefully describe the potential side effects to the patients and their families. Instruct them to seek medical care rapidly if side effects occur, especially dystonia, severe rigidity, seizures, and hypotension. Inform patients that antipsychotics in rare cases cause agranulocytosis, so they should be evaluated for any sign of even a minor infection, such as a fever.

EVALUATION AND MANAGEMENT

Give the appropriate emergency medical care.

DRUG TREATMENT

Decrease the antipsychotic dosage or discontinue the antipsychotic if necessary to eliminate severe side effects. Many side effects can be reduced by switching to another antipsychotic drug. Extrapyramidal side effects are easily treated with anticholinergic drugs. Anticholinergic side effects, hypotension, and the lowering of the seizure threshold can be decreased by changing to a higher-potency antipsychotic.

Cross-References:

Agitation; akathisia; akinesia; anxiety; cardiac arrhythmia; dystonia, acute; neuroleptic malignant syndrome.

---

82 / Impending Death of Psychogenic Origin

Medically healthy people can die as a result of overwhelming psychic stress. One proposed mechanism is that severe anxiety leads to massive central nervous system (CNS) autonomic discharges, which cause ventricular fibrillation. Another proposed mechanism is that the severe stress causes a shutdown of the hypothalamic-pituitary-adrenal axis, leading to shock and changes in the immune system. A patient who has suffered a major loss may become so hopeless that the will to live is lost.

CLINICAL FEATURES AND DIAGNOSIS

In voodoo cultures the effectiveness of a death curse is related to whether the intended victim believes in the power of the curse. The belief that one will die because of a curse may be enough to cause death. Patients may be dehydrated or in a state of starvation. Arrhythmias may be present.

INTERVIEWING AND PSYCHOTHERAPEUTIC GUIDELINES

Rapidly intervene with cognitive approaches. Involve the patient's family, or use other culturally appropriate interventions. Attempt to relieve or remove the stressor. Persons with cardiac arrhythmias should be advised to prepare themselves in advance for stressful situations and to anticipate anxiety-provoking events.

EVALUATION AND MANAGEMENT

In voodoo situations try to call on another person who is believed to have psychic powers to break the death curse. Patients with cardiac arrhythmias should be seen by the cardiologist in the emergency room. If impending death is not related to voodoo, try to identify other stressful life events.

DRUG TREATMENT

No specific drug treatment is needed, but severe anxiety may be relieved with benzodiazepines. Patients with known cardiac disease may benefit from agents that raise the electrical threshold of the heart or prevent a rapid heart rate. A cardiologist should be consulted.

Cross-References:
Agitation, anxiety, panic disorder.

---

83 / Impotence (Male Erectile Disorder)

Impotence is the inability to achieve penile erection. Although not usually a psychiatric emergency, impotence is a common complaint of men seen by physicians and can produce considerable anxiety and suffering for the patient.

CLINICAL FEATURES AND DIAGNOSIS

The immediate objective in evaluating a complaint of impotence is making a specific diagnosis, determined by whether (1) the patient is truly impotent (unable to achieve a functional erection under any circumstances); (2) the patient is impotent because of a medical condition, a drug, or alcohol (Table B.83–1 and Table B.83–2); (3) the impotence is primary (the patient never had an erection sufficient for coitus) or secondary (the patient has had an erection sufficient for coitus in the past); (4) factors have contributed to secondary impotence; and (5) conditions make the impotence selective (for example, only with the man's wife but not with his girlfriend). After a few episodes of impotence, anticipatory anxiety about being impotent again inevitably contributes to continued impotence. The diagnostic criteria for impotence (male erectile disorder) are given in Table B.83–3.

Primary impotence is uncommon (1 percent of men under age 35); secondary impotence is present in between 10 and 20 percent of all men. Prevalence increases with age, but, in the elderly, the availability of a sexual partner is more related to potency than is increasing age.

INTERVIEWING AND PSYCHOTHERAPEUTIC GUIDELINES

Impotence is a sensitive topic for most men. Interview the patient alone; later, interview the identified partner alone. Ask the patient about drugs, medications, and alcohol use. Does the patient have erections in the morning, while masturbating, or with other partners? The majority (50 to 80 percent) of patients complaining of impotence do not have an organic cause. They should usually be referred for psychotherapy, including individual, couples, and sex therapy.

Table B.83-1
Diseases Implicated in Erectile Dysfunction

Infectious and parasitic diseases
  Elephantiasis
  Mumps
	Neurological disorders
	  Multiple sclerosis
	  Transverse myelitis
	  Parkinson's disease

Cardiovascular diseases
  Atherosclerotic disease
  Aortic aneurysm
  Leriche's syndrome
  Cardiac failure
	Temporal lobe epilepsy
	  Traumatic or neoplastic spinal cord
	    disease
	  Central nervous system tumors
	  Amyotropic lateral sclerosis
	  Peripheral neuropathies

Renal and urological disorders
  Peyronie's disease
  Chronic renal failure
  Hydrocele or varicocele
	General paresis
	  Tabes dorsalis

Hepatic disorders
  Cirrhosis (usually associated with
    alcoholism)
	Pharmacological contributants (Table
	    B.83-2)
	  Alcohol and other addictive drugs (heroin,
	    methadone, morphine, cocaine,
	    amphetamines, and barbituates)

Pulmonary disorders
  Respiratory failure
	Prescribed drugs (psychotropic drugs,
	    antihypertensive drugs, estrogens, and
	    antiandrogens)

Genetics
  Klinefelter's syndrome
  Congenital penile vascular or structural
    abnormalities
	Poisoning
	  Lead (plumbism)
	  Herbicides

Nutritional disorders
  Malnutrition
  Vitamin deficiencies
	Surgical procedures
	  Perineal prostatectomy
	  Abdominal-perineal colon resection
	  Sympathectomy (frequently interferes with
	    ejaculation)

Endocrine disorders
  Diabetes mellitus
  Dysfunction of the pituitary-adrenal-testis
    axis
  Acromegaly
  Addison's disease
  Chromophobe ademona
  Adrenal neoplasias
  Myxedema
  Hyperthyroidism
	Aortoiliac surgery
	  Radical cystectomy
	  Retroperitoneal lymphadenectomy
	
	Miscellaneous
	  Radiation therapy
	  Pelvic fracture
	  Any severe systemic disease or debilitating
	    condition

Table from V A Sadock: Normal human sexuality and sexual dysfunctions. In *Comprehensive Textbook of Psychiatry* ed 5, H I Kaplan, B J Sadock, editors, p 1045. Williams & Wilkins, Baltimore, 1989. Used with permission.

EVALUATION AND MANAGEMENT

1. Rule out the use of drugs and alcohol.

2. Complete the patient's medical history. Could medical conditions (for example, diabetes mellitus) be the cause?

3. Determine the circumstances of the impotence—when, where, with whom, how frequent, how much effort was made. How anxious did the patient or the partner become?

4. If erections can ever be achieved (for example, in the morning, while masturbating, or with another partner), an organic cause is unlikely.

5. If drugs, alcohol, and medical conditions have been eliminated as possible causes, a sleep laboratory referral should be made to further evaluate the patient for organic causes. Spontaneous erections occur during rapid eye movement (REM) sleep, and their tumescence can be measured.

Some patients with mild organic impairments that cause impotence do have erections during REM sleep.

6. If no erections occur during several nights in which electroencephalogram (EEG)-documented REM periods have occurred, referral to a urologist is indicated. The next procedures to be done include an endocrine workup, penile doppler measurements of the blood flow, and nerve conduction studies.

Table B.83-2
Pharmacological Agents Inplicated In Male Sexual Dysfunction*

Drug	Impairs Erection	Impairs Ejaculation
Psychiatric drugs		
Tricyclic antidepressants†		
Imipramine (Tofranil)	+	+
Protriptyline (Vivactil)	+	+
Desmethylimipramine (Pertofrane)	+	+
Clomipramine (Anafranil)	+	+
Amitriptyline (Elavil)	+	+
Nortripytline (Aventyl)		
Monoamine oxidase inhibitors		
Tranylcypromine (Parnate)	+	
Mebanazine (Actomal)	+	+
Phenelzine (Nardil)	+	+
Pargyline (Eutonyl)	−	+
Isocarboxazid (Marplan)	−	+
Other mood-active drugs		
Lithium (Eskalith)	+	
Amphetamines	+	+
Antipsychotics		
Fluphenazine (Prolixin)	+	
Thioridazine (Mellaril)	+	+
Chlorprothixene (Taractan)	−	+
Mesoridazine (Serentil)	−	+
Perphenazine (Trilafon)	−	+
Trifluoperazine (Stelazine)	−	+
Butaperazine (Repoise)	−	+
Reserpine (Serpasil)	+	+
Haloperidol (Haldol)	−	+
Antianxiety Drugs§		
Chlordiazepoxide (Librium)	−	+
Antihypertensive drugs		
Clonidine (Catapres)	+	
Methyldopa (Aldomet)	+	+
Spironolactone (Aldactone)	+	−
Hydralazine (Apresoline)	+	−
Arramethidine (Ismelin)	+	+
Commonly abused drugs		
Alcohol	+	+
Barbituates	+	+
Cannabis	+	−
Cocaine	+	+
Heroin	+	+
Methadone	+	−
Morphine	+	+

continued

Table B.83–2—*continued*

Drug	Impairs Erection	Impairs Ejaculation
Miscellaneous drugs		
Antiparkinsonian agents	+	+
Clofibrate (Atromid-S)	+	−
Digoxin (Lanoxin)	+	−
Glutethimide (Doriden)	+	+
Indomethacin (Indocin)	+	−
Phentolamine (Regitine)	−	+
Propranolol (Inderal)	+	−

*Both increases and decreases in libido have been reported with psychoactive agents. It is difficult to separate those effects from the underlying condition or from improvement of the condition. Sexual dysfunction associated with the use of a drug disappears when the drug is discontinued.
†The incidence of erectile dysfunction associated with the use of tricyclic antidepressants is low.
§Benzodiazepines have been reported to decrease libido, but in some patients the diminution of anxiety caused by the drugs enhances sexual function.
Table from V A Sadock: Normal human sexuality and sexual dysfunctions. In *Comprehensive Textbook of Psychiatry,* ed 5, H I Kaplan, B J Sadock, editors, p 1045. Williams & Wilkins, Baltimore, 1989. Used with permission.

Table B.83–3
Diagnostic Criteria for Male Erectile Disorder

A. Either (1) or (2):
    (1) persistent or recurrent partial or complete failure in a male to attain or maintain erection until completion of the sexual activity
    (2) persistent or recurrent lack of a subjective sense of sexual excitement and pleasure in a male during sexual activity
B. Occurrence not exclusively during the course of another Axis I disorder (other than a sexual dysfunction), such as major depression.

Table from DSM-III-R *Diagnostic and Statistical Manual of Mental Disorders,* ed 3, revised. Copyright American Psychiatric Association, Washington, 1987. Used with permission.

7. Surgical placement of a penile prosthesis is a drastic course. Such prostheses are either semirigid or inflatable. Possible problems include infection, perforation, pain, and urinary retention. Often, the prostheses are not sexually satisfying for the partner.

8. Revascularization of the penis is an additional experimental treatment for impotence caused by vascular disease. Another proposed treatment is electrical stimulation of the penis.

DRUG TREATMENT

For impotence with an organic cause, invasive treatments can be considered, including the injection of vasoactive substances into the cavernosa of the penis. The drugs used most often are a combination of papaverine (Cerespan) and phentolamine (Regitine). Priapism and venous sclerosis are possible complications. Other drugs that have been considered are vasoactive intestinal polypeptide, phenoxybenzamine (Dibenzyline), and gonadotropin-releasing hormone (which is inhaled). Yohimbine (Yocon) may sometimes be of use in treating psychotropic-drug-induced impotence.

Cross-References:
Alcohol intoxication, anger, anxiety, depression, homosexual panic, marital crisis.

84 / Incest

Incest is sexual activity (for example, fondling and coitus) between close blood relatives or family members (father-daughter, mother-son, siblings, stepparent-stepchild).

CLINICAL FEATURES AND DIAGNOSIS

Incest victims are usually female. The most commonly reported type of incest is father-daughter (75 percent of cases). Sibling incest is reported less often but may be just as common. Mother-son incest is the least common. The true prevalence of incest is unknown because of underreporting, but more than 10 percent of all women may have been victims of sexual abuse or incest. Families of low socioeconomic status may be less able to conceal incest than are families of higher status. Coitus occurs in about half of all incest cases. Homosexual incest (father-son and mother-daughter) is very rare; in those cases the father may not be otherwise homosexual and may be having sex with a daughter, as well as with a son.

In virtually all societies, parent-child incest is a taboo and indicates a breakdown of normal social and moral behavior. Socialized taboos against incest protect against the biological expression of recessive pathological genes. However, in some societies, brother-sister marriages are sanctioned.

The clinical features associated with the initiators of incest include alcohol abuse, sociopathy, violence, overcrowding, increased physical proximity, rural isolation that prevents extrafamilial contacts, remarriage, intellectual deficiencies, and major mental disorders. Usually, the incestuous father is domineering, potentially violent, and feared, and the mother is passive or disabled and unable to interfere. The parents' relationship is often marked by preexisting sexual discord.

In the typical father-daughter case of incest, the eldest daughter has been close to the father, who begins to approach her sexually at about age 10. Incest is usually identified when the child is 9 to 13 years old and after the sexual relationship has been going on for two to four years. The father becomes alternately and unpredictably parental and sexual with the daughter, leading to confusion about familial roles. The mother may at times be competitive and often refuses to believe the daughter's reports that her father has been approaching her sexually. Her mother may have abandoned the family in some way, often through illness. The siblings sense the special role that the victim has with the father, and they treat her as an outsider. The father, fearful that the incest will be revealed, interferes with his daughter's development of normal social relationships. Girls who have experienced incest have a higher than usual rate of adolescent pregnancy, suicide, and running away. If the victim runs away, the father may begin a sexual relationship with the next youngest daughter.

INTERVIEWING AND PSYCHOTHERAPEUTIC GUIDELINES

If incest is suspected, always interview each family member alone, especially the abused child. Assure the child that he or she is safe and will be protected from possible retribution. The child should know that he or she can safely talk about the incest with professionals in a secure environment. Begin by approaching the topic indirectly. Ask about behaviors specifically, attempting to document precisely what happened. Usually, the parent denies the behavior. Elicit relevant data, including the level of privacy within the home, the nature of the parents' relationship, a parental childhood history of abuse, and embarrassment about the level of physical contact among family members.

Violence, depression, suicidality, somatic complaints, substance abuse, eating disorders, pregnancy, hypersexuality, personality disorders, and dissociative disorders may be related to incestuous experiences. Self-destructive behavior in a child may be a result of incest.

EVALUATION AND MANAGEMENT

1. The primary objective in incest cases is to reveal the fact that incest is occurring. Once the collusion, denial, and fear of other family members have been broken down, awareness and the fear of consequences usually prevent incest from recurring. Pay attention to suicide risk in all incest participants, particularly at the time of disclosure.

2. Examine the patient for bruising and trauma, and check for venereal disease. Follow protocols similar to rape-evidence collection.

3. Involve legal child-protective agencies early to counteract the considerable pressure that will be exerted on the child to recant the story.

4. Evaluate the family members for primary psychiatric disorders that need to be treated. Evaluate siblings for possible victimization.

5. Individual psychotherapy is the preferred treatment for victims; it can be an avenue for the ventilation of anger.

6. Family therapy may help reconstruct a fractured family.

7. Group therapy is sometimes helpful for the survivors of incest who are able to discuss the topic openly in a group. Some groups specifically for female incest survivors help reduce the associated shame and stigma. Other groups are for the mothers of children who were incest victims. Often, the incest led to divorce, and the mothers have prominent feelings of rage and guilt.

8. Teach children clearly and simply that their genitals are their private parts and should not be touched by others, including family members.

DRUG TREATMENT

No specific drug treatment is indicated, although some underlying psychiatric disorders may require drug treatment at a later date.

Cross-References:

Abuse: child, elder, and spouse; anger; homosexual panic; hypersexuality; marital crisis; rape and sexual abuse.

---

85 / Insomnia

Insomnia is difficulty in falling asleep, difficulty in maintaining sleep, or insufficient sleep.

CLINICAL FEATURES AND DIAGNOSIS

Insomnia is a nonspecific symptom, rather than a specific disorder. Although it is the most common complaint presented to any physician, insomnia usually does not receive an adequate workup. Typically, the complaint is rapidly treated with a hypnotic before a sufficient evaluation has been made. Insomnia can be a symptom of many different psychiatric disorders, including depression, mania, anxiety disorders, psychotic disorders, substance abuse, and primary sleep disorders. In the elderly, complaints of insomnia may be secondary to normal age-related changes in sleep architecture. The initial approach should be to describe the course and the severity of the insomnia and its relation to associated factors.

A complaint of insomnia is not clinically important unless there is associated impaired functioning (usually daytime sleepiness). People have individual differences in the amount of sleep they need, and some people are natural short sleepers, so a complaint of too few hours of sleep needs to be related to impaired daytime functioning to be significant. Furthermore, many patients who complain of insomnia, when monitored in a sleep laboratory, actually fall asleep rapidly.

INTERVIEWING AND PSYCHOTHERAPEUTIC GUIDELINES

Diagnose a disorder of initiating and maintaining sleep (DIMS) (Table B.85–1). Take the patient's history of substances taken, including alcohol, caffeine and other stimulants, sedative-hypnotics, and drugs of abuse, virtually all of which can cause insomnia. Prescribed medications, such as bronchodilators, can cause insomnia.

How long has the symptom been present, and what impairment has resulted? Is it related to some change in the environment? Does it occur only at home or only during the week?

Table B.85–1
DIMS: Disorders of Initiating and Maintaining Sleep (Insomnias)

Diagnosis	Signs and Symptoms	Comments	Treatment
Persistent psychophysiological insomnia	Persistent DIMS without drug use or gross psychopathology. Repeated awakenings, anxious dreams, increased muscle activity, rapid pulse rates. Patient may sleep well when away from work, on vacation, or in a new sleep environment.	May be the result of chronic tension, anxiety, negative conditioning to sleep environment, or a combination of the above. Usually diagnosed after eliminating all other possibilities.	Relaxation training, behavior modification, and inculcation of good sleep hygiene (regular bedtime, no stimulants before sleep, good sleep environment)
Insomnia related to anxiety or personality disorder	Persistent DIMS with a diagnosis of neurosis or personality disorder. EEG likely to reveal sleep fragmentation, with decreased slow-wave sleep (SWS) and, to a smaller extent, REM sleep.	Similar to the above, except that the psychiatric symptoms are more prominent. Often the insomnia parallels the severity of the psychiatric symptoms.	Sleep architecture improves with therapy of the underlying psychiatric symptoms. The above treatments may be helpful.
Insomnia related to depression	With diagnosis of depression. Restless, unsatisfying sleep, multiple awakenings, sometimes shortened REM latency. Frequent insomnia in the early morning hours (terminal insomnia). Some depressives, particularly of the bipolar or atypical depressive type, have hypersomnia. Reactive depressives usually have insomnia without shortened REM latency.	Insomnia is common among depressives, especially elderly depressives, who have little or no slow-wave sleep.	Treatments for depression tend to correct sleep architecture.
Insomnia related to mania	Very little sleep (2 to 4 hours), with or without refreshing daytime naps. May not sleep until physically exhausted.	Frequently, the worried family complain of the patient's reduced sleep time.	Treatment for mania tends to correct sleep architecture.
Insomnia related to exacerbation of schizophrenia or functional psychosis	Severe increased sleep-onset latency (SOL) with poor sleep continuity. Patient may not sleep until exhausted.	Sleep may be out of phase with the usual circadian rhythms (inversion of the sleep-wake cycle).	Treatment of the psychosis with antipsychotics tends to correct sleep architecture.

Insomnia related to central nervous system depressants	On drug—decreased ¾, REM, increased ½. Stage demarcations frequently blurred. After a few weeks of use, increased SOL, increased awakenings. On abrupt withdrawal—almost complete disruption of sleep. REM rebound (often nightmares).	Results from tolerance to or withdrawal from drug. More common in elderly or very young. Withdrawal accompanied by restlessness, increased muscle tension, nausea.	Physician-supervised drug withdrawal. In abrupt withdrawal, complete sleep disruption is likely. Disturbed sleep may continue long after drug withdrawal. REM rebound is common in the withdrawal period.
Insomnia related to stimulants	Increased SOL, decreased ¾, decreased REM. Disorders of excessive somnolence (DOES) may develop. The occasional crash is a classic symptom.	Caffeine ingestion late in the day is a common cause. Patient should be checked after complete withdrawal for other sleep pathologies.	Physician-supervised drug withdrawal. In abrupt withdrawal, crashing (hypersomnia) is likely.
Insomnia related to apnea or alveolar hypoventilation	10+-second cessations of breathing. Subsequent awakenings produce sleeplessness.	More commonly associated with DOES Three types: Central apnea—cessation of breathing effort. Upper blockage of airflow in upper air passages—severe snoring; patients often obese. Mixed—central in first stage followed by renewed respiratory effort against a temporary blockage.	Upper and mixed types can be successfully treated with weight loss or tracheostomy. A variety of drugs have been tried for central apnea, with little success. Hypnotic drugs can be detrimental to sleep apnea patients because of respiratory suppression.
Insomnia related to nocturnal myoclonus	Sleep-initiated periodic contractions in hip, leg, ankle, and foot, followed by partial or complete arousal. Episodes of 10+ seconds' duration. The EEG does not show seizure activity.	Must be differentiated from seizures and from hypnic jerks—gross-motor jerks when falling asleep that are not pathological. Restless legs syndrome may accompany and is characterized by a deep creeping feeling in the legs and the feet.	No wholly satisfactory treatment. Benzodiazepines may relieve symptoms when taken at bedtime. Carbamazepine for restless legs syndrome, but can depress bone marrow function. Oxycodone at bedtime, but is addictive.

Table B.85–1—*continued*

Diagnosis	Signs and Symptoms	Comments	Treatment
Insomnia related to alcohol	Unsatisfying, unrefreshing sleep. Stages 3 and 4 completely absent in chronic alcoholism. REM disrupted and short. Strong REM suppression is the most common characteristic. There may be hypersomnia or terminal insomnia, with increased awakenings in the latter part of the night.	Alcohol is frequently taken to hasten sleep onset, but it seriously disrupts REM, SWS, and sleep architecture.	Supervised withdrawal from alcohol.
Insomnia related to alcohol withdrawal	Dramatically increased SOL, decreased ¾, REM rebound, frequent awakenings, restlessness.	Delirium and hallucinations characteristic of alcohol withdrawal may be present.	Sleep pattern normalizes somewhat in 10 to 14 days. However, sleep may be disturbed (increased awakenings, decreased ¾) for months to years in sober alcoholics.
Insomnia related to medical, neurological, toxic, or environmental conditions	Vary in type and severity. In general, increased SOL, increased awakenings, increased restlessness, and decreased ¾.	Particularly associated with insomnia are conditions with pain, pruritis, fever, dyspnea, and those requiring enforced sleep position (e.g., orthopedic problems).	Treat the underlying disorder if possible. Hypnotics can be helpful for acute illnesses when respiratory suppression is not contraindicated. Long-term use of hypnotics leads to habituation and tolerance and eventually may exacerbate insomnia.

Table adapted from I Karacan, R L Williams, C A Moore: Sleep disorders. In *Comprehensive Textbook of Psychiatry*, ed 5, H I Kaplan, B J Sadock, editors, p 1105. Williams & Wilkins, Baltimore, 1989. Used with permission.

Interview the bed partner about when the patient actually falls asleep. Ask the partner or the patient about related symptoms, such as snoring, gastroesophageal reflux, restless legs, and myoclonic jerks. Does the patient have nocturia secondary to excessive evening fluid intake or urinary tract pathology?

Inquire about sleep hygiene. Is the room comfortable and quiet? Is the bed clean? Does the patient do distracting things in bed, such as watching television, eating, and reading? Are psychologically stimulating situations avoided just before bedtime? Large meals, strenuous exercise, and more than one or two alcoholic beverages should be avoided shortly before bedtime. Does the patient sleep late on weekends, only to be unable to fall asleep Sunday night? If so, that suggests a delayed sleep-wake cycle.

EVALUATION AND MANAGEMENT

1. Do a complete psychiatric evaluation to diagnose depression, mania, anxiety disorders, and psychotic disorders if any are present. The presence of a definitive psychiatric diagnosis suggests specific treatment; insomnia related to an acute exacerbation of schizophrenia is usually treated with antipsychotics, and mania is treated with lithium (Eskalith) or antipsychotics.

2. Could medical conditions be contributing to the insomnia?

3. Instruct patients to wake up at the same time every day, regardless of what time they went to sleep the night before. Although the patients will be sleepy the next day, they will fall asleep easily the next night. That is the best way to prevent delayed sleep-wake schedule disorder (characterized by sleeping late on the weekends).

4. If a definitive diagnosis is not obvious, consider a referral to a sleep laboratory, and have the patient complete a sleep diary over several weeks, including the time to bed, the time asleep, the time awake, naps, activity, and important events.

DRUG TREATMENT

In general, if the insomnia is brief (less than three weeks), a trial of hypnotics may be appropriate. If the insomnia is chronic, avoid hypnotics, and make a definitive diagnosis. The contraindications for hypnotics also include heavy snoring, other signs of sleep apnea, and possible dependence, tolerance, or abuse of sedative-hypnotics. If psychosis is present, consider prescribing an antipsychotic. Otherwise, benzodiazepines are usually the hypnotics of choice, because they have a wider therapeutic index, less enzyme induction, and lower dependence potential than do barbiturates.

The choice of benzodiazepine depends on the route of metabolism and the elimination half-life. Treat initial insomnia without daytime anxiety with short-acting benzodiazepines—for example, triazolam (Halcion) 0.125 mg, temazepam (Restoril) 15 mg, and estazolam (ProSom) 1 mg. Middle insomnia or early-morning awakening may require a long-acting benzodiazepine, such as those used to treat insomnia with prominent daytime anxiety—for example, diazepam (Valium) 5 mg, flurazepam (Dalmane) 15 mg, and quazepam (Doral) 7.5 mg.

Start with the lowest dose and increase the dosage until it produces an effect. Most patients respond to any benzodiazepine if the dosage is increased sufficiently. When an effective dosage is reached, do not increase it further. Loss of efficacy at that dosage indicates tolerance and requires a drug washout. Inform patients that, after stopping the drug, they will have one to two weeks of rebound insomnia, which is not an indication for continued drug treatment.

The frequency of hypnotic use should be not more than three out of four nights, and the duration of use should not exceed several months.

Cross-References:

Alcohol withdrawal, anxiety, cocaine intoxication and withdrawal, delusional disorder, depression, mania, opioid intoxication and withdrawal.

---

86 / Intermittent Explosive Disorder

Intermittent explosive disorder, also called episodic dyscontrol syndrome, is found in persons who have discrete episodes of loss of control of aggressive impulses, resulting in serious assaultive acts or the destruction of property.

CLINICAL FEATURES AND DIAGNOSIS

Sometimes the term "epileptoid personality" is used for the seizurelike quality of the aggressive episodes, which are not characteristic of the patient's usual behavior. Related symptoms and signs may include an aura, changes in the sensorium, increasing tension before the violent act, hypersensitivity to sound or light, amnesia, and nonspecific electroencephalographic (EEG) abnormalities.

Intermittent explosive disorder is more common in men than in women, and it usually begins before age 30. The men are often described as physically large but psychologically dependent, with threatened masculinity. The patient often witnessed parental violence in childhood. Usually, a history of family instability includes such problems as alcohol abuse, promiscuity, a poor work history, child abuse, and spouse abuse. The patient may have a history of pathological alcohol intoxication or disinhibition after taking other central nervous system (CNS) depressants.

The diagnostic criteria for intermittent explosive disorder are given in Table B.86–1.

Table B.86–1
Diagnostic Criteria for Intermittent Explosive Disorder

A. Several discrete episodes of loss of control of aggressive impulses resulting in serious assaultive acts or destruction of property.

B. The degree of aggressiveness expressed during the episodes is grossly out of proportion to any precipitating psychosocial stressors.

C. There are no signs of generalized impulsiveness or aggressiveness between the episodes.

D. The episodes of loss of control do not occur during the course of a psychotic disorder, organic personality syndrome, antisocial or borderline personality disorder, conduct disorder, or intoxication with a psychoactive substance.

Table from DSM-III-R, *Diagnostic and Statistical Manual of Mental Disorders,* ed 3, revised. Copyright American Psychiatric Association, Washington, 1987. Used with permission.

INTERVIEWING AND PSYCHOTHERAPEUTIC GUIDELINES

The patient is usually remorseful about the episode and should be approached with support and understanding. Focus on the explosive episodes as specific targets of treatment.

Psychotherapy with these patients is difficult, dangerous, and often unrewarding, as the therapist may have difficulties with countertransference and limit setting. Group psychotherapy may be of some help, as may family therapy, particularly when the explosive patient is an adolescent or a young adult.

EVALUATION AND MANAGEMENT

Rule out antisocial and borderline personality disorders, organic personality disorder and other organic mental disorders, psychotic disorders, conduct disorder, mental retardation, and intoxication. In personality disorders, maladaptive behaviors are present between episodes. Psychotic disorders are usually easily differentiated from intermittent explosive disorder by psychotic symptoms and other mental status abnormalities. Conduct disorder shows a repeated pattern, rather than distinct episodes. Organic mental disorders—including brain tumor, epilepsy, and metabolic disorders—must be ruled out. Intoxication with alcohol or sedative-hypnotics can lead to disinhibition and episodic violence. Intoxication with hallucinogens, cocaine, and other psychostimulants must also be considered.

DRUG TREATMENT

In the midst of an aggressive episode, the patient must be physically restrained. Administer an antipsychotic medication—for example, fluphenazine (Prolixin), trifluoperazine (Stelazine), thiothixene (Navane), or haloperidol (Haldol), all given at 5 mg by mouth or intramuscularly, repeated in 30 minutes if necessary.

There is no general consensus about drug treatment. Anticonvulsants, antipsychotics, antidepressants, and lithium (Eskalith) have all been reported to be helpful. Benzodiazepines have also been used but may cause disinhibition through a paradoxical reaction. Propranolol (Inderal) has also been used.

Cross-References:

Abuse: child, elder, and spouse; borderline personality disorder; epilepsy; hospitalization; intoxication; violence.

---

87 / Intoxication

Intoxication is defined as maladaptive behavior—such as belligerence, impaired judgment, or impaired social or occupational functioning—associated with recent substance ingestion.

CLINICAL FEATURES AND DIAGNOSIS

A substance-specific syndrome may be observed in some patients that will help in making the diagnosis. See Table B.87–1 for the diagnostic criteria for intoxication.

INTERVIEWING AND PSYCHOTHERAPEUTIC GUIDELINES

The mental status of intoxicated patients changes as the substance is cleared. But potentially dangerous patients require immediate evaluation, even though they may be completely different several hours later. Always consider the possibility that multiple substances have been taken. Assume that the patient is minimizing the amount of substance taken and the frequency and the duration of substance abuse.

Be reassuring and give the patient the sense that the environment is under control and that limits have been set, at least temporarily, on their use of alcohol or drugs.

Constantly consider possible medical complications of either acute or chronic intoxication (for example, central nervous system [CNS] or respiratory depression after the use of opioids, barbiturates, or sedative-hypnotics and seizures and cardiac arrhythmias after the use of cocaine).

EVALUATION AND MANAGEMENT

1. Obtain the patient's vital signs.

2. Look for other obvious signs of intoxication, including ataxia, dysarthria, nystagmus, pupillary changes, CNS depression, and agitation.

3. Consider the possibility of an overdose. Assume that the amount of substance taken has been underrepresented. Also consider the possibility of polysubstance intoxication or overdose.

4. Look for withdrawal symptoms. Patients who are intoxicated on alcohol or a sedative-hypnotic may also have withdrawal symptoms if the amount taken on an ongoing basis has been recently decreased.

Table B.87–1
Diagnostic Criteria for Intoxication

A. Development of a substance-specific syndrome due to recent ingestion of a psychoactive substance. (**Note:** More than one substance may produce similar or identical syndromes.)

B. Maladaptive behavior during the waking state due to the effect of the substance on the central nervous system (e.g., belligerence, impaired judgment, impaired social or occupational functioning).

C. The clinical picture does not correspond to any of the other specific organic mental syndromes, such as delirium, organic delusional syndrome, organic hallucinosis, organic mood syndrome, or organic anxiety syndrome.

Table from DSM-III-R, *Diagnostic and Statistical Manual of Mental Disorders,* ed 3, revised. Copyright American Psychiatric Association, Washington, 1987. Used with permission.

5. Rapidly assess the patient for dangerousness, and prevent harm to the patient and to others. Physical restraints and involuntary hospitalization are sometimes necessary. Restraints should be used with caution, particularly in phencyclidine (PCP) intoxication, in which patients are at risk for rhabdomyolysis.

6. Evaluate and treat the patient's medical problems.

7. Provide an environment appropriate to the substance ingested—for example, minimize stimulation after PCP use but provide interactive support after lysergic acid diethylamide (LSD) use.

8. Allow the substance to clear, and reevaluate when the patient is no longer intoxicated. A patient intoxicated on multiple substances with different pharmacokinetic actions may be clearing one substance (such as alcohol) while the blood level of another substance (such as a barbiturate) is rising.

DRUG TREATMENT

Drug treatment depends on the substances taken and the patient's clinical needs. If tranquilization is needed, benzodiazepines are preferable to antipsychotics; benzodiazepines raise the seizure threshold, but antipsychotics lower the seizure threshold. In general, avoid medications of any type if possible.

Cross-References:

Alcohol intoxication; barbiturate and similarly acting sedative, hypnotic, or anxiolytic intoxication and withdrawal; blackouts; cannabis intoxication; cocaine intoxication and withdrawal; hallucinogen hallucinosis; opioid intoxication and withdrawal; phencyclidine or similarly acting arylcyclohexylamine intoxication; psychotropic drug withdrawal.

88 / Jaundice

Jaundice (also called icterus) is a yellow pigmentation of the skin caused by deposits of bilirubin.

CLINICAL FEATURES AND DIAGNOSIS

Jaundice may be detected as yellowing of the sclera or as darkening of the urine. In patients who are taking chlorpromazine (Thorazine), another phenothiazine, or a cyclic antidepressant, obstructive jaundice may be an allergic reaction to the drug.

Some phenothiazines reported to cause jaundice include chlorpromazine, promazine (Sparine), thioridazine (Mellaril), prochlorperazine (Compazine), and fluphenazine (Prolixin). Nonphenothiazine antipsychotics, such as haloperidol (Haldol), have not been associated with jaundice.

Jaundice develops during the first month of drug treatment and is often preceded by a flulike syndrome. The liver is not inflamed, and liver function tests indicate a cholestatic type of jaundice (increased direct-indirect bilirubin ratio, increased alkaline phosphatase, and absence of prominent elevation of serum glutamic-oxaloacetic transaminase [SGOT] and serum glutamic-pyruvic transaminase [SGPT]). The syndrome usually resolves after several weeks, but it can in rare cases have a long-term course.

INTERVIEWING AND PSYCHOTHERAPEUTIC GUIDELINES

Reassure the patient that the symptom is probably due to the drug, that it will resolve within a few weeks, and that a complete return to normal is expected.

EVALUATION AND MANAGEMENT

1. Consider other causes of jaundice, such as hepatitis. Perform a physical examination, including the liver. Obtain blood tests, including a complete blood count (CBC), and liver function tests. The CBC often shows eosinophilia in chlorpromazine-induced jaundice.

2. Check the result of baseline liver function tests if they are available.

3. Get a medical consultation to rule out other possible causes of jaundice.

4. Discontinue the drug. Patients with jaundice should avoid alcohol.

DRUG TREATMENT

If the patient still requires medication for a psychiatric condition, consider changing to a different drug. Nonphenothiazine antipsychotics may be substituted for phenothiazines. Jaundice requires no specific drug treatment.

Cross-References:

Alcohol intoxication, schizophrenia, volatile nitrates, Wernicke's encephalopathy.

89 / Korsakoff's Syndrome

Korsakoff's syndrome (also called alcohol amnestic disorder) is an amnestic syndrome caused by thiamine (vitamin B₁) deficiency related to long-standing severe alcohol dependence and general nutritional deficiency. It often follows an acute episode of Wernicke's encephalopathy (confusion, ataxia, nystagmus, ophthalmoplegia), which is also due to thiamine deficiency. Wernicke's encephalopathy, the acute stage of the syndrome, usually has an abrupt onset; Korsakoff's syndrome has a slow onset and a chronic course. Once Korsakoff's syndrome emerges, the prognosis is poor; only 20 percent of patients make a substantial recovery. Thus, any manifestation of Wernicke's encephalopathy must be treated immediately.

CLINICAL FEATURES AND DIAGNOSIS

In Korsakoff's syndrome the patient has an irreversible short-term memory impairment in the presence of a clear sensorium. The syndrome is associated with confabulation (the filling in of memory deficits with false information). Since the disorder usually occurs in persons who have been drinking heavily for many years, it rarely occurs before the age of 35. Postmortem brain biopsies often reveal bilateral structural lesions in the mamillary bodies.

INTERVIEWING AND PSYCHOTHERAPEUTIC GUIDELINES

The patients are generally alert and cooperative but completely disoriented, not knowing the place, the time, or in some cases even their own identities. Be calm, supportive, and empathic, as the patients can be severely confused and vulnerable.

EVALUATION AND MANAGEMENT

1. Prompt diagnosis and treatment is crucial.
2. Thiamine treatment improves the ocular symptoms, the ataxia, and the confusional symptoms within days.
3. The administration of carbohydrates (including IV dextrose) before thiamine replacement has been reported to worsen the patient's symptoms. Therefore, give thiamine first to all alcoholic and nutritionally deficient patients before starting any other treatment.
4. Institute an adequate diet.

DRUG TREATMENT

Treatment includes immediate thiamine supplementation—often 50 mg intravenously (IV) and 50 mg intramuscularly (IM), followed by 50 to 100 mg IM or by mouth each day until the patient is eating regularly.

No specific drug treatment is indicated other than thiamine. If severe agitation or confusion makes the patient unmanageable, a short-acting benzodiazepine—for example, lorazepam (Ativan) 0.5 to 1 mg by mouth or IM—or a high-potency antipsychotic—for example, haloperidol (Haldol) or fluphenazine (Prolixin), both given at 1 to 2 mg by mouth or IM—may be used.

Cross-References:

Alcohol dementia, amnesia, confusion, Wernicke's encephalopathy.

90 / Leukopenia and Agranulocytosis

Both leukopenia and agranulocytosis are characterized by a decreased number of white blood cells (WBC) in the peripheral blood. *Leukopenia* is defined as fewer that 3,500 WBC per cubic millimeter, with a granulocyte count of fewer than 1,500 per cubic millimeter (granulocytopenia). *Agranulocytosis* is defined as fewer than 500 granulocytes per cubic millimeter.

CLINICAL FEATURES AND DIAGNOSIS

Leukopenia is a relatively common and benign side effect of drugs, but agranulocytosis is potentially fatal, as the patient is vulnerable to bacterial infection. Patients taking psychotropic drugs in whom leukopenia develops should be monitored closely for continued decreases in the WBC count that can lead to agranulocytosis.

Drugs that can cause leukopenia and agranulocytosis include antipsychotics, tricyclic antidepressants, and carbamazepine (Tegretol). Many patients taking those drugs have their WBC fall to between 3,500 and 5,000 and then fluctuate. That condition is usually clinically benign.

Drug-induced leukopenia and agranulocytosis usually resolve after the causative drug has been discontinued. The key objective is to identify the problem early, before the patient is overcome by infections. Often, patients with agranulocytosis present with high fever and are severely ill with pharyngitis and oral or perianal ulcerations. In those patients the offending drug must be discontinued, and the patient must be referred for a medical consultation immediately.

Phenothiazines

Between 5 and 15 percent of patients treated with phenothiazines experience leukopenia, which is usually benign but requires monitoring. About 1 of every 1,000 patients taking phenothiazines have agranulocytosis. The risk is greatest for the elderly and for women. Phenothiazine-induced agranulocytosis usually occurs in the first three to five weeks of treatment, and 90 percent of cases occur in the first eight weeks.

Clozapine

Clozapine-induced agranulocytosis is not related to the dosage or to the patient's age. It is rare in the first four weeks of treatment and is most likely to occur between the 5th and the 25th week of treatment. That fact suggests that patients can be given a four-week trial of clozapine with only a minimal risk of agranulocytosis. Only patients who are improving should be continued into the period of increased risk. Patients taking clozapine should have their WBC measured weekly, even if they have no leukopenia.

INTERVIEWING AND PSYCHOTHERAPEUTIC GUIDELINES

Patients with possible leukopenia or agranulocytosis must understand that those conditions are potentially dangerous side effects of their medications. Encourage them to seek medical attention and to have a complete blood count (CBC) for even minor infections, such as a cold. Do not allow the patients to minimize the significance of the problem. Engage the patients' family members, if necessary, to ensure cooperation with medical follow-up.

EVALUATION AND MANAGEMENT

1. If the WBC falls below 3,500, follow the WBC with a differential white blood cell count three times a week.

2. Monitor the patient closely for signs of infection. Check the CBC in any antipsychotic-treated patient who has a fever or a sore throat during the first eight weeks of treatment (the period when the effect usually occurs with phenothiazines).

3. In cases of leukopenia, immediately discontinue clozapine and other drugs. Usually, leukopenia does not progress to agranulocytosis.

4. Consult a hematologist. Bone marrow biopsy may help if the cause of the agranulocytosis is unclear or if it continues after the offending drug has been discontinued.

5. If the WBC falls below 1,000 or if the granulocytes count falls below 500, place the patient in reverse isolation—that is, protected from infection.

DRUG TREATMENT

Use antibiotics to treat the infections as indicated by culture and sensitivity results. Institute other supportive treatment as necessary. If drug treatment is absolutely necessary for behavioral control, use a short-acting benzodiazepine—for example, lorazepam (Ativan) 1 to 2 mg by mouth or intramuscularly (IM), oxazepam (Serax) 10 to 30 mg by mouth, or alprazolam (Xanax) 0.5 to 1 mg by mouth, all given every four hours as needed.

Cross-Reference:

Schizophrenia.

91 / Lithium Toxicity

Lithium toxicity is produced by an excess of lithium (Eskalith). The toxic state affects the central nervous system (CNS), thyroid, kidneys, gastrointestinal (GI) system, and metabolic system.

CLINICAL FEATURES AND DIAGNOSIS

Peak serum lithium levels are reached about two hours after ingestion (four hours after ingesting controlled-release preparations); consequently, the peak is usually over by the time the patient comes to clinical attention. The elimination half-life of lithium is about 22 hours, and excretion is almost completely renal.

Lithium levels are increased by dehydration, low salt intake, decreased fluid intake, thiazide diuretics, and many nonsteroidal anti-inflammatory drugs. Lithium side effects are common, but most do not lead to emergencies. The side effects include mild tremor, hypothyroidism, polyuria, polydipsia, nausea, vomiting, diarrhea, weight gain, leukocytosis, acne, psoriasis, hypercalcemia, elevated serum magnesium, and hyperparathyroidism. Long-term administration of lithium can cause impaired renal concentrating ability, diabetes insipidus, and possibly renal failure.

INTERVIEWING AND PSYCHOTHERAPEUTIC GUIDELINES

Reassure the patient that mild lithium toxicity is usually benign. Questions concerning fluid and salt intake may clarify the cause of mild toxicity. However, lithium overdose in a suicide attempt is a toxicological emergency that may require dialysis. Immediately estimate the dose of lithium taken. When the amount taken was considerably more than the patient's daily dose, get an immediate blood lithium level and a medical consultation if the level is more than 2.0 mEq/L or if the patient shows signs of deterioration in mental functioning.

EVALUATION AND MANAGEMENT

1. Obtain a serum lithium level, and test for electrolytes, blood urea nitrogen (BUN), creatinine, complete blood count, and thyroid functions, including thyroid-stimulating hormone (TSH). Obtain two blood lithium levels over several hours to assess whether the levels are rising or falling.

2. Perform a neurological examination. The acute toxic effects of lithium primarily affect the brain. The early signs include dysarthria, ataxia, a mild fine tremor, and neuromuscular irritability. Severe intoxication may produce a severe tremor, delirium, impaired consciousness, seizures, coma, and death.

3. For mild cases, consider decreasing the lithium dosage or changing the schedule of drug administration.

4. Check the results of thyroid function tests, including TSH, and examine the patient for goiter. Mild abnormalities in thyroid function without clinical hypothyroidism (chemical hypothyroidism) are common. Whether those abnormalities should be treated is controversial. Clinical hypothyroidism can be treated with supplemental thyroid hormone.

5. If polyuria is present (daily urine output greater than three liters), determine if lithium-induced diabetes insipidus is present. Maintain adequate fluid intake, decrease the lithium dosage, change the dosage schedule to a single bedtime dose, and consider treatment with a thiazide or potassium-sparing diuretic (which will treat the diabetes insipidus).

6. Hydration (intravenous normal saline) and diuresis with osmotic or loop diuretics (for example, furosemide [Lasix] or ethacrynic acid [Edecrin]) may be effective for mild cases of intoxication.

7. Hemodialysis is rapidly effective in reducing the serum lithium level but may need to be repeated, since tissue stores of lithium may cause a rebound in the serum lithium level. Clinical improvement may lag for days after hemodialysis.

8. Electrocardiographic (ECG) monitoring is indicated in severe cases. Lithium generally causes only mild reversible ECG abnormalities (for example, inverted or isoelectric T waves), but arrhythmias and conduction delays have been reported.

9. Evaluate for lithium overdose secondary to a suicide attempt.

DRUG TREATMENT

Decrease the lithium dosage or discontinue lithium if side effects are a clinical problem. Generally, try to obtain the lowest possible lithium level that is still effective. Changing the drug schedule to a single dose at bedtime may create peak serum levels during sleep that make mild side effects less bothersome.

If thiazide diuretics are needed, use a low lithium dosage, and follow the lithium levels and electrolytes closely. Tremor can be treated with β-blockers—for example, propranolol (Inderal).

Cross-References:

Mania, tremor.

92 / Malingering

Malingering is the voluntary production of false or grossly exaggerated symptoms to achieve some clearly identifiable objective.

CLINICAL FEATURES AND DIAGNOSIS

The external motivations for malingering can be put into three categories: (1) to avoid responsibility, danger, or punishment; (2) to receive compensation, free room and board, or drugs; and (3) to retaliate after a loss. Malingering can be differentiated from factitious disorders by the presence in malingering of a clearly definable objective for the symptoms. In factitious disorders, the symptoms are intentionally produced to assume the sick role in the absence of other clearly defined objectives. With somatoform and conversion disorders, the symptoms are not produced intentionally.

Malingering is common, especially in such settings as prisons, the military, and industrial settings. Malingering may be more common in men than in women; it is common in adults with antisocial personality disorder and in children and adolescents with conduct disorder.

The first goal is to recognize malingering, so that unnecessary treatments are avoided. Malingering should be suspected in any patient who presents in a medicolegal situation, who has a marked discrepancy between the subjective complaints and the objective findings, who is noncompliant with diagnostic procedures or treatment, or who has antisocial personality disorder.

The symptoms are often vague, subjective, poorly localized, and impossible to measure objectively. Typical symptoms include pain in the head, the neck, the chest, or the back; dizziness; amnesia; loss of vision or sensation; fainting; seizures; and hallucinations and other psychotic symptoms. The patient often becomes angry if the doctor questions the symptom. Malingerers may also cause self-inflicted injuries, may stage an injury or an accident to obtain compensation, and may tamper with data or records to support a false complaint. Malingerers may show *Vorbeireden*, in which they give approximate answers to questions when feigning psychiatric illness (for example, $2 + 2 = 5$ or identifying a blue chair as red).

Sometimes, patients with true disease feign more severe symptoms than they actually have, which makes the proper identification difficult (Table B.92-1).

INTERVIEWING AND PSYCHOTHERAPEUTIC GUIDELINES

With suspected malingerers, maintain a neutral attitude, and avoid being confrontational. Give the patients at least the same evaluation and respect that you would give any other patient. In fact, when you suspect malingering, your initial response should be to make a careful clinical evaluation to verify your suspicions and to rule out any genuine disease. Casually observing the patients may reveal behavior that is inconsistent with their complaints (for example, they may easily bend at the waist, despite complaints of severe back pain, or they may laugh and joke with other patients, despite somber complaints of depression during the interview).

Table B.92-1
Features of Malingering Usually Not Found in Genuine Illness

Symptoms are vague, ill-defined, overdramatized, and not in conformity with known clinical conditions.

The patient seeks addicting drugs, financial gain, the avoidance of onerous (e.g., jail) or other unwanted conditions.

History, examination, and evaluative data do not elucidate complaints.

The patient is uncooperative and refuses to accept a clean bill of health or an encouraging prognosis.

The findings appear compatible with self-inflicted injuries.

History or records reveal multiple past episodes of injury or undiagnosed illness.

Records or test data appear to have been tampered with (e.g., erasures, unprescribed substances in urine).

Table by Arthur T. Meyerson, M.D.

EVALUATION AND MANAGEMENT

1. Begin by assuming that the complaints are genuine, and rule out medical and psychiatric diseases.

2. Be suspicious of patients presenting in medicolegal situations and patients who have been noncompliant with treatment.

3. Order laboratory tests and other diagnostic tests as appropriate for the complaints.

4. If malingering is suspected, be sure that a legitimate condition has not been overlooked before confronting the patient.

5. Attempt to make a definitive psychiatric diagnosis. Often, malingerers fulfill the diagnostic criteria for antisocial personality disorder, borderline personality disorder, or psychoactive substance abuse disorder. They should be differentiated from patients with somatoform disorders and factitious disorders.

6. When sufficient data have been collected, tell the patient that no medical intervention is indicated. Many patients leave at that point. Suggest that the symptoms are a way of dealing with some other problem in the patient's life, and offer help in coping.

7. Do not treat a condition that does not exist or give in to a malingerer's demands for verification of a desired diagnosis. Do not offer any type of placebo treatment (for example, vitamins), since doing so only leads to further complications. Avoid admitting malingerers to the hospital, since hospitalization only reinforces the behavior. However, if it appears that the malingerer will escalate into truly dangerous self-destructive acts unless hospitalized, hospitalization should be considered.

DRUG TREATMENT

No drug treatment is indicated in this condition.

Cross-References:

Blindness, borderline personality disorder, group hysteria.

93 / Mania

Mania is a distinct episode of abnormally and persistently elevated, expansive, or irritable mood. The abnormal mood has led to impaired judgment and has caused a marked impairment in the patient's functioning. The most important task in treating a manic episode is to recognize it.

CLINICAL FEATURES AND DIAGNOSIS

Psychotic symptoms may be present. If they are present, the patient's delusions are often grandiose or paranoid and may also be mood-incongruent. The diagnostic criteria for mania are given in Table B.93–1.

Mania usually occurs in the context of bipolar disorder, schizoaffective disorder, and organic mood disorders. Unipolar mania is less common than bipolar disorder. Mania can be precipitated by electroconvulsive therapy, antidepressant medications, and other medications. In a single clinical evaluation of a psychotic patient, mania may be indistinguishable from schizophrenia, and the proper diagnosis must be based on the patient's history.

The lifetime prevalence of bipolar disorder is about 1 percent, and the disorder is found equally in men and women. Without treatment, a manic episode usually lasts from three to six months.

INTERVIEWING AND PSYCHOTHERAPEUTIC GUIDELINES

Manic patients may be initially entertaining and charming, but they can become annoying, irritating, and inescapable. Their behavior may be unpredictable, and violence can occur. Set firm limits early with manic patients, and do not allow them to exploit or take advantage of you. Manic patients are highly distractable; therefore, provide a nonstimulating environment for the interview.

EVALUATION AND MANAGEMENT

1. Maintain a secure environment that will prevent flight, and be sure that enough staff members are available if restraint is required.

2. Take the patient's vital signs. Agitation from other causes (such as an organic disorder) may be mistaken for mania. Manic patients may also have medical conditions as a result of their poor judgment. Intoxication with drugs or withdrawal from alcohol may be present.

3. Observe the patient for signs of organic disorders, drug intoxication, or the side effects of prescribed medications. Antipsychotic-induced akathisia may cause restlessness or agitation.

4. Order laboratory tests, including a complete blood count (CBC), thyroid function tests, a urine toxicology screen, a chemistry profile, hepatic

Table B.93–1
Diagnostic Criteria for Manic Episode

Note: A manic syndrome is defined as including criteria A, B, and C below. A hypomanic syndrome is defined as including criteria A and B, but not C (i.e., no marked impairment).

A. A distinct period of abnormally and persistently elevated, expansive, or irritable mood.

B. During the period of mood disturbance, at least three of the following symptoms have persisted (four if the mood is only irritable) and have been present to a significant degree:
  (1) inflated self-esteem or grandiosity
  (2) decreased need for sleep (e.g., feels rested after only three hours of sleep)
  (3) more talkative than usual or pressure to keep talking
  (4) flight of ideas or subjective experience that thoughts are racing
  (5) distractibility (i.e., attention too easily drawn to unimportant or irrelevant external stimuli)
  (6) increase in goal-directed activity (either socially, at work or school, or sexually) or psychomotor agitation
  (7) excessive involvement in pleasurable activities which have a high potential for painful consequences (e.g., the person engages in unrestrained buying sprees, sexual indiscretions, or foolish business investments)

C. Mood disturbance sufficiently severe to cause marked impairment in occupational functioning or in usual social activities or relationships with others, or to necessitate hospitalization to prevent harm to self or others.

D. At no time during the disturbance have there been delusions or hallucinations for as long as two weeks in the absence of prominent mood symptoms (i.e., before the mood symptoms developed or after they have remitted).

E. Not superimposed on schizophrenia, schizophreniform disorder, delusional disorder, or psychotic disorder NOS.

F. It cannot be established that an organic factor initiated and maintained the disturbance. **Note:** Somatic antidepressant treatment (e.g., drugs, ECT) that apparently precipitates a mood disturbance should not be considered an etiologic organic factor.

Table from DSM-III-R, *Diagnostic and Statistical Manual of Mental Disorders,* ed 3, revised. Copyright American Psychiatric Association, Washington, 1987. Used with permission.

and renal function tests (blood urea nitrogen [BUN] and creatinine), and an electrocardiogram (ECG).

5. Perform a mental status examination and obtain a psychiatric history. Focus on identifying clear previous episodes of mania and depression to determine the presence of bipolar disorder. If psychotic symptoms were present for two or more weeks with no disturbance in mood, consider a diagnosis of schizoaffective disorder.

6. Correct thyroid problems and other medical problems if present. A complete, detailed physical examination should be performed as soon as the patient can cooperate.

DRUG TREATMENT

Lithium (Eskalith) is the treatment of choice for acute mania. However, lithium requires 7 to 10 days before it is effective. Carbamazepine (Tegretol) and valproic acid (Depakene) are also effective. Antipsychotics are rapidly effective and commonly used, but their use should be discouraged because of their side effects, such as tardive dyskinesia. Carbamazepine has an onset of action comparable to that of the antipsychotics. Benzodiazepines—for example, lorazepam (Ativan) and clonazepam (Klonopin)—are also effective and may be used for acute agitation or to augment the antipsychotics.

The drug treatment of mania should provide behavioral control. Lithium, carbamazepine, and valproic acid are used for maintenance, but they are usually not initiated in emergency settings because of their delayed onset, the need for baseline laboratory data, and the need for the patient's cooperation.

If agitation or hyperactivity requires tranquilization, avoid antipsychotics. Start with a benzodiazepine—for example, lorazepam 1 to 2 mg by mouth or intramuscularly (IM) as needed or clonazepam 1 to 2 mg by mouth as needed. Repeat the benzodiazepine as needed until the patient's agitation is reduced or until the signs of benzodiazepine intoxication occur (ataxia, slurred speech, nystagmus). Disinhibition caused by benzodiazepines may be indistinguishable from worsening mania. If the patient becomes increasingly agitated, discontinue the benzodiazepine immediately. Manic patients who are also substance abusers may be particularly nonresponsive to benzodiazepines or may require very high doses.

If the patient is benzodiazepine-intoxicated and still agitated or otherwise appears to be unresponsive to the benzodiazepine, discontinue that drug and give an antipsychotic. All the antipsychotics are equal in terms of their eventual antimanic efficacy. Many psychiatrists prefer to use high-potency antipsychotics—for example, fluphenazine (Prolixin) or haloperidol (Haldol), both given at 5 mg by mouth three times a day or 5 mg IM every four hours as needed—because those drug cause few anticholinergic and hypotensive side effects. Titrate the dosage according to the patient's response. Antipsychotics, other than clozapine (Clozaril), may be augmented with benzodiazepines for acute agitation to avoid exposure to high dosages of antipsychotics. If the patient is already taking lithium and is in outpatient treatment, check with the outpatient physician. If a current or recent lithium level is below the therapeutic level, consider discharging the patient back to outpatient care after raising the lithium dosage and giving the patient adjunctive medication—for example, lorazepam 1 to 2 mg by mouth every four to six hours. Use that treatment only in patients who are firmly engaged in outpatient follow-up and who have adequate support systems.

Cross-References:

Agitation, anxiety, chronic schizophrenia in acute exacerbation, cocaine intoxication and withdrawal, depression, hospitalization, intoxication, lithium toxicity, restraints.

---

94 / Marital Crisis

A *marital crisis* is a serious conflict in which one or both members of a marriage present for help.

CLINICAL FEATURES AND DIAGNOSIS

The common precipitants of marital crisis include the discovery of an extramarital affair, the announcement of an intended divorce, separation, financial problems, work problems, alcohol or drug abuse, depression or other mental illnesses, and physical illnesses. The precipitants may affect either spouse or a child.

The goals are a thorough evaluation of the spouses and a referral for appropriate treatment.

INTERVIEWING AND PSYCHOTHERAPEUTIC GUIDELINES

Interview each member of the couple individually, in addition to seeing them together. Other family members may provide other information. In addition to evaluating the marital problem, screen both spouses for individual psychiatric disorders that may be factors in the marital problem.

EVALUATION AND MANAGEMENT

1. Interview each spouse separately.

2. Perform a complete mental status examination. Obtain a psychiatric history for each spouse, and identify any psychiatric conditions present. Depression, dementia, psychosis, or a medical illness in one spouse may be a precipitant of marital crisis.

3. Obtain a detailed marital, sexual, and financial history. Inquire about both heterosexual and homosexual extramarital affairs. Ask about sexual problems in the marriage, financial conflicts, and disagreements about child rearing and other tasks requiring decision making. Ask about the family and personal histories of divorce, the ages and situations of the children (are any leaving home?), and any chronic or acute medical problems that have destabilized the marital relationship. Complaints of impotence or anorgasmia usually suggest deeper problems. How are conflicts between the spouses resolved? How well do the spouses communicate?

4. Evaluate the couple for domestic violence and suicidality.

5. Refer one or both spouses for appropriate treatment of individual conditions.

6. Determine whether the marital problem is related to a specific circumscribed stress or conflict (for example, child rearing) or is a ubiquitous problem in communication. Well-circumscribed problems in a basically good marriage may be suitable for marriage counseling; pervasive problems require marital therapy. Marital therapy focuses on restructuring the relationship between the partners, improving communication, and exploring the psychodynamics of each spouse. Many types of marital therapies are available, including individual, conjoint (both partners present), four-way (with two therapists), group (with several other couples), and combinations of those types.

DRUG TREATMENT

No specific drug treatment is indicated. Patients with anxiety, depression, psychosis, or psychoactive substance abuse may require specific drug treatment.

Cross-References:

Abuse: child, elder, and spouse; agitation; anxiety; depression; grief and bereavement; impotence; incest; intermittent explosive disorder; rape and sexual abuse.

---

95 / Mercury Poisoning

Mercury poisoning is an organic mental disorder produced by long-term exposure to mercury or the ingestion of a large quantity of mercury. Long-term exposure can lead to personality changes, such as irritability, quarrelsomeness, loss of temper, depression, and chronic fatigue.

CLINICAL FEATURES AND DIAGNOSIS

Mercury poisoning causes an encephalopathy with a predilection for the cerebellum. Ataxia, tremor, and involuntary movements may be prominent and are usually permanent. Peripheral neuritis may also appear. When ingested, mercury is highly corrosive and can produce severe inflammation of the mouth, pharynx, and larynx; abdominal cramps; nausea; vomiting; and a severe enteritis, with bloody diarrhea. Hepatic injury is a delayed effect. Poisoning can also occur after the inhalation of mercury vapors. Mercury is concentrated in the kidneys and causes renal failure. The ingestion of 0.1 g of mercury can cause toxic symptoms, and the ingestion of 0.5 g is usually fatal.

INTERVIEWING AND PSYCHOTHERAPEUTIC GUIDELINES

High-risk groups include thermometer workers, photoengravers, ore workers, laboratory workers, fingerprinters, chemical workers, repairers of electrical meters, and workers in the felt hat industry. The long-term use of mercury-containing vaginal douches is another source of exposure. Explain to the patient that appropriate treatment measures will be taken which are often effective.

EVALUATION AND MANAGEMENT

1. After ingestion, remove mercury by gastric lavage.
2. Blood mercury levels of more than 0.03 μg/mL or urine mercury levels of more than 25 μg/L are abnormal and suggest exposure to mercury. Blood

levels of more than 1.0 μg/mL cause symptoms of acute poisoning in most patients.

DRUG TREATMENT

Chelating agents bind mercury, form nontoxic stable molecules, and are excreted safely through the kidneys. Rapidly treat acute mercury poisoning with British anti-Lewisite (BAL). In chronic mercury poisoning, N-acetyl-penicillamine, which binds mercury selectively without depleting copper, is the drug of choice and can be administered orally.

Cross-References:

Bromide intoxication, confusion, delirium, delusions.

---

96 / Mitral Valve Prolapse

Mitral valve prolapse is a bulging of the mitral valve into the left atrium during systole.

CLINICAL FEATURES AND DIAGNOSIS

Mitral valve prolapse produces a midsystolic click and a systolic murmur (systolic click-murmur syndrome). The condition is associated with symptoms of panic disorder. It is more common in females than in males, especially between the ages of 14 and 30 years; the patients are often tall and thin. Asymptomatic mitral valve prolapse may be present in as many as 10 percent of the females between 14 and 30 years. It is commonly found in patients with connective tissue diseases, such as Marfan's syndrome. It is usually a benign finding, but it may be associated with mitral regurgitation that is significant enough to cause ventricular hypertrophy.

The symptoms of mitral valve prolapse are similar to those of panic disorder and include chest pain, palpitations, tachycardia, dyspnea, extrasystoles, weakness, fatigue, dizziness, syncope, and anxiety. Perhaps up to one half of all patients who have panic disorder have mitral valve prolapse. The symptoms are thought to be related to arrhythmias. Treatment includes β-blockers and antiarrhythmics if arrhythmias are present.

The diagnosis is confirmed by echocardiography. An electrocardiogram (ECG) typically shows biphasic or inverted T waves in leads II, III, and aVF. Mitral valve prolapse is considered to be an associated feature of panic disorder, although some cardiologists consider it the cause of panic disorder. However, in some patients, the mitral valve prolapse is caused by hemodynamic factors associated with panic attacks. In those patients, when the panic disorder is treated, the mitral valve prolapse also resolves.

INTERVIEWING AND PSYCHOTHERAPEUTIC GUIDELINES

Mitral valve prolapse and panic disorder may be indistinguishable from the patient's history alone. In fact, many patients have both conditions. Consider mitral valve prolapse in the differential diagnosis of paniclike symptoms, and proceed with an appropriate medical workup, even though the patient may be young and generally healthy. Anxiety is usually prominent. Be calm and reassuring. The disorder need not interfere with any of the patient's activities of daily living. Anxiety superimposed on a cardiac condition can increase the possibility of arrhythmias and angina.

EVALUATION AND MANAGEMENT

1. Consult a cardiologist. An electrocardiogram and an echocardiogram are noninvasive parts of the workup.

2. Order thyroid function tests—triiodothyronine (T_3), thyroxine (T_4), T_3 resin uptake (T_3RU), and thyroid stimulating hormone (TSH). Thyrotoxicosis can produce symptoms identical to those of mitral valve prolapse.

3. Obtain the patient's vital signs, and order screening tests—complete blood count (CBC), a chemistry profile, and liver and renal function tests—before initiating any drug treatments.

4. Behavioral treatment, such as in vivo exposure, is effective in panic disorder.

DRUG TREATMENT

β-Blockers—for example, propranolol (Inderal)—are helpful in mitral valve prolapse but are usually not completely effective in panic disorder. Many mitral valve prolapse patients also fulfill the diagnostic criteria for panic disorder. Panic disorder can be treated with benzodiazepines (for example, alprazolam [Xanax] and clonazepam [Klonopin]), tricyclic antidepressants (for example, imipramine [Tofranil]), monoamine oxidase inhibitors (MAOIs) (for example, phenelzine [Nardil]), and serotonergic agents.

Cross-References:

Anxiety, cardiac arrhythmia, panic disorder, syncope.

97 / Mutism

Mutism is the absence of speech in a person capable of speaking. Elective mutism is an uncommon childhood disorder in which the child refuses to speak in certain settings. However, the common emergency presentation of mutism is in adults, in whom it can be symptomatic of a wide range of disorders, including malingering.

CLINICAL FEATURES AND DIAGNOSIS

The diagnosis of elective mutism in children is relatively straightforward, as the parents report that the child is able to talk normally at home. The child may follow directions or give other evidence of comprehension in the clinical setting, even if the child remains mute with the examiner.

The onset of mutism in children is usually between ages 5 and 6 years. Girls are affected more often than boys. The children typically talk only with the nuclear family at home.

In adults, mutism may be one aspect of severe psychomotor retardation in depression. The mute patients often visibly struggle to produce responses, then seemingly tire and abandon the effort. When the attempted interview is terminated, they may cling imploringly to the examiner and try again. They may lack the energy to express thoughts or have slowed thinking.

Schizophrenia may also present with mutism. As with depression, the patients may exhibit poverty of thought or a lack of energy or motivation. Schizophrenic persons may be too frightened of others to speak, may be completely preoccupied by internal stimuli, may have bizarre grandiose beliefs about themselves that entail silence, or may be paralyzed by ambivalence.

Other involuntary causes include certain drug intoxications, notably phencyclidine (PCP) and hallucinogens. Mutism may also occur as a symptom of a conversion disorder.

Mutism may be voluntarily produced to gain admission to a hospital or to delay release from a hospital. Particularly with patients from other cultures, the combination of a language barrier, unusual behavior in public, mistrust, the wish to avoid psychiatric attention or labeling, and perhaps personality factors may result in mutism with no other mental disorder.

INTERVIEWING AND PSYCHOTHERAPEUTIC GUIDELINES

The mute patient is likely to be frustrating. Time and patience is the key to obtaining data from mute patients. It may take hours or days to identify a patient, contact collateral sources of information, or otherwise obtain a history. Try a variety of approaches to find something about which the patient is able or willing to converse. Frequent brief contacts may be more useful than long frustrating interviews. In general, simple concrete questions yield more information than do complex open-ended questions. Providing food or fluids gives the opportunity for social contact, a demonstration of concern, and observation. The nursing and social work staff members may be less threatening and more successful than the physicians. Surreptitious observation is important, as patients often socialize with peers, seeming to be normal until the examiner appears.

EVALUATION AND MANAGEMENT

1. The management of mutism depends on the cause. Depressed patients require support for nourishment and hydration. Schizophrenic patients may require encouragement for basic self-care. Catatonic patients should be

closely observed, as dangerous periods of excitement may suddenly occur. Restraints may be necessary in such cases.

2. If mute patients require admission to a hospital, they usually require involuntary admission, as competence cannot be established. For patients who are voluntarily mute, the condition usually ceases to be a problem at some point simply because of the difficulty of remaining mute.

DRUG TREATMENT

Mute depressed patients may be psychotically depressed. Psychotic depression often requires both antipsychotic and antidepressant medications. The antipsychotic drugs, such as fluphenazine (Prolixin), trifluoperazine (Stelazine), or haloperidol (Haldol), all given at 2 to 5 mg a day, may be used. Explain the prescribed treatment, even if the patient is unresponsive. If the patient passively accepts treatment, that is probably adequate. If the patient actively refuses medication, involuntary treatment may be necessary.

Drug psychoses may also be managed with benzodiazepines; lorazepam (Ativan) 1 to 2 mg by mouth or intramuscularly (IM) or oxazepam (Serax) 10 to 30 mg by mouth may be given at one-hour intervals.

If no progress is made with other techniques and sufficient time has elapsed to reduce the likelihood of malingering, an amobarbital (Amytal) interview may yield results.

Cross-References:

Aphasia, brief reactive psychosis, catatonia, catatonic schizophrenia, confusion, depression, malingering, restraints, schizophrenia.

---

98 / Narcolepsy

Narcolepsy is characterized by the symptom tetrad of (1) excessive daytime somnolence, (2) cataplexy, (3) sleep paralysis, and (4) hypnagogic hallucinations.

CLINICAL FEATURES AND DIAGNOSIS

Excessive daytime somnolence is considered the primary symptom of narcolepsy. It is distinguished from fatigue by irresistible sleep attacks of short duration—that is, less than 15 minutes.

Cataplexy is brief (seconds to minutes) episodes of muscle weakness or paralysis with no loss of consciousness. It is often triggered by laughter or anger.

Sleep paralysis is a temporary partial or complete paralysis that most commonly occurs on awakening. The patient is conscious but unable to move. Sleep paralysis generally lasts less than one minute.

Hypnagogic hallucinations are dreamlike experiences during the transition from wakefulness to sleep.

INTERVIEWING AND PSYCHOTHERAPEUTIC GUIDELINES

Explain the disorder to the patient, especially the relation between sleep attacks and strong emotion. Memory problems may occur, and the patient needs reassurance that the disorder is treatable.

EVALUATION AND MANAGEMENT

1. Many people are chronically sleepy because they do not get enough nocturnal sleep.
2. A multiple sleep latency test is used as a diagnostic tool.
3. Differentiate narcolepsy from (1) sleep apnea, (2) nocturnal movement disorders (myoclonus and restless legs syndrome), (3) the effects of drugs and alcohol, and (4) atypical depressions.
4. Advise the patient to have a regular bedtime and to take daytime naps.
5. Safety considerations, such as driving cautiously and avoiding sharp edges on furniture, are also advised.

DRUG TREATMENT

Tricyclics and monoamine oxidase inhibitors are used for rapid eye movement (REM)-related symptoms, mainly cataplexy.

Stimulants for daytime sleepiness are also used, such as dextroamphetamine (Dexedrine) 10 to 40 mg a day by mouth or methylphenidate (Ritalin) 10 to 40 mg a day by mouth.

Cross-References:

Cataplexy, catatonia, hallucinations, syncope, temporal lobe epilepsy.

---

99 / Neologisms (New Words)

A *neologism* is a new word created by the patient. Neologisms are often condensations of two or more other words.

CLINICAL FEATURES AND DIAGNOSIS

Neologisms occur in patients with such psychotic disorders as schizophrenia and in patients with aphasia.

Neologisms are a single symptom and must be placed in the context of a complete mental status examination. Schizophrenic patients often have neologisms that are fixed and consistent. The error in language may reflect a fixed delusional system and, thus, may not change over time and may not be associated with other language abnormalities. In contrast, a patient with Wernicke's aphasia frequently develops new neologisms and has other language comprehension impairments.

INTERVIEWING AND PSYCHOTHERAPEUTIC GUIDELINES

Thoroughly evaluate the patient's overall language functioning. Perform a mental status examination, and assess the patient for such psychotic symptoms as hallucinations and delusions, which may help confirm a diagnosis of a psychotic disorder.

EVALUATION AND MANAGEMENT

1. Determine whether the symptoms and any associated psychotic symptoms are new or old.

2. If the symptoms are new, is there an identifiable stressor or precipitant?

3. Is there reason to suspect an organic cause (for example, drug intoxication, head trauma, central nervous system [CNS] lesion, or epilepsy)?

4. Do other signs suggest a functional psychotic disorder?

5. Usually, neologisms are not a specific complaint of the patient but, rather, are noticed by others. The definitive treatment is based on the diagnosis.

DRUG TREATMENT

Drug treatment depends on the definitive diagnosis.

Cross-References:

Aphasia, chronic schizophrenia in acute exacerbation, delusional disorder, hallucinations, illusions.

---

100 / Neuroleptic Malignant Syndrome

Neuroleptic malignant syndrome is an uncommon but dangerous toxic syndrome associated with antipsychotic treatment. Its symptoms include muscle rigidity, dystonia, akinesia, mutism, obtundation, and agitation.

CLINICAL FEATURES AND DIAGNOSIS

Neuroleptic malignant syndrome is characterized by fever (up to 107°F), marked to severe lead-pipe rigidity, autonomic instability (tachycardia, labile blood pressure, diaphoresis), and impaired consciousness. Severe rigidity can lead to rhabdomyalosis and subsequent myoglobinuria and renal failure. Other complications include venous thrombosis, pulmonary embolism, shock, and death. The mortality may be as high as 20 percent.

Neuroleptic malignant syndrome usually occurs within the first few days of starting an antipsychotic or increasing the dosage. The majority of cases occur in the first 10 days of antipsychotic treatment. Neuroleptic malignant syndrome may be most likely in patients taking high dosages (or rapidly increasing dosages) of high-potency antipsychotics. Other risk factors include dehydration, a young age (20 to 40 years), being male, malnourishment, and the use of restraints. The full syndrome usually develops within 48 hours of its onset. Incidence estimates range from 1 to 10 in 10,000 episodes of antipsychotic treatment. The disorder can also occur when the patient is withdrawn from dopaminergic agonists—for example, carbidopa (Sinemet), levodopa (Larodopa, Dopar), amantadine (Symmetrel), and bromocriptine (Parlodel). Concomitant treatment with lithium (Eskalith) and an antipsychotic has been associated with several cases of neuroleptic malignant syndrome.

INTERVIEWING AND PSYCHOTHERAPEUTIC GUIDELINES

Patients with neuroleptic malignant syndrome are in the midst of a medical emergency and may require admission to an intensive care unit (ICU). The patient's consciousness is impaired. Apprise friends and family members of the patient's progress.

EVALUATION AND MANAGEMENT

1. Consider neuroleptic malignant syndrome as a possibility in any patient taking an antipsychotic who has fever and rigidity.

2. If the patient's mild rigidity does not respond to conventional anticholinergic agents—for example, benztropine (Cogentin) 2 mg by mouth or intramuscularly (IM)—and if the fever does not have an obvious origin, a provisional diagnosis of neuroleptic malignant syndrome is warranted.

3. Discontinue the patient's prescribed antipsychotic immediately.

4. Monitor the patient's vital signs frequently.

5. Order the needed laboratory tests. Creatine phosphokinase (CPK) is usually markedly elevated and is directly related to the severity of the neuroleptic malignant syndrome. Leukocytosis is also common. Also order routine blood tests, including a complete blood count (CBC) with differential white blood count, a chemistry profile, a test for blood urea nitrogen (BUN) and creatinine, and liver function tests.

6. Emergency cooling with an ice bath or evaporative cooling helps reduce the patient's fever. Antipyretics are not usually useful.

7. Vigorous hydration may prevent shock and decrease the likelihood of renal impairment.

8. Neuroleptic malignant syndrome usually lasts about 15 days. After recovery, the difficult decision remains of whether to reinstitute an antipsychotic agent. Conventional clinical wisdom suggests trying an antipsychotic of a different class and potency, but the benefits must be weighed against the risk of not using the original antipsychotic, which may have been effective.

DRUG TREATMENT

Anticholinergics and benzodiazepines are generally not effective in neuroleptic malignant syndrome. Dantrolene (Dantrium) 1 mg per kilogram four times a day or 1 to 5 mg per kilogram intravenously (IV) directly prevents the contraction of the skeletal muscles and may prevent rigidity and myoglobinuria. Bromocriptine—2.5 to 5 mg by mouth three times a day through a nasogastric tube and repeated if not effective, up to 60 mg a day—is a dopaminergic agonist that may help reduce the severity of the syndrome. Other supportive treatments and close monitoring are indicated. The patient often needs treatment in an intensive care unit.

Cross-References:

Catatonia, catatonic schizophrenia, coma, hyperthermia, serotonin syndrome.

---

101 / Nitrous Oxide Intoxication

Inhaling nitrous oxide produces euphoria. Nitrous oxide (laughing gas) is used by anesthesiologists, nurse anesthetists, and dentists as an anesthetic. It is also used to provide the pressure needed for whipped cream, so it can be inhaled from whipped cream cans, and it can be purchased at restaurant supply stores in the small pressurized canisters (whippets) used to make whipped cream. Nitrous oxide is not a controlled drug.

CLINICAL FEATURES AND DIAGNOSIS

The typical abuser of nitrous oxide usually falls into one of two categories: (1) an anesthesiologist, an anesthetist, a dentist, a nurse, or a paraprofessional who has access to nitrous oxide tanks used for anesthesia; and (2) an adolescent who inhales nitrous oxide from whippets or whipped cream cans. The abusers may use nitrous oxide occasionally, with only minimal or no impairment in functioning.

The abuser exhales as much air as possible, inhales as much nitrous oxide as possible in a full breath, and then holds it in as long as possible. Masks are used to breathe in nitrous oxide from tanks; whipped cream cans are held upright without shaking to allow the gas to be released; and whippets are opened in a special device that releases the gas into a balloon or a bottle, from which the gas is inhaled.

The onset of the euphoria is rapid and is associated with a tingling throughout the entire body and, eventually, numbness. The effects usually wear off within several minutes. Nitrous oxide is often abused with cannabis or alcohol. Repeated rapid inhalation can lead to the loss of consciousness, but that effect usually requires a constant supply from a tank, a mask, or someone to hold the mask in place as the abuser passes out.

INTERVIEWING AND PSYCHOTHERAPEUTIC GUIDELINES

Patients are rarely intoxicated by the time they come to clinical attention. Carefully evaluate the patient for the use of other drugs and alcohol. Evaluate the patient for possible personality disorders and other psychiatric disorders.

EVALUATION AND MANAGEMENT

1. Obtain the patient's history of the frequency and the quantity of nitrous oxide taken and the use of other drugs of abuse, such as alcohol, cannabis, cocaine, and intravenous drugs. Physicians and nurses should be asked about the use of pharmaceutical drugs (for example, prescription opioids, stimulants, barbiturates, and benzodiazepines), which may have been taken from the hospital's supplies.

2. Evaluate the patient for other psychiatric conditions.

3. The nitrous oxide intoxication resolves rapidly, and usually no further short-term treatment is necessary.

4. Detoxification and drug rehabilitation are usually not needed unless other drugs are also being abused.

DRUG TREATMENT

No specific drug treatment is available.

Cross-References:

Intoxication, toluene and other inhalant intoxication and withdrawal, volatile nitrates.

---

102 / Nocturia

Nocturia is excessive urination at nighttime.

CLINICAL FEATURES AND DIAGNOSIS

Occasional awakening to urinate may be normal, but nocturia can be caused by any medical condition in which urinary output exceeds bladder capacity and by some psychiatric and neurological conditions. Any medical condition that can cause polyuria can cause nocturia, including diabetes mellitus, diabetes insipidus (including lithium-induced nephrogenic diabetes insipidus), primary polydipsia (excessive water drinking), drugs (for example, diuretics), and many types of renal disease. Polyuria that is not due to excessive water intake implies impaired renal-concentrating ability. Seizure disorders can cause nighttime incontinence.

INTERVIEWING AND PSYCHOTHERAPEUTIC GUIDELINES

The two most important clinical objectives are to identify the possible presence of renal disease and to determine if primary polydipsia is the cause of the polyuria. Patients who voluntarily drink excessive amounts of water daily may be difficult to differentiate from patients with diabetes insipidus. Explain to the patient that this condition is treatable.

EVALUATION AND MANAGEMENT

1. Order laboratory tests, including routine urinalysis, urine osmolality, blood chemistries, complete blood count, serum osmolality, thyroid function tests, electrocardiogram, and electroencephalogram.

2. Identify the drugs the patient is taking. Lithium (Eskalith), phenytoin (Dilantin), and propoxyphene (Darvon) can cause nephrogenic diabetes insipidus.

3. Obtain a medical consultation.

4. Perform a complete psychiatric evaluation of patients in whom a clear medical cause is not identified. Primary polydipsia may be a sign of a psychotic disorder (for example, certain schizophrenic patients suffer from water intoxication), obsessive-compulsive disorder, or an organic disorder.

5. Advise the patient to stop drinking anything four hours before bedtime if nocturia is due to excessive nocturnal fluid intake.

DRUG TREATMENT

No specific drug treatment exists. Some patients benefit from imipramine (Tofranil) 50 to 100 mg at bedtime because of its anticholinergic side effects.

Cross-References:

Bed-wetting, chronic schizophrenia in acute exacerbation, obsessions and compulsions.

---

103 / Nutmeg Intoxication

Nutmeg contains myristicin, an hallucinogen. It may be taken by adolescents seeking intoxication. Occasionally, *nutmeg intoxication* occurs accidentally when excessive amounts of nutmeg are used in baking a pie.

CLINICAL FEATURES AND DIAGNOSIS

Nutmeg intoxication is characterized by agitation, severe headaches, hallucinations, flushing, palpitations, and numbness in the extremities that occur after the ingestion of a large amount of nutmeg.

INTERVIEWING AND PSYCHOTHERAPEUTIC GUIDELINES

Reassure the patient that the symptoms of intoxication will resolve in several hours.

EVALUATION AND MANAGEMENT

1. Take the patient's vital signs. If the results are elevated, follow the patient until the signs are normal.

2. Evaluate the patient fully for signs of the abuse of other drugs, although such signs are unlikely in cases of accidental overdose.

3. The symptoms usually resolve without treatment after several hours, but observation may be needed if the patient's vital signs do not return to normal.

DRUG TREATMENT

No specific drug treatment is available. Severe anxiety or agitation may be treated with a benzodiazepine—for example, alprazolam (Xanax) 0.5 to 1 mg by mouth, lorazepam (Ativan) 1 to 2 mg by mouth or intramuscularly (IM), oxazepam (Serax) 10 to 30 mg by mouth, or estazolam (ProSom) 0.5 to 1 mg by mouth.

Cross-References:

Agitation, anxiety, hallucinations, intoxication.

---

104 / Obsessions and Compulsions

An *obsession* is a pathological, persistent, recurrent, and irresistible idea, thought, or impulse that cannot be eliminated from consciousness by logic or reasoning. A *compulsion* is a pathological, repetitive, and unwanted need to perform an act, often in response to an obsession. The failure to perform a compulsive act leads to anxiety.

CLINICAL FEATURES AND DIAGNOSIS

Common obsessions include disgust with bodily wastes and secretions, dirt, germs, contamination, or toxins; the fear that something terrible may happen; the need for symmetry, order, or exactness; excessive praying or religious thoughts; the belief in lucky and unlucky numbers; and forbidden sexual thoughts. Common compulsions include excessive hand washing, showering, bathing, toothbrushing, and grooming; repeated rituals; checking doors, locks, stove, and car brakes; cleaning to remove contaminants; touching; ordering and arranging; counting; hoarding and collecting; and measures to prevent harm to oneself or others.

The diagnostic criteria for obsessive-compulsive disorder are given in Table B.104–1.

INTERVIEWING AND PSYCHOTHERAPEUTIC GUIDELINES

Focus on the patient's specific obsessional thoughts and compulsive behaviors. Ask about the frequency of the compulsive behavior, the time spent obsessing, and the consequent impairments. Inquire about related obsessions and compulsions that are different from the one initially identified; many patients have multiple related obsessions and compulsions. Patients recognize the irrationality of their obsessions and compulsions and see them as a source of anxiety, so address the patients directly and openly. Reassure the patients that they are not going crazy and that treatment is available.

EVALUATION AND MANAGEMENT

1. Quantify the obsessions and the compulsions in terms of their type, number, and frequency; the time spent obsessing or doing compulsive behaviors; and the impaired functioning.

2. Complete a mental status evaluation to screen for other disorders, including depression (present in 50 percent of patients with obsessive-compulsive disorder), schizophrenia, and phobias. The differential diagnosis between phobias and obsessive-compulsive disorder is often difficult, but phobic patients are usually much more successful at avoiding the stimulus than are obsessive-compulsive patients.

3. Behavior therapy is thought to be the treatment of choice, with in vivo exposure (flooding), desensitization, thought stopping, implosion therapy, and aversive conditioning as possible choices. Behavior therapy requires considerable commitment on the part of the patient. Often, the patient is forcibly prevented from carrying out the compulsive act and learns that the consequent anxiety or panic will eventually lessen.

4. Insight-oriented psychotherapy is used by some clinicians for obsessive-compulsive disorder but usually in combination with medication.

5. Family therapy helps the patient's family cope with the patient's impaired functioning and can minimize the usual marital stress.

6. For patients who do not respond to any other treatments, psychosurgery (bilateral leukotomies that produce lesions in the thalamofrontal connections) may be effective.

DRUG TREATMENT

Clomipramine (Anafranil), a tricyclic antidepressant, is a potent inhibitor of serotonin reuptake and is a drug of first choice. Fluoxetine (Prozac), paroxetine (Paxil), and sertraline (Zoloft) are also effective. The medications should be prescribed in connection with ongoing treatment and are unlikely to be initiated in the emergency room. If the patient comes to the emergency room or doctor's office in an acutely anxious state, a benzodiazepine—for example, alprazolam (Xanax) 0.25 to 1 mg by mouth, clonazepam (Klon-

Table B.104–1
Diagnostic Criteria for Obsessive-Compulsive Disorder

A. Either obsessions or compulsions:

Obsessions: (1), (2), (3), and (4):
(1) recurrent and persistent ideas, thoughts, impulses, or images that are experienced, at least initially, as intrusive and senseless (e.g., a parent's having repeated impulses to kill a loved child, a religious person's having recurrent blasphemous thoughts)
(2) the person attempts to ignore or suppress such thoughts or impulses or to neutralize them with some other thought or action
(3) the person recognizes that the obsessions are the product of his or her own mind, not imposed from without (as in thought insertion)
(4) if another Axis I disorder is present, the content of the obsession is unrelated to it (e.g., the ideas, thoughts, impulses, or images are not about food in the presence of an eating disorder, about drugs in the presence of a psychoactive substance use disorder, or guilty thoughts in the presence of a major depression)

Compulsions: (1), (2), and (3):
(1) repetitive, purposeful, and intentional behaviors that are performed in response to an obsession, or according to certain rules or in a stereotyped fashion
(2) the behavior is designed to neutralize or to prevent discomfort or some dreaded event or situation; however, either the activity is not connected in a realistic way with what it is designed to neutralize or prevent, or it is clearly excessive
(3) the person recognizes that the behavior is excessive or unreasonable (this may not be true for young children; it may no longer be true for people whose obsessions have evolved into overvalued ideas)

B. The obsessions or compulsions cause marked distress, are time-consuming (take more than an hour a day), or significantly interfere with the person's normal routine, occupational functioning, or usual social activities or relationships with others.

Table from DSM-III-R, *Diagnostic and Statistical Manual of Mental Disorders,* ed 3, revised. Copyright American Psychiatric Association, Washington, 1987. Used with permission.

opin) 0.5 to 1 mg by mouth, or lorazepam (Ativan) 1 to 2 mg by mouth, all given every four hours as needed—may help reduce the acute anxiety.

Cross-References:

Anxiety, depression, panic disorder, paranoia, phobia.

105 / Opioid Intoxication and Withdrawal

I. OPIOID INTOXICATION

Opioid intoxication follows the recent ingestion, inhalation, or injection of an opioid. It is characterized by drowsiness, euphoria, analgesia, slurred speech, impaired attention, anorexia, decreased sex drive, and hypoactivity.

CLINICAL FEATURES AND DIAGNOSIS

Opioid intoxication can lead to opioid overdose, which can be a life-threatening emergency.

The lifetime risk of opioid dependence is 0.7 percent in the United States. The opioids include opium derivatives and synthetic drugs: opium, morphine, diacetylmorphine (heroin, smack, horse, dope), methadone, codeine, oxycodone (Percodan, Percocet), hydromorphone (Dilaudid), levorphanol (Levo-Dromoran), pentazocine (Talwin), meperidine (Demerol), and propoxyphene (Darvon). Table B.105–1 lists the duration of action of several opioids.

The route of administration depends on the drug. Opium is smoked. Heroin is typically injected (intravenously [IV] or subcutaneously) or snorted; it may be combined with stimulants (cocaine or amphetamine) for intravenous injection (speedball) to reduce sedation and increase euphoria. When injected, opioids have an onset of action in approximately five minutes and produce symptoms for up to 30 minutes. Pharmaceutical opioids are typically taken orally. Although injectable pharmaceutical opioids are available, they are less frequently abused than are street drugs because of better monitoring and control of parenteral drug supplies.

The dose of heroin (and other street opioids) is difficult to estimate accurately because the percent concentration of heroin purchased on the street varies unpredictably. Furthermore, the subjective experience of euphoria is influenced by many factors other than drug dosage. The patient may grossly overstate the dose in order to get more methadone.

Typical patients who abuse opioids fall into several categories: the heroin addict is poorly nourished and poorly groomed, antisocial, and often dependent on cocaine, as well as heroin; the opium addict may have been smoking opium for years; the professional patient has gone to many doctors to receive multiple prescriptions for opioids; and the health care professional has access to pharmaceutical opioids.

INTERVIEWING AND PSYCHOTHERAPEUTIC GUIDELINES

In evaluating a patient who has possibly overdosed, initiate medical treatment immediately. When interviewing the patient or family and friends later, remember that the amount (dose) of the drug taken is very unreliable. An overdose commonly occurs when the user unknowingly obtains some heroin that is markedly more potent than were previous batches. Always consider the possibility of an overdose on multiple drugs.

EVALUATION AND MANAGEMENT

1. Take the patient's vital signs.
2. Obtain a complete drug history, including the use of alcohol, prescribed drugs, over-the-counter drugs, and street drugs.
3. Check for past and present medical problems related to drug abuse: For parenteral users, check for acquired immune deficiency syndrome (AIDS), hepatitis, sepsis, cellulitis, osteomyelitis, scars from subcutaneous or intravenous (IV) injection, endocarditis, pulmonary edema, and thrombophlebitis; look for old and new track marks all over the body, including all extremities. For intranasal snorters, check for nasal septum deviation and perforation, nosebleeds, and rhinitis.

Table B.105–1
Duration of Action of Opioids

Drug	Duration of Action
Heroin	3–4 hours
Meperidine	2–4 hours
Morphine, hydromorphone	4–5 hours
Methadone	12–24 hours
Propoxyphene	12 hours
Pentazocine	2–3 hours

4. Obtain a toxicology screen to evaluate the patient for polysubstance abuse.

5. Avoid giving opioids in the emergency room or your office exclusively for the treatment of opioid withdrawal unless absolutely necessary. Distributing opioids in the emergency room or your office rapidly leads to a long line of malingering patients presenting with identical symptoms.

6. Look for objective signs of opioid intoxication, including central nervous system (CNS) depression, decreased gastrointestinal (GI) motility, respiratory depression, analgesia, nausea and vomiting, slurred speech, hypotension, bradycardia, pupillary constriction, and seizures (in overdose). Tolerant patients still have pupillary constriction and constipation.

7. Consider polydrug intoxication and overdose, particularly with alcohol and such sedative-hypnotics as barbiturates and benzodiazepines. In a polydrug overdose, the opioids may be reversed by opiate receptor antagonists—for example, naloxone (Narcan)—leaving just an overdose of alcohol and sedative-hypnotics to be treated. Cocaine intoxication may complicate the clinical picture, but cocaine intoxication is usually brief (several hours).

8. Assess the patient for suicidality and resulting intentional overdose.

9. Admit the patient to an intensive care unit (ICU) for overdose. Give supportive treatments (for example, give IV fluids and maintain the patient's vital signs). If suicidal, the patient may require constant observation to prevent another attempt.

DRUG TREATMENT

If CNS depression, respiratory depression, or other signs of moderate intoxication are present, consider a possible overdose. Give naloxone 0.8 mg IV (0.01 mg per kilogram for neonates), and wait 15 minutes. If the patient shows no response, give another 1.6 mg IV, and wait 15 minutes. If the patient still shows no response, give 3.2 mg IV, and suspect another diagnosis. If the opioid overdose is successfully reversed, continue the naloxone at 0.4 mg an hour IV. If the patient is opioid-addicted, keep the dosage of naloxone to a minimum once the patient is awake to avoid precipitating withdrawal (which recedes when the naloxone wears off). An intentional heroin overdose in a suicide attempt can be potentially fatal, but a more common history is one of accidental overdose, in which the abuser received a bag that was 15 percent heroin instead of the usual 5 percent received for months. An accidental overdose may also occur in naive users and in previously abstinent experienced users who are no longer tolerant.

II. OPIOID WITHDRAWAL

Opioid withdrawal occurs after the cessation or the decrease in the dose of opioid taken by a long-term user. Withdrawal is characterized by a craving for the drug, pupillary dilation, piloerection, sweating, fever, hypertension, insomnia, yawning, and a flulike syndrome with nausea and vomiting, muscle aches, malaise, lacrimation and rhinorrhea, and diarrhea. The presence of opioid withdrawal implies opioid dependence.

CLINICAL FEATURES AND DIAGNOSIS

Opioid withdrawal, although uncomfortable, is not dangerous in patients who are otherwise healthy, although patients in withdrawal may vehemently and dramatically demand that they be treated with opioids.

The objective signs of opioid withdrawal include piloerection, pupillary dilation, tremor, and elevated vital signs (Table B.105–2). The flulike symptoms of withdrawal—myalgias, arthralgias, rhinorrhea, lacrimation, weakness, nausea, and vomiting—are easily faked and are difficult to evaluate objectively. Withdrawal symptoms are more severe for short-acting opioids (for example, heroin and meperidine) than for long-acting drugs (for example, methadone). The onset of withdrawal is directly related to the duration of action of the drug abused. For example, methadone withdrawal begins one to three days after the last dose and lasts 10 to 14 days; heroin withdrawal begins in six to eight hours, peaks at two to three days, and lasts 7 to 10 days (Table B.105–3).

INTERVIEWING AND PSYCHOTHERAPEUTIC GUIDELINES

Patients in opioid withdrawal are agitated and may be confused and demanding. Reassure the patients that their symptoms can be controlled with appropriate medications and that they will not be allowed to suffer or experience pain. Most patients respond to such reassurance. Do not admonish or blame the addicts for bringing on the symptoms by the abusive use of drugs.

EVALUATION AND MANAGEMENT

1. Rely on objective findings (for example, piloerection, pupillary changes, and hypertension), when determining whether withdrawal is present.

2. The main objectives in treating opioid withdrawal are the prevention of medical complications (for example, in medically ill patients) and the reduction of withdrawal symptoms to avoid a return to continued opioid abuse.

Table B.105–2
Diagnosis and Treatment of Opioid Withdrawal

Objective signs of opioid withdrawal
    Pulse 10 beats/min over baseline* or >90 in the absence of a history of tachycardia if the
      baseline is unknown
    Systolic blood pressure >10 mm Hg over baseline or >160/95 in the absence of known
      hypertension
    Dilated pupils
    Sweating, gooseflesh, rhinorrhea, or lacrimation

Treatment
    Administer methadone, 10 mg by mouth every four hours as needed when two of the four
      criteria above are met; decrease by 5 mg/day to zero

*Baseline refers to the patient's vital signs one hour after receiving 10 mg of methadone. For a
patient who has received no methadone, the baseline vital signs should be estimated according
to what one would expect from the patient's age, sex, and general health.
Table from R D Weiss, S M Mirin: Intoxication and withdrawal syndromes. In *Manual of
Psychiatric Emergencies,* ed 2, S E Hyman, editor, p 234. Little, Brown, Boston, 1988. Used with
permission.

Table B.105–3
Withdrawal from Opioid Preparations

	Morphine or Heroin	Meperidine	Methadone
First onset of symptoms (anxiety, drug seeking)	6–8 hours	2–4 hours	1–3 days
Peak withdrawal symptoms	2nd or 3rd day	8–12 hours	Gradual
Duration of withdrawal	7–10 days	4–5 days	10–14 days

Table from P Gillig: Drug abuse. In *Manual of Clinical Emergency Psychiatry,* J R Hillard, editor,
p 221. American Psychiatric Press, Washington, 1990. Used with permission.

    3. Methadone maintenance is the primary long-term treatment for opioid
dependence, and most patients can be maintained on less than 60 mg a
day. Blood methadone levels are helpful in determining the appropriate
dosage. Patients taking methadone may feign symptoms of depression and
request amitriptyline (Elavil), which, when taken with methadone, can produce euphoria.

    4. Naltrexone (Trexan), a long-acting opioid antagonist, can be taken
orally for up to two months to help patients maintain their abstinence from
opioids.

    5. Therapeutic communities (for example, Phoenix House), drug reha-
bilitation programs, and group therapy are all helpful for the rehabilitation
of opioid-dependent patients.

DRUG TREATMENT

    Determine that the objective signs of withdrawal are present and that
the benefits of reducing those signs outweigh the risks of dispensing more
opioids. If so, give methadone 10 mg by mouth, and repeat every four to
six hours if the signs of withdrawal are still present. The total dosage in 24
hours should equal the dosage for the next day (seldom more than 40 mg).

Decrease the dosage by 5 mg daily for heroin withdrawal. Detoxification from methadone may require a slower decrease in the dosage.

Pentazocine-dependent patients should be detoxified on pentazocine because of its mixed agonist-antagonist effects on various opioid receptors.

Clonidine (Catapres) is a centrally acting α_2-agonist that is used primarily for hypertension that may help relieve the patient's nausea, vomiting, and diarrhea. Give 0.1 to 0.2 mg every three hours as needed, but do not exceed 0.8 mg a day; titrate according to the patient's symptoms; and taper over two weeks. Do not give clonidine if the patient's blood pressure is less than 90/60. Clonidine may cause hypotension, is short-acting, and is not habit-forming.

Cross-References:

Anxiety, depression, intoxication, malingering, psychotropic drug withdrawal, suicide.

106 / Pain

Pain is a complex symptom consisting of an unpleasant sensation underlying a potential physical disease and an associated emotional state. *Chronic pain* is pain that persists for more than six months.

CLINICAL FEATURES AND DIAGNOSIS

Pain is a subjective experience that cannot be objectively measured and that is greatly influenced by many factors other than the degree of physical disease or injury. Those factors include the patient's psychological makeup; the presence of depression, anxiety, or psychotic disorders; the reactions elicited in the family, health care providers, the employer, and the rest of the patient's environment; stressors; and the level of distraction by other stimuli. Pain may serve simultaneously as a symptom of stress and as a defense against stress.

A physiological classification of pain is given in Table B.106–1.

Differentiating somatic pain from psychogenic pain is often complex (Table B.106–2). Somatic pain varies with time, the situational stress, the patient's emotional state, and the use of analgesics. A constant pain that is unaffected by anything is often psychogenic. A sudden, dramatic presentation suggests histrionic and borderline personality disorders. If the course of the pain parallels that of depression, psychosis, or anxiety, those psychiatric diagnoses should be made and those conditions treated. If litigation is an issue, reliably evaluating how much of the pain is somatic and how much is psychogenic may not be possible. Malingering, factitious disorders, and drug-seeking behavior in substance abusers must always be ruled out.

Table B.106–1
Physiological Classification of Pain

Type	Subtypes	Examples	Comments
Nociceptive	Somatic Visceral	Bone metastasis Intestinal obstruction	Caused by activation of pain-sensitive fibers; usually aching or pressure
Deafferentiation	Peripheral Central Somatic Visceral Sympathetic- dependent Nonsympathetic- dependent	Causalgia Thalamic pain Causalgia Visceral pain in paraplegics Postherpetic pain Phantom pain	Caused by interruption of afferent pathways. Pathophysiology poorly understood, with most syndromes probably involving both peripheral and central nervous system changes. Usually dysesthetic, often burning and lancinating
Psychogenic	Somatization disorder Psychogenic pain Hypochondriasis Specific pain diagnoses, with organic contribution	Low back pain Atypical facial pain Chronic headache	Does not include factitious disorders—i.e., malingering and Munchausen syndrome

Table from R Berkow editor: *Merck Manual,* ed 15. Merck Sharp & Dohme Research Laboratories, Rahway, N J, 1987. Used with permission.

Table B.106–2
Characteristics of Somatic and Psychogenic Pain

Somatic pain
  Nociceptive stimulus usually evident
  Usually well localized: visceral pain may be referred
  Similar to other somatic pains in patient's experience
  Relieved by anti-inflammatory or narcotic analgesics

Neuropathic pain
  No obvious nociceptive stimulus
  Often poorly localized
  Unusual, dissimilar from somatic pain
  Only partially relieved by narcotic analgesics

Table from E Braunwald, K Isselbacher, R G Petersdorf, J D Wilson, J B Martin, A S Fauci: *Harrison's Principles of Internal Medicine II, Companion Handbook.* McGraw-Hill, New York, 1988. Used with permission. Modified by R Maciewicz, J B Martin.

INTERVIEWING AND PSYCHOTHERAPEUTIC GUIDELINES

Examine the effects that the pain has caused on the patient and the patient's environment. Have family members responded by increasing their care and nurturing? Has the primary physician responded by strengthened efforts to diagnose an unidentified medical condition? Does litigation depend on the patient's disability? Does the patient need to have pain to receive health care attention? Does the administration of analgesics depend on the patient's proving that pain is present, thus causing a battle between the patient and the nursing staff?

Regardless of the quality of the complaint, assume that a somatic cause is present and perform a medical workup.

If the pain appears to be psychogenic, help the patient move past placing the responsibility on the physician to find the cause of the pain. Help the patient take some responsibility for coping with the pain through rehabilitation. Pain patients are sensitive to any implications that the pain is all in their heads, so the approach should be one of focusing on the pain as genuine and working out strategies to cope with the stress created by the pain.

EVALUATION AND MANAGEMENT

1. Perform a complete medical evaluation.

2. Obtain a detailed history of the pain, including the frequency and the duration of past episodes of the pain and the factors that exacerbate or relieve the pain.

3. Administer a complete mental status examination, and obtain a psychiatric history. Evaluate the patient for symptoms of depression, anxiety disorders, psychotic disorders, personality disorders, malingering, and drug-seeking behavior. Evaluate the patient for suicidality, since chronic pain increases the risk of suicide.

4. When medical and psychiatric causes have been ruled out, switch to a rehabilitation approach. Start by discussing the neurophysiological substrates of pain, and work toward explaining how those factors can cause stress, influence behavior, and lead to impairments in functioning.

5. Chronic pain programs are usually best suited for treating patients with chronic pain; they provide medical and psychiatric treatment, individual therapy, group therapy, and rehabilitation programs. Referral to chronic pain programs minimizes the treating physician's frustration and reduces direct conflicts with the patient.

6. Cognitive therapy is often useful. Conventional folk wisdom dictates, "If you think about your pain all the time, you'll make it worse." The cognitive approach expands on that concept. Use relaxation, visual imagery, and other techniques to distract the patient from the pain.

7. Individual psychotherapy is fraught with many obstacles but may be useful in some patients. A short-term problem-oriented supportive approach should focus on bolstering the patient's ego strengths and avoiding conflicts and anxiety.

8. Family therapy is often useful. The family almost always plays an important role in shaping the patient's behavior. Family therapy should focus on changing the pattern of responses to reinforce positive behavior and to ignore negative behavior.

9. Group therapy is helpful and places responsibility on the patient for the management of the pain. However, avoid creating situations in which group members compete to see who can be sicker or learn sick-role behaviors from each other.

10. Use physical therapy as needed.

Table B.106–3
Drugs Used to Relieve Pain

Nonnarcotic analgesics; equivalent doses and intervals

Generic name	Dose (mg)	Interval
Aspirin	750–1250	Every 3 hours
Phenacetin	750–1000	Every 3 hours
Acetaminophen	600–800	Every 3 hours
Phenylbutazone	200–400	Every 4 hours
Indomethacin	50–75	Every 4 hours
Ibuprofen	200–400	Every 4 hours
Naproxen	250–500	Every 4 hours

Narcotic analgesics compared with 10 mg morphine sulfate (MS)

Generic name	IM dose (mg)	Oral dose (mg)	Differences from MS
Oxymorphine	1	6	None
Hydromorphone	1.5	7.5	Shorter acting
Levorphanol	2	4	Good oral-IM potency
Heroin	4		Shorter acting
Methadone	10	20	Good oral-IM potency
Morphine	10	60	
Oxycodone	15	30	Shorter acting
Meperidine	75	300	None
Pentazocine	60	180	Agonist-antagonist
Codeine	130	200	More toxic

Anticonvulsants

Generic name	Oral dose (mg)	Interval
Phenytoin	100	Every 6–8 hours
Carbamazepine	200	Every 6 hours
Clonazepam	1	Every 6 hours

Antidepressants

Generic name	Oral dose (mg)	Range (mg/day)
Doxepin	200	75–400
Amitriptyline	150	75–300
Imipramine	200	75–400
Nortriptyline	100	40–150
Desipramine	150	75–300
Amoxapine	200	75–300
Trazodone	150	50–600

Table from R Maciewicz, J B Martin: Pain: Pathophysiology and management. In E Braunwald, K Isselbacher, R G Petersdorf, J D Wilson, J B Martin, A S Fauci: *Harrison's Principles of Internal Medicine II.* McGraw-Hill, New York, 1988. Used with permission.

11. Use increased sensory stimulation, such as massage, acupuncture, and transcutaneous nerve stimulation.

12. Use biofeedback and relaxation techniques.

13. Nerve blocks differentiate central sources of pain from peripheral sources of pain. Chemical or surgical ablation may follow.

14. Neurosurgery is a last resort, but it has helped some patients, although the relief from pain may also have been caused by the relief of severe depression or a change in personality.

DRUG TREATMENT

Base the drug treatment on as accurate a diagnosis as possible. Undertake drug treatment with the agents in Table B.106–3 as part of a comprehensive, ongoing treatment plan; therefore, the mediations should not be given in the emergency room or your office. Before beginning any drug treatment, decide unequivocally that drug treatment is clearly indicated. Avoid ambivalence in ordering pain medications to minimize undermedicating the patient or setting up situations in which the patient must struggle to receive medication.

In conditions with paroxysmal pain, such as trigeminal neuralgia, try such anticonvulsants as carbamazepine (Tegretol) first, and prescribe the anticonvulsant on a standing basis.

Tricyclic antidepressants are often helpful in chronic pain, regardless of whether they are being used to treat depression or insomnia. The dosage of antidepressant needed is often much less than that typically used for depression—for example, imipramine (Tofranil) or amitriptyline (Elavil), both given at 25 to 100 mg at bedtime.

Nonnarcotic analgesics, such as aspirin and nonsteroidal anti-inflammatory drugs—for example, ibuprofen (Motrin)—are useful and should be given on a standing basis to achieve therapeutic blood levels.

Opioids are effective analgesics but produce rapid tolerance and dependence and should be limited to short-term use. However, if the decision is made to use opioids, a sufficient dosage should be prescribed—that is, a dosage sufficient to cause analgesia. Some chronic pain patients become dependent on opioids and later require detoxification.

Do not give placebos without the patient's agreement. Although placebo analgesic effects have been documented, a more effective treatment should not be withheld, and deception of the patient undermines trust in the physician.

Cross-References:

Agitation, anxiety, depression, headache, hypochondriasis, malingering, opioid intoxication and withdrawal.

---

107 / Panic Disorder

Panic disorder is an anxiety disorder characterized by spontaneous, episodic, and intense periods of anxiety, usually lasting about 30 minutes. These panic attacks usually occur twice a week.

CLINICAL FEATURES AND DIAGNOSIS

The symptoms of panic attacks include palpitations, sweating, shaking, dizziness, shortness of breath, and fear of dying, going crazy, or losing control (Table B.107–1). The lifetime prevalence of panic disorder is be-

Table B.107–1
Diagnostic Criteria for Panic Disorder

A. At some time during the disturbance, one or more panic attacks (discrete periods of intense fear or discomfort) have occurred that were (1) unexpected (i.e., did not occur immediately before or on exposure to a situation that almost always caused anxiety) and (2) not triggered by situations in which the person was the focus of others' attention.

B. Either four attacks, as defined in criterion A, have occurred within a four-week period, or one or more attacks have been followed by a period of at least a month of persistent fear of having another attack.

C. At least four of the following symptoms developed during at least one of the attacks:
   (1) shortness of breath (dyspnea) or smothering sensations
   (2) dizziness, unsteady feelings, or faintness
   (3) palpitations or accelerated heart rate (tachycardia)
   (4) trembling or shaking
   (5) sweating
   (6) choking
   (7) nausea or abdominal distress
   (8) depersonalization or derealization
   (9) numbness or tingling sensations (paresthesias)
   (10) flushes (hot flashes) or chills
   (11) chest pain or discomfort
   (12) fear of dying
   (13) fear of going crazy or of doing something uncontrolled

   Note: Attacks involving four or more symptoms are panic attacks; attacks involving fewer than four symptoms are limited symptom attacks (see agoraphobia without history of panic disorder).

D. During at least some of the attacks, at least four of the C symptoms developed suddenly and increased in intensity within 10 minutes of the beginning of the first C symptom noticed in the attack.

E. It cannot be established that an organic factor initiated and maintained the disturbance (e.g., amphetamine or caffeine intoxication, hyperthyroidism).

Note: Mitral valve prolapse may be an associated condition, but does not preclude a diagnosis of panic disorder.

Table from DSM-III-R, *Diagnostic and Statistical Manual of Mental Disorders,* ed 3, revised. Copyright American Psychiatric Association, Washington, 1987. Used with permission.

tween 1.5 and 2 percent of the population; the disorder is more common in women than in men. The onset is typically in young adulthood.

Agoraphobia, the fear of being in situations from which escape may be difficult if symptoms of anxiety develop, is a common associated syndrome that can occur after repeated panic attacks have left the patient incapacitated or embarrassed.

Mitral valve prolapse is an associated cardiac condition that often presents with symptoms similar to panic disorder. Physical findings in mitral valve prolapse include a midsystolic click and murmur. Mitral valve prolapse is present in up to 50 percent of panic disorder patients.

Panic disorder can be disabling. It may lead to agoraphobia so severe that the patient cannot leave the home. Repeated unsuccessful attempts to seek treatment can lead to depression and a feeling of hopelessness and can place panic disorder patients at increased risk for suicide.

Identify panic disorder as early as possible when patients present with physical symptoms. In the typical case the patient has repeatedly presented to emergency rooms or a doctor's office with physical complaints (for example, chest pain and fainting) only to be told that the findings of the medical workup were normal and that no definitive diagnosis can be made and no treatment recommended.

Panic attacks are believed to be biological events related to excessive noradrenergic discharge from the locus ceruleus. Panic attacks can be provoked by the infusion of lactate, the inhalation of carbon dioxide (CO_2), the administration of yohimbine (Yocon), and other physiological maneuvers. Panic disorder has a genetic component, and first-degree relatives of panic disorder patients have about a 10 times greater chance of having panic disorder than do the general population.

The first few panic attacks are often spontaneous and are not related to any identified stressor, although increased stress during the period preceding the onset of symptoms can often be identified. The panic attack begins with a rapid onset of physical symptoms, leading to a crescendo of overwhelming fear and subsequent behavior to leave the situation and seek help. The entire attack is usually over in about 30 minutes.

After multiple attacks, the patient learns to anticipate the attacks and avoids situations that may precipitate panic (agoraphobia). The avoidance can become crippling, since many of the situations avoided are necessary for normal work and social functioning. Panic disorder patients eventually suffer from the triad of panic attacks, anticipatory anxiety (that is, worrying about having another attack), and agoraphobic avoidance. As a result, they are anxious most of the time.

INTERVIEWING AND PSYCHOTHERAPEUTIC GUIDELINES

Reassure the patient that a diagnosis and a treatment plan can be made. The patients are often demoralized from repeated unsuccessful efforts to seek help. Inform them that help is forthcoming and that the disorder is not imaginary. Emphasize the need for compliance with medication and the benefit from behavioral and other therapies. Encourage the patients to limit or decrease their avoidant behavior, which can escalate rapidly, leading to increased dysphoria.

EVALUATION AND MANAGEMENT

1. Rule out possible medical causes for panic symptoms (Table B.107-2). Include a detailed physical examination; electrocardiogram (ECG); a complete chemistry profile, including electrolytes, calcium, and magnesium; thyroid function tests; a urine toxicology screen; a complete blood count; and liver and renal function tests. An echocardiogram may help diagnose mitral valve prolapse. Order other tests as indicated.

2. Obtain a detailed history of all the patient's medications and drugs, especially caffeine, alcohol, sedative-hypnotics, nicotine, and bronchodilators. Drugs that are central nervous system (CNS) stimulants can precipitate panic attacks, as can withdrawal from drugs that are CNS depressants. Many panic disorder patients also self-medicate with alcohol or sedative-hypnotics.

Table B.107-2
Organic Causes of Panic or Anxiety Symptoms Listed in DSM-III-R

Hyperthyroidism or hypothyroidism
Pheochromocytoma
Fasting hypoglycemia
Hypercortisolism
Intoxication with caffeine, cocaine, amphetamine
Withdrawal from sedative-hypnotics
Seizure of the diencephalon
Pulmonary embolus
Chronic obstructive pulmonary disease (COPD)
Aspirin intolerance
Collagen-vascular diseases
Brucellosis
Vitamin B_{12} deficiency
Multiple sclerosis
Heavy metal intoxication

Table from J R Hillard: Anxiety disorders. In *Manual of Clinical Emergency Psychiatry*, J R Hillard, editor, p 241. American Psychiatric Press, Washington, 1990. Used with permission.

3. Perform a full psychiatric evaluation. Carefully examine the patient for symptoms of depression and for other anxiety disorders (for example, phobias, generalized anxiety disorder, obsessive-compulsive disorder, and posttraumatic stress disorder).

4. Refer the patient for appropriate treatment. If panic disorder is the definitive diagnosis, make a referral to a psychiatrist experienced in the treatment of anxiety disorders. A wide range of approaches are effective.

5. Behavior therapy is an effective treatment for panic disorder, but some patients do not choose that modality because of the high level of commitment required and the high degree of anxiety present during the treatment. The treatment involves repeatedly exposing the patient to those situations that provoke the panic (in vivo exposure) and having the patient endure the symptoms to learn that panic is self-limited. The patient learns strategies to cope other than fleeing the situation. Relaxation techniques may also be of help.

6. Insight-oriented psychotherapy, group therapy, and family therapy are often helpful.

DRUG TREATMENT

Benzodiazepines such as alprazolam (Xanax), clonazepam (Klonopin), and lorazepam (Ativan) are effective in stopping the panic attacks. Start with a low dosage (for example, alprazolam 0.25 to 0.5 mg or lorazepam 1 to 2 mg, both given by mouth every four hours), and increase the dosage as needed until it is clearly effective.

Show the patient early that an effective treatment is available. Many patients carry a benzodiazepine tablet with them and derive considerable relief from simply knowing that it is there, even if they never take it.

The dosage range needed for panic disorder may be relatively higher than the range needed for other conditions (for example, alprazolam 4 to 6 mg a day for panic disorder). Tricyclic antidepressants—for example, imipramine (Tofranil)—are effective, as are monoamine oxidase inhibitors (MAOIs)—for example, phenelzine (Nardil)—and serotonergic agents. Those medications are usually initiated in the context of an ongoing outpatient treatment program, rather than in the emergency room. Buspirone (BuSpar) is not effective for panic disorder.

Cross-References:

Agitation; agoraphobia; alcohol withdrawal; anxiety; barbiturate and similarly acting sedative, hypnotic, or anxiolytic intoxication and withdrawal; depression; hyperventilation; intoxication; mitral valve prolapse; obsessions and compulsions; pain; suicide.

108 / Paranoia

Paranoia is a general term used to describe a range of thinking and behavior, from normal suspiciousness to systematized persecutory delusions.

CLINICAL FEATURES AND DIAGNOSIS

Paranoia is a nonspecific symptom that can be present in personality disorders, delusional disorders, other psychotic disorders, (for example, schizophrenia, mania, and psychotic depression), and other acute psychotic states (for example, toxic and other organic psychoses and brief reactive psychosis). Paranoid patients are potentially dangerous, since they may act out violently against someone they perceive to be a threat.

Determine the course of the paranoid ideation in addition to its severity. Paranoid personality disorder and delusional disorder of the persecutory type typically have paranoid ideation that has been relatively constant over long periods of time. Those two diagnoses are differentiated by the absence of delusions in paranoid personality disorder and by the prominent delusions that are the major defining clinical feature in delusional disorder. Paranoia in the context of mania or depression is present only during acute episodes. Schizophrenia is usually identified by the presence of other symptoms, such as hallucinations and thought disorders.

The objectives in treating the paranoid patient are to immediately evaluate the patient's potential dangerousness, to make a definitive psychiatric diagnosis, and to initiate an appropriate treatment plan based on the diagnosis.

INTERVIEWING AND PSYCHOTHERAPEUTIC GUIDELINES

Do not directly challenge the paranoid patient's beliefs, regardless of how implausible they seem. When testing the extent of the patient's paranoid ideation, be cautious, and avoid alienating the patient. Try asking,

"What do other people say when you tell them that the FBI is against you?" and "How do you respond to that?" Paranoid patients may have already encountered surprise or disbelief from others, so that line of questioning may be less threatening than directly challenging their beliefs.

The patient may be paranoid about you. Do not interview the patient in a potentially dangerous situation, such as alone in an office with the door closed. Be sure that help is rapidly available if the patient becomes violent. Maintain a formal stance, as paranoid patients view overfamiliarity with suspicion.

EVALUATION AND MANAGEMENT

1. Take the patient's vital signs. They may provide clues to a possible organic disorder.

2. Laboratory screening tests should include a complete blood count (CBC); a complete chemistry profile, including electrolytes, liver function tests, renal function tests, and tests for calcium and magnesium; a urine toxicology screen; thyroid function tests; and blood levels of any drugs being taken.

3. A complete psychiatric evaluation should lead to a diagnosis. Neuropsychological testing, electroencephalography (EEG), and structural brain imaging by a computed tomography (CT) scan or magnetic resonance imaging (MRI) may help identify any underlying organic conditions.

4. Hospitalization, even involuntary commitment, may be needed if the patient is dangerous. Question the patient in detail about any plans for suicide or homicide. Directly ask what the patient may do to those perceived to be against him or her. Inquire about previous acts of violence, including suicide attempts.

DRUG TREATMENT

In the emergency room or office, anxiety or agitation in paranoid patients is treated according to the diagnosis. If the patient is already taking an antipsychotic medication, give another dose of that drug. In general, psychotic paranoid patients can be given haloperidol (Haldol), thiothixene (Navane), fluphenazine (Prolixin), or trifluoperazine (Stelazine), all at a dose of 2 to 5 mg by mouth or intramuscularly (IM) as needed. Paranoid conditions caused by intoxication or withdrawal from drugs can be managed with lorazepam (Ativan) 1 to 2 mg by mouth or IM. Severely anxious paranoid patients can also be treated with lorazepam. Paranoia with agitation that is caused by delirium or dementia can be managed with haloperidol 1 to 5 mg by mouth or IM.

Cross-References:

Agitation, anxiety, chronic schizophrenia in acute exacerbation, delusional disorder, homosexual panic, hospitalization, ideas of reference, mania, marital crisis, schizoaffective disorder, schizophrenia, violence.

109 / Parkinsonism

Parkinsonism is an extrapyramidal syndrome characterized by brady-kinesia, tremor, and masked facies.

CLINICAL FEATURES AND DIAGNOSIS

Parkinsonism is also characterized by cogwheel rigidity, a flattened affect, drooling, and a shuffling gait. The tremor is greatest at rest; it often affects the hands, giving them a pill-rolling motion. Parkinsonism may be due to Parkinson's disease (idiopathic), may be a side effect of antipsychotic medication (most commonly with high-potency antipsychotics), may follow head trauma or exposure to such toxins as N-methyl-4-phenyl-1,2,3,6-tetrahydropyridine (MTPT, an illicit opioid of abuse), or may be due to other neurological conditions.

Parkinson's disease occurs in the elderly; antipsychotic-induced parkinsonism (in which the tremor is usually bilateral) is associated with taking antipsychotics and usually begins shortly after starting the medication or increasing the dosage; MTPT-induced parkinsonism is associated with a history of intravenous (IV) drug abuse; and parkinsonism caused by head trauma is likely only after a history of repeated trauma, as in boxers.

The primary mechanism in parkinsonism is believed to be a decrease in dopaminergic activity in the nigrostriatal pathway. In Parkinson's disease, MTPT use, and head trauma, the decrease in dopaminergic activity is due to the loss of dopaminergic cells. In antipsychotic-induced parkinsonism, the decrease is due to the blockade of dopaminergic receptors by the antipsychotic. Treatments of parkinsonism are based either on increasing the stimulation of dopaminergic receptors or decreasing the stimulation of cholinergic receptors. Dopaminergic and cholinergic activity are in a balance; decreasing cholinergic activity is another way to compensate for decreased dopaminergic activity.

INTERVIEWING AND PSYCHOTHERAPEUTIC GUIDELINES

The patient's degree of distress varies according to the specific syndrome causing the parkinsonism. Antipsychotic-induced parkinsonism may be associated with acute dystonia, which can be a frightening experience for the patient. Reassure the patient that an effective treatment is readily available. Patients with Parkinson's disease are commonly depressed and may also be demented.

EVALUATION AND MANAGEMENT

1. Make a definitive diagnosis that accounts for the cause of the parkinsonism. Look for stiffness, cogwheeling, decreased arm swing, and other features of parkinsonism.

2. Unless the parkinsonism is obviously antipsychotic-induced, perform a neurological examination, looking for focal neurological findings. Examine the patient taking an antipsychotic agent for dystonia and neuroleptic malignant syndrome, particularly if the rigidity is severe.

3. Conduct a full psychiatric mental status examination, and obtain the patient's history, looking for depression, dementia, and psychosis.

4. Evaluate the patient's present antipsychotic drug regimen (if any) and consider whether (a) the dose is sufficient, (b) the duration of treatment is sufficient, (c) the patient has responded, (d) a change of drug or a change in dosage could be made, and (e) dopaminergic agonists or cholinergic antagonists are indicated.

5. For antipsychotic-induced parkinsonism, consider lowering the antipsychotic dosage, changing to a low-potency antipsychotic, or adding an anticholinergic drug.

6. A surgical treatment involving the brain implantation of tissue from the adrenal medulla has helped some patients.

DRUG TREATMENT

Antipsychotic-induced parkinsonism is a common side effect of high-potency antipsychotics—for example, haloperidol (Haldol) and fluphenazine (Prolixin). A dosage reduction may decrease the risk of parkinsonism, but usually the patient requires rapid relief, which can be given with anticholinergic drugs, such as benztropine (Cogentin) 1 to 2 mg by mouth twice a day (Table B.109–1). Benztropine 1 to 2 mg is also rapidly effective when given intramuscularly (IM) or intravenously (IV) if the patient is in acute distress. The benztropine should then be given on a standing basis.

Usually, the target symptoms for antipsychotic treatment should be evaluated to decide whether a dosage decrease is possible. If the high-potency antipsychotic is ineffective or if its side effects are severe enough to warrant its discontinuation, the drug should be changed to a low-potency antipsychotic, such as chlorpromazine (Thorazine) or thioridazine (Mellaril). Those drugs are not likely to cause extrapyramidal side effects, such as parkinsonism, and they have strong anticholinergic effects. Amantadine (Symmetrel) 100 to 300 mg a day increases dopaminergic activity and is sometimes useful. However, a problem with amantadine is its possible precipitation of psychotic symptoms. It may be a good alternative to anticholinergics for the elderly and for other patients who are particularly susceptible to anticholinergic toxicity. Another alternative is clozapine (Clozaril), which may not cause any extrapyramidal side effects.

Parkinson's disease is usually treated with L-dopa (levodopa [Larodopa, Dopar]), which is a dopamine precursor. L-dopa is sometimes combined with carbidopa (Sinemet); carbidopa is a dopa decarboxylase inhibitor that further increases brain dopamine levels. Amantadine and deprenyl (a selective inhibitor of monoamine oxidase type B that selectively catabolizes dopamine) have also been used.

Table B.109–1
Antiparkinson Agents

Generic Name	Trade Name	Type of Drug	Usual Drug Range (mg per day)	Injectable
Amantadine	Symmetrel	Dopamine agonist	100 to 300	No
Benztropine	Cogentin	Antihistamine and anticholinergic	1 to 6	Yes
Biperiden	Akineton	Anticholinergic	2 to 6	Yes
Diphenhydramine	Benadryl	Antihistamine and anticholinergic	25 to 100	Yes
Ethopropazine	Parsidol	Antihistamine and anticholinergic	50	No
Orphenadrine	Disipal, Norflex	Antihistamine	300	No
Procyclidine	Kemadrin	Anticholinergic	6 to 20	No
Trihexyphenidyl	Artane	Anticholinergic	5 to 15	No

Table from S C Schoonover, A J Gelenberg: Emergency presentations related to psychiatric medication. In *Emergency Psychiatry,* E L Bassuk, A W Birk, editors, p 187. Plenum, New York, 1984. Used with permission.

Depression in Parkinson's disease should be treated with antidepressants. Electroconvulsive therapy (ECT) can be considered in refractory cases.

Cross-References:

Akinesia; catatonia; dementia; L-dopa intoxication; dystonia, acute; head trauma; neuroleptic malignant syndrome; perioral (rabbit) tremor; tremor.

110 / Perioral (Rabbit) Tremor

Perioral (rabbit) tremor is a focal tremor that is often associated with facial grimacing and that produces a rabbitlike appearance. It is caused by long-term antipsychotic treatment.

CLINICAL FEATURES AND DIAGNOSIS

Perioral (rabbit) tremor differs from other extrapyramidal side effects in that it typically occurs only after prolonged treatment, although it is considered a variant of parkinsonism. The syndrome may be misdiagnosed as a negative symptom of schizophrenia (flattened affect).

EVALUATION AND MANAGEMENT

Patients with the syndrome should be evaluated for other antipsychotic-induced side effects, such as tardive dyskinesia. If the patient is not taking antipsychotics, consider other diagnoses in consultation with a neurologist.

INTERVIEWING AND PSYCHOTHERAPEUTIC GUIDELINES

Focus on obtaining a history of the onset of the syndrome in relation to antipsychotic exposure. Reassure the patient, explaining the cause of the syndrome and its treatability.

DRUG TREATMENT

Drug treatment is the same as for other antipsychotic-induced parkinsonian side effects and typically involves anticholinergic drugs—for example, benztropine (Cogentin) 1 to 2 mg by mouth two times a day—a decrease in the antipsychotic dosage, or a change to a low-potency antipsychotic, such as thioridazine (Mellaril).

Cross-References:

Akinesia; dystonia, acute; neuroleptic malignant syndrome; parkinsonism; tardive dyskinesia; tremor.

---

111 / Phencyclidine or Similarly Acting Arylcyclohexylamine Intoxication

---

Phencyclidine (PCP) intoxication consists of a constellation of signs, symptoms, and maladaptive behavior after the use of PCP.

CLINICAL FEATURES AND DIAGNOSIS

PCP is a hallucinogen belonging to the class of arylcyclohexylamines that were once called dissociative anesthetics. In addition to hallucinations and delusions, PCP produces belligerence, assaultiveness, agitation, impulsiveness, unpredictability, nystagmus (vertical or horizontal), hypertension, tachycardia, numbness or diminished response to pain, ataxia, dysarthria, muscle rigidity, hyperacusis, echolalia, staring into space, anticholinergic effects, and, in large doses, hyperthermia, seizures, extrapyramidal movement disorders, myoglobinuria, renal failure, delirium, and death. The degree of intoxication is dose-dependent.

PCP commonly causes paranoid ideation and unpredictable violence that brings the abuser to medical attention. PCP-induced psychotic states may be long-lasting in vulnerable persons. A delusional state may emerge one week after an overdose. The patient often has amnesia for the acute psychotic episode, which may be followed by an episode of depression. The psychosis can be persistent. Tolerance and a withdrawal syndrome consisting of lethargy, drug craving, and depression have been reported. Delirium can emerge up to a week after PCP is discontinued, possibly because of PCP's release from fat stores.

PCP is used as a veterinary anesthetic, and it also produces anesthesia in humans, which makes PCP-intoxicated patients prone to injure themselves and those nearby, since the patients feel no pain. Abuse is widely prevalent because PCP is easily synthesized in illegal laboratories.

PCP may be administered orally, by sniffing, or intravenously (IV), although usually it is smoked in a tobacco or cannabis cigarette (a laced joint). Sometimes patients take PCP inadvertently by drinking PCP-containing punch at a party or by unknowingly smoking a laced joint, which can cause sudden, unpredicted behavior. Street names include PCP, peace pill, angel dust, crystal, peace, peace weed, supergrass, and superweed. A dose of PCP is impossible to assess accurately, and the dose in one cigarette may range from 1 to 250 mg. PCP is sometimes marketed as LSD, mescaline, or cannabis.

Intoxication symptoms can begin within five minutes of smoking or injecting and one hour after oral intake. Intoxication usually lasts three to six hours, although a full recovery may require one or two days. PCP is detectable in the patient's urine for more than a week after its use.

INTERVIEWING AND PSYCHOTHERAPEUTIC GUIDELINES

Do not try to talk down or reassure a PCP-intoxicated patient, who may be completely out of touch with the environment. Reduce the stimulation of the patient to a minimum. Provide psychiatric and medical treatment for potential behavioral and physiological complications.

EVALUATION AND MANAGEMENT

1. Take the patient's vital signs.

2. Assess whether PCP has been taken, using whatever history is available.

3. Determine if the patient appears to be psychotic, agitated, or out of contact with the environment.

4. Conduct a physical examination and a medical evaluation for such complications as hypertension, seizures, and vomiting.

5. Isolate the patient in a dark, quiet area—alone, if possible. Limit the number of staff members in the room unless the patient is potentially dangerous and requires physical intervention. Do not overstimulate the patient.

6. Avoid restraints if at all possible, since patients may injure themselves or others during the process of putting on the restraints and may also injure themselves in attempting to fight against limb restraints. Anesthetized PCP-intoxicated patients can break their own limbs trying to fight against limb restraints. They are also at risk for rhabdomyolysis.

7. If PCP was recently taken orally, gastric lavage may be of use in a patient who is relatively cooperative, although you should consider the risk of vomiting and aspiration.

8. Hospitalization may be needed for the medical, behavioral, or psychological sequelae of PCP intoxication.

DRUG TREATMENT

Acidification of the urine, which increases the renal excretion of PCP, is usually done with large doses (1 to 2 g) of ascorbic acid (vitamin C) or cranberry juice. However, PCP is stored in fatty tissues (including the brain), where it has usually been deposited by the time the patient comes for treatment, so increasing renal clearance may not bring about clinical improvement; nonetheless, it is common clinical practice, since it is relatively devoid of complications.

Benzodiazepines—for example, lorazepam (Ativan) 1 to 2 mg given intramuscularly (IM), diazepam (Valium) 5 to 10 mg by mouth or IV, oxazepam (Serax) 10 to 30 mg by mouth, and estazolam (ProSom) 0.5 to 1 mg by mouth—are the drugs of choice for agitation, since they raise the seizure threshold and do not cause anticholinergic effects. The dose may be repeated as necessary unless signs of benzodiazepine toxicity are present (for example, worsened dysarthria or ataxia).

Antipsychotics are also a possibility, especially after several doses of benzodiazepines have been ineffective. High-potency antipsychotics—for example, fluphenazine (Prolixin), thiothixene (Navane), and haloperidol (Haldol), all given at 2 to 5 mg IM—are preferable because they cause fewer anticholinergic effects than do low-potency antipsychotics. Since PCP itself can cause anticholinergic effects or seizures, low-potency antipsychotics should be avoided.

A combination of a benzodiazepine and an antipsychotic (for example, lorazepam 2 mg and haloperidol 5 mg) has also been used with some success. Some clinicians believe that the combination is more effective than either drug alone.

Cross-References:

Agitation, amphetamine or similarly acting sympathomimetic intoxication and withdrawal, anxiety, cocaine intoxication and withdrawal, delusional disorder, hallucinations, hospitalization, intoxication, self-mutilation, violence.

---

112 / Phenylpropanolamine Toxicity (Diet Pill)

Agitation, paranoia, psychosis, anxiety, headache, dizziness, insomnia, restlessness, tachycardia, and hypertension may be induced by an excessive dose of phenylpropanolamine.

CLINICAL FEATURES AND DIAGNOSIS

Phenylpropanolamine is found in over-the-counter cold medications and appetite suppressants. It is most commonly used as a decongestant. Phenylpropanolamine is a sympathomimetic amine with properties similar to those of ephedrine. A moderate dose does not usually cause signs of intoxication.

INTERVIEWING AND PSYCHOTHERAPEUTIC GUIDELINES

Reassure the patient that the symptoms are induced by the drug and will resolve as the drug is cleared, usually in four to six hours. Educate the patient about the importance of avoiding an excessive dose. With patients taking phenylpropanolamine for appetite suppression, evaluate the patient for a possible eating disorder.

EVALUATION AND MANAGEMENT

1. Discontinue the medication containing the phenylpropanolamine.
2. Evaluate the patient for possible toxic drug interactions with monoamine oxidase inhibitors (MAOIs), anticholinergics, and caffeine.

DRUG TREATMENT

Benzodiazepines—for example, lorazepam (Ativan) 0.5 to 1 mg by mouth, diazepam (Valium) 5 to 10 mg by mouth, oxazepam (Serax) 10 to 30 mg by mouth, chlordiazepoxide (Librium) 10 to 25 mg by mouth, and alprazolam (Xanax) 0.5 to 1 mg by mouth, all given every three to four hours as needed—may be used for severe restlessness, anxiety, or insomnia.

Cross-References:

Agitation, anorexia nervosa, anxiety, bulimia nervosa.

---

113 / Phobia

A *phobia* is an irrational fear of a specific object, activity, or situation that leads to avoidance. The failure to avoid the stimulus causes severe anxiety. The patient realizes that the fear is unrealistic, and the entire experience is dysphoric.

CLINICAL FEATURES AND DIAGNOSIS

The patient experiences severe anxiety or panic related to a specific object, activity, or situation. Specific types of phobias include social phobia—in which the patient is fearful of public humiliation, such as what may be encountered when speaking or performing in public, eating alone in a restaurant, or urinating in a public bathroom—and agoraphobia, in which the patient is afraid of being in public places or situations if escape from the situation may be difficult or embarrassing or if help would not be available should an embarrassing or incapacitating symptom suddenly develop.

In social phobia the focus of the fear is on public humiliation; in agoraphobia the focus of the fear is on the inability to escape.

Simple phobias are unrealistic fears of specific stimuli, such as spiders, snakes, animals, heights, storms, illness, injury, being alone, death, and contamination.

Phobic symptoms may be caused by intoxication with psychostimulants or hallucinogens and, rarely, by an organic disorder, such as a small brain tumor or a cerebrovascular disease. Those causes can usually be identified by a physical examination and laboratory tests.

Alcohol dependence is common in phobic patients, who may medicate their anxiety with alcohol. Subsequent withdrawal from alcohol may exacerbate the anxiety.

Schizophrenic patients may have delusional fears about specific stimuli, but they do not realize that the fear is unrealistic, and they have other signs of schizophrenia.

Phobic disorders may be difficult to differentiate from obsessive-compulsive disorder, in which obsessive thoughts about the stimulus may lead to compulsive behavior to relieve the anxiety.

The severe anxiety that is present in patients with phobias may produce physiological symptoms, as well as psychological symptoms. Manifestations of anxiety include restlessness, diarrhea, dizziness, palpitations, hyperhidrosis, tremor, syncope, tachycardia, and urinary symptoms.

Some patients show counterphobic behavior, in which the feared stimulus is sought out intentionally and encountered repeatedly in an attempt to overcome the fear. Examples include such risky behaviors as hang gliding, sky diving, and mountain climbing.

INTERVIEWING AND PSYCHOTHERAPEUTIC GUIDELINES

Since the patients realize that the phobia is irrational, address the fear directly. Inquire about the severity of the avoidant behavior and how impaired the patient's functioning has become as a result of trying to avoid the phobic stimulus. Also inquire about other anxiety symptoms—including panic, symptoms of posttraumatic stress disorder (for example, flashbacks and startle reactions), obsessions, and other associated phobias—and about depression, psychosis, and substance abuse. The patients may be embarrassed, feel foolish, or believe that they are going crazy. Take their fears seriously, and reassure them. Tell them about the availability of effective treatments.

EVALUATION AND MANAGEMENT

1. Take the patient's vital signs.

2. Order a urine toxicology screen, a detailed physical examination, thyroid function tests, and routine laboratory screening tests.

3. Obtain a detailed history of the specific phobic stimulus, the duration and severity of the impairment, and the presence of other associated phobic

stimuli. Obtain a history of any environmental changes that have made avoidance difficult or impossible.

4. Complete a psychiatric evaluation to identify the presence of other anxiety disorders (for example, obsessive-compulsive disorder, panic disorder, generalized anxiety disorder), depression, psychotic disorders, and drug or alcohol use.

5. The primary treatment is behavior therapy (for example, systematic desensitization and imaginal or in vivo flooding), but such therapy requires considerable effort and a commitment on the part of the patient. The patient must repeatedly encounter the phobic stimulus without the possibility of avoiding it and must learn to cope with the consequent anxiety. The treatment may begin by desensitizing the patient progressively to more and more anxiety-provoking stimuli. For example, patients who are phobic about elevators may start by imagining that they are in an elevator and slowly and repeatedly imagine that the elevator is going to higher and higher floors. The imagining is then replaced by actually getting into an elevator and then gradually going to higher and higher floors.

6. Refer the patient to supportive psychotherapy and family therapy to help both the patient and the patient's family cope with any impairments related to the phobia.

7. Refer the patient to group therapy, especially if the members of a group have a common phobia that they can help each other overcome together (for example, flying in airplanes).

8. Recommend hypnosis as an adjunct to psychotherapy.

DRUG TREATMENT

Benzodiazepines, tricyclic antidepressants, and monoamine oxidase inhibitors (MAOIs) are all helpful for phobic patients, although most of the available research is on the treatment of social phobia. The patient can also take β-blockers—for example, propranolol (Inderal)—before encountering the phobic stimulus; β-blockers are helpful for social phobia (for example, stage fright). Extremely anxious phobic patients can be given a small supply of lorazepam (Ativan) 1 to 2 mg by mouth three times a day, oxazepam (Serax) 10 to 30 mg a day by mouth, or clonazepam (Klonopin) 0.5 to 1 mg by mouth in the morning and at bedtime—to be taken until their first outpatient appointment.

Premedication with lorazepam 1 to 2 mg by mouth, intramuscularly (IM), or intravenously (IV) or diazepam (Valium) 5 to 10 mg by mouth, IM, or IV may be needed before medical procedures that are phobic stimuli (for example, a claustrophobic patient undergoing magnetic resonance imaging [MRI] or venipuncture in a patient with a needle phobia).

Cross-References:

Agitation, agoraphobia, anxiety, chronic schizophrenia in acute exacerbation, delusional disorder, depression, obsessions and compulsions, panic disorder, paranoia, school phobia and school refusal.

114 / Photosensitivity

Photosensitivity is characterized by easy and sometimes severe sunburning that occurs as a side effect of antipsychotic medication, most commonly phenothiazines. It is reportedly most common with low-potency antipsychotics, although high-potency antipsychotics have also been implicated.

CLINICAL FEATURES AND DIAGNOSIS

Severe sunburn in a patient taking a phenothiazine may include maculopapular, urticarial, edematous, and petechial lesions that develop after only brief exposure (as brief as several minutes) to direct bright sunlight. Photosensitivity is caused by ultraviolet radiation (290 to 400 nm wavelength), usually from the sun. It requires sufficient skin concentration of the drug and appropriate wavelengths of ultraviolet light. The proper medical term is "cutaneous photosensitivity," which is subdivided into phototoxic reactions and photoallergic reactions. Phenothiazine-induced photosensitivity is of the phototoxic type and can occur after only several minutes of exposure to bright sunlight and does not require previous exposure to the sun (as is necessary for photoallergic reactions).

A gray-blue hyperpigmentation in patients taking a phenothiazine can develop in areas often exposed to sunlight. That skin hyperpigmentation is sometimes associated with eye changes, described as brown granular deposits in the anterior lens and posterior cornea that do not impair vision. Those eye changes are usually found only in patients who have taken high dosages of chlorpromazine (Thorazine) for many years. The eye changes are unrelated to the retinitis pigmentosa that can be caused by high dosages of thioridazine (Mellaril) and that can lead to blindness. Dosages of thioridazine of more than 800 mg a day should be avoided.

INTERVIEWING AND PSYCHOTHERAPEUTIC GUIDELINES

Educate patients that the skin effects are an interaction of the antipsychotic medication and exposure to sunlight.

EVALUATION AND MANAGEMENT

1. Consider other possible causes of erythema (for example, contact dermatitis).
2. Minimize the patient's exposure to the sun.
3. Treat the sunburn if needed.
4. Consult a dermatologist if needed.
5. Consider changing to a nonphenothiazine antipsychotic if possible.

DRUG TREATMENT

Use sunscreens with a high sun protection factor (SPF). Local dermatological treatment and systemic analgesics or anti-inflammatory drugs may increase the patient's comfort. However, the phenothiazine-induced photosensitivity reaction may not be prostaglandin-mediated, so anti-inflammatory drugs that inhibit prostaglandin synthesis—for example, indomethacin (Indocin)—may not be effective in reducing the erythema.

Cross-References:

Dermatitis, self-inflicted; pigmentary retinopathy.

---

115 / Pigmentary Retinopathy

Pigmentary retinopathy is characterized by retinal infiltrations. It is similar to retinitis pigmentosa and can be caused by the long-term use of thioridazine (Mellaril) at dosages of 1,600 mg a day or higher.

CLINICAL FEATURES AND DIAGNOSIS

An ophthalmological examination reveals retinal pigmentation and visual impairment in a patient who has been taking thioridazine for a long time.

Thioridazine can conjugate with the melanin of the pigment layer of the retina, resulting in degeneration of the outer layers of the retina and leading to impaired vision or even blindness. The condition may not resolve even after the drug is discontinued. Patients who have been taking thioridazine at dosages greater than 800 mg a day should be evaluated by an ophthalmologist. Complaints of impaired vision in patients taking thioridazine must be thoroughly evaluated.

INTERVIEWING AND PSYCHOTHERAPEUTIC GUIDELINES

Educating the patient is the priority. Make the patient aware that pigmentary retinopathy is a potential side effect of thioridazine and is dose-related. Most patients with the problem have either chronic psychotic disorders (for example, schizophrenia and schizoaffective disorder) or chronic behavioral problems (for example, agitation associated with dementia of the Alzheimer's type and other organic disorders).

Emphasize the clinical benefits of thioridazine, and discuss possible alternatives, such as other antipsychotics. Inform the patient that all antipsychotics have some side effects in addition to their desired clinical effects.

EVALUATION AND MANAGEMENT

1. Request an ophthalmology consultation.
2. Early pigmentary retinopathy can be best detected by using small colored objects to test the patient's central visual field.

DRUG TREATMENT

Discontinue thioridazine or lower the dosage. If antipsychotics are still needed, consider changing to an antipsychotic of a different class. In general, thioridazine should not be used at dosages greater than 800 mg a day.

Cross-Reference:

Photosensitivity.

---

116 / Postpartum or Puerperal Psychosis

Postpartum or *puerperal psychosis* is an acute psychotic episode in a woman that appears shortly after she has given birth.

CLINICAL FEATURES AND DIAGNOSIS

Postpartum psychosis can occur within one year after giving birth. Most often, it begins within the first week of childbirth. Most patients have no previous psychiatric problems. However, the incidence is greatest in patients with a history of bipolar disorder, previous postpartum psychiatric disorders (psychosis and depression), and a family history of postpartum psychiatric disorders. The disorder occurs after 0.1 to 0.2 percent of all pregnancies and is much less common than postpartum depression.

Manic symptoms are the most common; depression with psychotic features is also common. Typical symptoms include agitation, restlessness, and a labile mood, including elation, insomnia, crying spells, confusion, and eventually the development of a full-blown psychotic episode with features of mania and delirium. Suicide or infanticide occurs in up to 10 percent of untreated cases. Obsessions are common and often focus on an impulse to hurt or kill the infant.

INTERVIEWING AND PSYCHOTHERAPEUTIC GUIDELINES

Postpartum psychotic patients are potentially dangerous, so make appropriate provisions to prevent their flight or sudden violence. Often, new mothers are discharged from the postpartum obstetric ward several days after giving birth, and they experience the onset of postpartum psychosis days or weeks after leaving the obstetric ward. Be alert for the condition, and use the family to provide the patient's history.

If hospitalization is indicated, reassure the patient and her family that in most cases the condition is brief and that recovery can be expected. Involve the family in the evaluation and treatment, exploring the effects that the episode is having, especially on the father, siblings, and grandparents.

EVALUATION AND MANAGEMENT

1. Consider the high potential risk for infanticide or suicide, and be prepared to hospitalize the patient. A full medical evaluation and workup for possible organic causes is indicated.

2. Follow-up counseling is important and should include help with child rearing and observing the patient for subsequent mania, depression, or other psychiatric syndromes.

3. Family therapy can help explore and process the effects that the episode had on the family and can help the family cope with possible subsequent episodes. The family may be needed to provide child care.

4. Antipsychotics may be needed. If antipsychotics are ineffective, electroconvulsive therapy (ECT) is an alternative treatment that may be combined with antipsychotics.

DRUG TREATMENT

The patient may require a brief course of antipsychotic medication, such as haloperidol (Haldol) or fluphenazine (Prolixin), both given at 2 to 5 mg by mouth three times a day. For agitation, the patient may require 2 to 5 mg intramuscularly (IM) of a high-potency antipsychotic. Breast feeding should be prohibited during drug treatment. Because of the high incidence of postpartum psychosis in women with bipolar disorder, lithium (Eskalith) prophylaxis during the third trimester or shortly after giving birth should be considered. Antidepressants should be used in patients with suicidal depression.

Cross-References:

Confusion, delirium, delusions, grandiosity, hallucinations, homicidal and assaultive behavior, hospitalization, mania, obsessions and compulsions, suicide.

---

117 / Posttraumatic Stress Disorder (PTSD)

Posttraumatic stress disorder is a syndrome of anxiety, autonomic instability, emotional numbing, and reexperiencing of the traumatic experience after a physical or emotional stress that is beyond the realm of what can be reasonably expected and that would be traumatic for most people.

CLINICAL FEATURES AND DIAGNOSIS

The diagnostic criteria for posttraumatic stress disorder are given in Table B.117–1.

The prevalence of posttraumatic stress disorder is 0.5 percent in males and 1.2 percent in females. The most common stressor in men is wartime combat experience. In women the most common stressor is an assault or rape. Although the disorder does affect all ages, the majority of patients are young adults, because that age group has the greatest exposure to the precipitating stressors.

Posttraumatic stress disorder can develop at any time after the stressor; delayed posttraumatic stress disorder may develop as late as 30 years after the trauma. A minority of patients go on to have chronic posttraumatic stress disorder. The prognosis is good for patients who have symptoms shortly after the stressor, have a brief duration of symptoms, have good premorbid functioning and a social support system, and are free of other medical and psychiatric problems.

Many patients present with symptoms after stresses ranging from a minor car accident in which no one was injured to physical or sexual abuse, threats, fires, and other disasters.

The factors affecting the development of posttraumatic stress disorder include the severity of the stressor and the vulnerability of the patient. Children and the elderly are more vulnerable than young adults, presumably because children do not yet have coping mechanisms for severe stress and because the elderly may be rigid in their coping mechanisms and are poorly suited to adapt to an unexpected stress.

A wide range of associated features may be present, including drug and alcohol abuse or dependence, prominent guilt feelings, insomnia, depression, illusions or hallucinations, dissociation, panic attacks, aggression, poor impulse control, violence, and impaired memory and concentration.

INTERVIEWING AND PSYCHOTHERAPEUTIC GUIDELINES

The diagnosis of posttraumatic stress disorder is missed if the clinician is not looking for it. Patients may present with signs of substance abuse, depression, generalized anxiety disorder, panic disorder, and dissociative disorders. Focus on reducing the patient's denial of the stress (if present) and on reviewing and processing the feelings brought on by reexperiencing the stress. Address any guilt and feelings of responsibility for the trauma.

Some patients are knowledgeable about posttraumatic stress disorder. The symptoms are difficult to measure objectively; consequently, they are often feigned by malingerers who are attempting to obtain medications or admission to a hospital. While weeding out the malingerers, do not miss the true cases. At least initially, accept the patient's symptoms as presented.

Table B.117-1
Diagnostic Criteria for Posttraumatic Stress Disorder

A. The person has experienced an event that is outside the range of usual human experience and that would be markedly distressing to almost anyone (e.g., serious threat to one's life or physical integrity; serious threat or harm to one's children, spouse, or other close relatives and friends; sudden destruction of one's home or community; or seeing another person who has recently been, or is being, seriously injured or killed as the result of an accident or physical violence).

B. The traumatic event is persistently reexperienced in at least one of the following ways:
   (1) recurrent and intrusive distressing recollections of the event (in young children, repetitive play in which themes or aspects of the trauma are expressed)
   (2) recurrent distressing dreams of the event
   (3) sudden acting or feeling as if the traumatic event were recurring (includes a sense of reliving the experience, illusions, hallucinations, and dissociative [flashback] episodes, even those that occur upon awakening or when intoxicated)
   (4) intense psychological distress at exposure to events that symbolize or resemble an aspect of the traumatic event, including anniversaries of the trauma

C. Persistent avoidance of stimuli associated with the trauma or numbing of general responsiveness (not present before the trauma), as indicated by at least three of the following:
   (1) efforts to avoid thoughts or feelings associated with the trauma
   (2) efforts to avoid activities or situations that arouse recollections of the trauma
   (3) inability to recall an important aspect of the trauma (psychogenic amnesia)
   (4) markedly diminished interest in significant activities (in young children, loss of recently acquired developmental skills such as toilet training or language skills)
   (5) feeling of detachment or estrangement from others
   (6) restricted range of affect (e.g., unable to have loving feelings)
   (7) sense of a foreshortened future (e.g., does not expect to have a career, marriage, children, or a long life)

D. Persistent symptoms of increased arousal (not present before the trauma), as indicated by at least two of the following:
   (1) difficulty falling or staying asleep
   (2) irritability or outbursts of anger
   (3) difficulty concentrating
   (4) hypervigilance
   (5) exaggerated startle response
   (6) physiologic reactivity upon exposure to events that symbolize or resemble an aspect of the traumatic event (e.g., a woman who was raped in an elevator breaks out in a sweat when entering any elevator)

E. Duration of the disturbance (symptoms in B, C, and D) of at least one month

Specify delayed onset if the onset of symptoms was at least six months after the trauma.

Table from DSM-III-R, *Diagnostic and Statistical Manual of Mental Disorders,* ed 3, revised. Copyright American Psychiatric Association, Washington, 1987. Used with permission.

EVALUATION AND MANAGEMENT

1. Establish the diagnosis by using the diagnostic criteria.

2. Evaluate the patient for substance intoxication or withdrawal, and treat it as needed.

3. Evaluate the patient for possible head injury and other physical traumas sustained if the traumatic stress involved physical injury. Physical and neurological examinations are mandatory. Further diagnostic testing, such as computed tomography (CT) or magnetic resonance imaging (MRI) or an electroencephalogram (EEG), is indicated if the neurological examination findings are abnormal or if the patient has a history of neurological symptoms.

4. Attempt to gain the patient's trust, and engage the patient in talking about the experience in some detail. That approach applies especially to rape victims.

5. Engage the patient's family and friends, educate them about post-traumatic stress disorder, and encourage them to be supportive and understanding of the patient.

6. Group therapy with other posttraumatic stress disorder patients may be useful.

DRUG TREATMENT

Start drug treatment only in the context of an ongoing therapeutic relationship, especially since substance abuse is common in posttraumatic stress disorder patients.

Antidepressant treatment of posttraumatic stress disorder remains controversial. Other drugs that have been used in the disorder include benzodiazepines, lithium (Eskalith), and β-blockers—for example, propranolol (Inderal), clonidine (Catapres), and carbamazepine (Tegretol). Those drugs are generally prescribed as part of an ongoing treatment plan, with the exception of the benzodiazepines—for example, estazolam (ProSom) 0.5 to 1 mg by mouth, oxazepam (Serax) 10 to 30 mg by mouth, diazepam (Valium) 5 to 10 mg by mouth, clonazepam (Klonopin) 0.25 to 0.5 mg by mouth, or lorazepam (Ativan) 1 to 2 mg by mouth or intramuscularly (IM)—which may also be used in the emergency room or office to treat the acute anxiety and the agitation that may accompany posttraumatic stress disorder.

Cross-References:

Alcohol intoxication, alcohol withdrawal, anxiety, borderline personality disorder, delusional disorder, depression, disaster survivors, hallucinations, illusions, insomnia, intoxication, malingering, opioid intoxication and withdrawal, panic disorder, psychotropic drug withdrawal, rape and sexual abuse, violence.

118 / Pregnancy

Pregnancy is the condition that exists from conception until the birth of the baby.

CLINICAL FEATURES AND DIAGNOSIS

The diagnosis can be obtained from the patient's history and physical examination. In early or doubtful cases, the diagnosis can be confirmed or ruled out by urine and blood pregnancy tests. The blood test—human chorionic gonadotropin (HCG)—is more sensitive than the urine test, but it is also more expensive and takes longer than the urine test.

Pregnancy is always a significant stress to both the prospective mother and her family. Many factors can increase the stressfulness of the situation. Those factors include pregnancy as the result of rape or incest, teenage pregnancy, pregnancy in families with insufficient resources, alcohol or drug dependence in the expectant mother, pregnancy in the context of marital conflict, and other adverse environmental conditions.

INTERVIEWING AND PSYCHOTHERAPEUTIC GUIDELINES

The reaction of the patient and her family to the pregnancy can vary, depending on the circumstances and the psychological makeup of the patient and her family members. The reactions to the pregnancy are greatly influenced by cultural factors and should be evaluated according to what is appropriate for the patient's culture. Determine whether the patient's family members and her friends from the same culture feel that her thoughts and behavior are abnormal. Do not impose your cultural beliefs, values, or judgments on the patient, whose reactions should be explored and understood.

EVALUATION AND MANAGEMENT

1. In teenage pregnancy the patient may want an abortion while the patient's parents do not. In general, crisis-intervention approaches should be used to try to negotiate an agreement between the patient and her parents. When no agreement is possible, most states consider the teenager to be capable of making her own informed decision and do not allow the parents to prevent the abortion.

2. In pregnancy caused by rape or incest, abortion is frequently recommended. Victims of rape and incest require psychiatric evaluation and treatment.

3. Heavy alcohol use during pregnancy has been associated with low birth weight (although that finding is confounded by cigarette smoking) and fetal alcohol syndrome. The safe level of alcohol consumption during pregnancy is not known, so alcohol should be avoided completely during pregnancy.

4. The use of illicit drugs during pregnancy has a wide range of deleterious effects on the fetus and the newborn. Those effects include dependence on and withdrawal from opioids, sedative-hypnotics, and cocaine. Opioid withdrawal in pregnancy can lead to a miscarriage. If opioid withdrawal is planned during pregnancy, it is safest during the second trimester. Methadone and probably other opioids used during pregnancy have been associated with intellectual development problems in the child. Cocaine use may cause spontaneous abortion during early pregnancy and premature labor during late pregnancy.

5. False pregnancy (also called pseudocyesis and hysterical pregnancy) is the presence of the physical symptoms of pregnancy—including abdominal distention, the cessation of the menses, nausea, breast enlargement and hyperpigmentation, and sometimes even labor—in a patient who is not

pregnant. The patient believes that she is pregnant. Sometimes, a negative pregnancy test convinces the woman, but often the patient is seriously ill and requires extensive treatment, primarily psychotherapy that explores the psychological need to be pregnant.

6. Sexual intercourse during pregnancy is permitted by most obstetricians until the last four or five weeks antepartum.

DRUG TREATMENT

Drug treatment should be avoided unless the patient is clearly psychotic, unmanageable, and a danger to herself or her baby or others. In those cases a high-potency antipsychotic—for example, fluphenazine (Prolixin) or halo-peridol (Haldol), both given at 0.5 to 2 mg by mouth or intramuscularly (IM) as needed—may be used.

The approach to take with medications is to compare the risk to the fetus of giving the medication with the risk to the mother of not giving the medication. In general, avoid giving medications during pregnancy, since they can be teratogenic or cause other toxic effects to the fetus or the newborn by passing across the placenta or in the breast milk. The two most teratogenic drugs in the psychopharmacopeia are lithium and anticonvulsants. Lithium administration during pregnancy is associated with a high incidence of birth abnormalities, including Ebstein's malformation, a serious abnormality in cardiac development. Other psychoactive drugs (antidepressants, antipsychotics, and anxiolytics), although less clearly associated with birth defects, should also be avoided during pregnancy if at all possible.

Cross-References:

Delusional disorder, depression, hypersexuality, incest, marital crisis, postpartum or puerperal psychosis, rape and sexual abuse.

---

119 / Psychotropic Drug Withdrawal

The symptoms of *psychotropic drug withdrawal* are associated with the abrupt discontinuation or the rapid decrease in the dosage of a psychotropic medication that has been taken steadily for weeks or longer.

CLINICAL FEATURES AND DIAGNOSIS

The common symptoms include insomnia, anxiety, agitation, weakness, chills, and pain. Withdrawal from psychotropic drugs capable of producing tolerance and dependence (for example, benzodiazepines and other seda-tive-hypnotics) can produce delirium and seizures. Withdrawal from antipsychotics can cause withdrawal dyskinesias and may unmask or worsen tardive dyskinesia. Withdrawal from antipsychotics or antidepressants with prominent anticholinergic effects (or from anticholinergic drugs themselves) can cause sinus tachycardia, ventricular arrhythmias, and cholinergic rebound, causing flulike symptoms.

Psychotropic drug withdrawal does not refer only to true withdrawal syndromes, like those encountered with substances that cause pharmacological dependence. Rather, the term is used to describe any syndrome that can develop when a drug is decreased or discontinued.

Discontinuation of the drug may be necessary because of side effects, allergic reactions, or other toxic effects. Although most psychotropic drugs do not cause pharmacological dependence and withdrawal, symptoms of rebound often occur. Since most psychotropic drugs are central nervous system (CNS) depressants, the most common symptoms of psychotropic drug withdrawal are insomnia and anxiety.

INTERVIEWING AND PSYCHOTHERAPEUTIC GUIDELINES

Reassure the patient that the symptoms of psychotropic drug withdrawal are neither proof that the drug is absolutely necessary nor proof that drug dependence has become a problem. Inform the patient that the symptoms are usually self-limited, will be over in a few days, and can be reduced by a slower lowering of the drug dosage.

EVALUATION AND MANAGEMENT

1. Determine what drugs the patient is taking, including prescribed drugs, over-the-counter drugs, alcohol, and drugs of abuse.

2. Consider whether the patient is pharmacologically dependent on alcohol, benzodiazepines, barbiturates, or other sedative-hypnotics. Withdrawal from those substances is potentially dangerous and requires active intervention. The severity of the withdrawal from benzodiazepines is related to the drug's pharmacokinetics (Table B.119–1). Dependence on benzodiazepines with short elimination half-lives can lead to abrupt and severe withdrawal symptoms.

3. Determine whether the psychotropic drug must be discontinued immediately or whether a slow taper over a period of weeks is possible. If a slow taper of the drug is possible, the withdrawal symptoms may disappear altogether.

4. If necessary, treat the withdrawal symptoms with other medications, as described below.

DRUG TREATMENT

Withdrawal from alcohol, benzodiazepines, barbiturates, and other sedative-hypnotics is usually treated with long-acting benzodiazepines, although some psychiatrists prefer to detoxify benzodiazepine-dependent patients by using the drug on which they are dependent.

Sinus tachycardia and ventricular arrhythmias after the abrupt discontinuation of antidepressants or highly anticholinergic antipsychotics can be

Table B.119–1
**Commonly Observed Withdrawal Symptoms
(Benzodiazepine Withdrawal Syndrome)**

Anxiety
Irritability
Insomnia
Fatigue
Headache
Muscle twitching or aching
Tremor, shakiness
Sweating
Dizziness
Concentration difficulties

*Nausea, loss of appetite
*Observable depression
*Depersonalization, derealization
*Increased sensory perception (smell, sight, taste, touch)
*Abnormal perception or sensation of movement

Table from P P Roy-Byrne, D Hommer: Benzodiazepine withdrawal: Overview and implications for the treatment of anxiety. Am J Med *84:* 1041, 1988. Used with permission.
*Symptoms likely to represent true withdrawal, rather than an exacerbation or the return of the original anxiety.

treated with anticholinergic drugs, including atropine and oral anticholinergics—for example, benztropine (Cogentin) 1 to 2 mg by mouth twice a day.

Withdrawal syndromes that develop when antipsychotics or antidepressants are suddenly discontinued can be minimized if the drug is gradually tapered over a period of several weeks.

Cross-References:

Agitation; alcohol withdrawal; anxiety; barbiturate and similarly acting sedative, hypnotic, or anxiolytic intoxication and withdrawal; insomnia; tardive dyskinesia.

120 / Rape and Sexual Abuse

Rape is the forceful coercion of an unwilling victim to engage in a sexual act, usually sexual intercourse, although anal intercourse and fellatio can also be acts of rape.

Like other acts of violence, rape is a psychiatric emergency that requires immediate appropriate intervention. Rape victims may suffer sequelae that persist for a lifetime. Rape is a life-threatening experience in which the victim has almost always been threatened with physical harm, often with a weapon.

In addition to rape, other forms of sexual abuse include genital manipulation with foreign objects, infliction of pain, and forced sexual activity.

CLINICAL FEATURES AND DIAGNOSIS

Clinicians must have a high degree of suspicion for unreported rape, since about 50 percent of rapes are not reported. Patients' hesitation or anxiety when you are exploring their sexual histories should be a clue.

Rape is fundamentally an act of violent humiliation, rather than an act of sexual intimacy, and the basic interaction between rapist and victim is one of physical domination and submission. Some rapists are impotent during the rape; only a minority are sexually aroused by the victim's pain and suffering.

The overwhelming majority of rapists are male, and a majority of victims are female. However, male rape does occur, often in institutions where men are detained (for example, prisons). Women between the ages of 16 and 24 years are in the highest risk category, but female victims as young as 15 months and as old as 82 years have been raped. More than a third of all rapes are committed by rapists known to the victim, 7 percent by close relatives. A fifth of all rapes involve more than one rapist (gang rape).

With the patient's written consent, collect evidence, such as semen and pubic hair, that may be used to identify the rapist. Take photographs of the evidence if possible. The medical record may be used as evidence in criminal proceedings; therefore, meticulous objective documentation of all aspects of the evaluation is essential. Do not write "rape" as a diagnosis on the chart, since rape is a legal determination.

Typical reactions in both rape and sexual abuse victims include shame, humiliation, anxiety, confusion, and outrage. Many victims wonder whether they are partly responsible and somehow invited the assault. In fact, victim behavior is less important in precipitating a rape than it is in precipitating a homicide or a robbery.

INTERVIEWING AND PSYCHOTHERAPEUTIC GUIDELINES

If possible, a female clinician should evaluate the patient, since the victim may find it easier to talk with a woman than with a man. The evaluation should take place in private. When rape or sexual abuse has not been acknowledged openly, be alert to the fact that many victims are hesitant to discuss the assault and avoid the topic. If the patient appears to be anxious when questioned about sexual history and avoids the discussion, do not validate the patient's avoidance by avoiding the topic yourself. Recognize that the rape victim has undergone an unanticipated life-threatening stress. It is legally and therapeutically important to take a detailed and complete history of the attack.

Rape and sexual abuse victims are often confused during the period after the assault. Be reassuring, supportive, and nonjudgmental. Educate the patient about the availability of medical and legal services and about rape crisis centers that provide multidisciplinary services.

EVALUATION AND MANAGEMENT

1. Offer appropriate medical, gynecological, and police services. Immediately refer the patient for the treatment of injuries sustained in the assault. If pregnancy is a possible consequence, consider giving progesterone or diethylstilbestrol by mouth for five days to prevent implantation. Provide treatment, including a course of antibiotics, for possible sexually transmitted diseases. Test for human immunodeficiency virus (HIV) at an appropriate time.

2. Offer crisis-intervention-oriented therapy. The objective is to minimize the psychological sequelae of the assault in the victim. Offer the victim supportive psychotherapy. Encourage the victim to talk about the rape or sexual abuse and to ventilate in a safe environment.

3. Encourage the patient to pursue the arrest and conviction of the rapist or sexual abuser. Reassure the patient that social support networks are available for the victims of rape and sexual abuse. Assess the availability of supportive friends and relatives.

4. Evaluate the patient for possible posttraumatic stress disorder. The disorder may not develop immediately, so educate the patient about the possible sequelae. Many rape and sexual abuse victims have symptoms that continue for years. The symptoms may include reliving the experience (flashbacks), preoccupation with the experience, feeling unable to make themselves clean, fear of being followed or of being alone, fear of returning to the site of the assault (often in the victim's home or neighborhood), nightmares, insomnia, and altered eating patterns. Such somatic symptoms as headaches, nausea and vomiting, and malaise are also common. In addition, the patient may avoid future sexual relationships or may experience such sexual symptoms as vaginismus.

5. Refer the patient for ongoing psychotherapy, which should focus on reestablishing the patient's sense of control over the environment, reducing feelings of helplessness and dependence, and addressing and processing obsessional thoughts about the rape or abusive experience.

6. Evaluate the patient for psychiatric conditions (for example, schizophrenia, substance dependence, and personality disorder) that may cause impaired judgment and place the patient in danger of rape or sexual abuse. If a psychiatric disorder is present, refer the patient for treatment of the underlying psychiatric disorder.

7. Refer the patient to group therapy for the victims of rape or sexual abuse. The groups are extremely helpful.

DRUG TREATMENT

Usually, no drug treatment is indicated. Some patients may experience overwhelming anxiety after the rape or sexual abuse. In those situations, short-term treatment with a benzodiazepine such as alprazolam (Xanax) 0.5 to 1 mg by mouth three times a day, lorazepam (Ativan) 1 to 2 mg by mouth three times a day, or oxazepam (Serax) 10 to 30 mg by mouth three times a day may be needed.

Insomnia can be treated with the medications listed above or with temazepam (Restoril) 15 to 30 mg by mouth at bedtime or flurazepam (Dalmane) 15 to 30 mg by mouth at bedtime.

Cross-References:

Abuse: child, elder, and spouse; homicidal and assaultive behavior; homosexual panic; hypersexuality; incest; intoxication; posttraumatic stress disorder; pregnancy; violence.

121 / Restraints

The physical restraint of patients may be necessary to prevent violence.

CLINICAL FEATURES AND DIAGNOSIS

Impending violence requires immediate intervention. Patients who are agitated, threatening violence, so severely disorganized that there is a risk of injury, or attempting to injure themselves must be restrained if they are not amenable to verbal intervention.

Physical restraint is an important, useful, and often necessary intervention. Although the experience can be humiliating, frustrating, and confusing for the patient, the stress is only temporary. The consequences of uncontained violence may be irreversible. Many patients feel more in control after they have been restrained and know that clear limits to their behavior are imposed.

INTERVIEWING AND PSYCHOTHERAPEUTIC GUIDELINES

Always begin by offering the patient a chance to stop the behavior that is leading to potential restraint. Speak authoritatively, and direct the patient to stop the behavior. Try to provide a quiet space alone (under visual observation), where the patient can try to calm down. Repeatedly explain that the continued behavior will lead to physical restraint. Offer the patient an opportunity to take medication that may avoid the necessity of physical restraint. However, do not negotiate with the patient. Simply identify which specific behaviors warrant physical restraint, and, if they continue, proceed with restraint. Do not let the patient feel that there is any doubt in your mind regarding what interventions are necessary.

EVALUATION AND MANAGEMENT

1. Leave physical restraint to those who are specifically trained to do it. Applying physical restraints is among the most hazardous of activities in mental health care. Improper restraint can lead to the injury of a staff member or the patient and even to patient death.

2. Have a sufficient number of staff members available to safely restrain the patient. If physical restraint is a possibility, call in sufficient staff members early. It is better to have an excess number of staff members waiting in the area than to have insufficient staff members at the moment that restraint is required. Sometimes, simply the presence of a number of staff members and the perception that restraint is inevitable produce a change in the patient's behavior.

3. Offer a chemical restraint before implementing physical restraint.

4. In choosing a restraint, use a type with which the staff members have been trained and are familiar. The improper use of restraints can lead to injury. Avoid restraining only one limb, since thrashing can cause a sprain or a fracture in the patient (Table B.121–1).

5. Once the patient is restrained, offer medication again if the patient has not yet complied. Patients who remain agitated in restraints should be medicated until they are calm.

6. Continue to monitor the patient's vital signs every half hour while the patient is in restraints.

7. Constantly reevaluate the need for restraints by an objective assessment of the patient's behavior as frequently as possible, preferably every 15 to 30 minutes.

8. Document the reasons for placing the patient in restraints.

DRUG TREATMENT

The vast majority of patients who require physical restraint benefit from medication that can provide chemical restraint and may reduce the need for physical restraint. It is probably more distressing to the patient to be physically subdued than to receive an injection. The three classes of drugs used most often are antipsychotics, benzodiazepines, and barbiturates. All can provide rapid behavioral control.

The choice of drug is based on what medication (if any) the patient is already taking, the drug's undesirable side effects, the patient's concomitant medical problems and other contraindications, and the availability of parenteral preparations for intramuscular (IM) administration. Drug dependence is a relative contraindication for benzodiazepines and barbiturates, since the dosages of those drugs required for dependent patients may be high and their use may lead to continued abuse. The presence of psychosis supports the use of antipsychotics, although the desired effect is immediate tranquilization, rather than a true antipsychotic effect, which takes days to weeks.

Most restrained patients comply with the oral administration of a liquid medication, but an IM injection is usually effective more rapidly.

If a patient is taking an antipsychotic, give an additional dose of the antipsychotic already being taken—for example, haloperidol (Haldol) 5 mg IM or 10 mg by mouth, perphenazine (Trilafon) 5 mg IM or 8 mg by mouth, or chlorpromazine (Thorazine) 10 to 25 mg IM or 50 to 100 mg by mouth. If the patient is taking an antipsychotic for which there is no parenteral

Table B.121-1
Use of Restraints

1. Preferably five or a minimum of four persons should be used to restrain the patient. Leather restraints are the safest and the surest type of restraints.
2. Explain to the patient why he or she is going into restraints.
3. A staff member should always be visible and reassuring the patient who is being restrained to help alleviate the patient's fear of helplessness, impotence, and loss of control.
4. Patients should be restrained with legs spread-eagled and one arm restrained to one side and the other arm restrained over the patient's head.
5. Restraints should be placed so that intravenous fluids can be given if necessary.
6. The patient's head is raised slightly to decrease the patient's feelings of vulnerability and to reduce the possibility of aspiration.
7. The restraints should be checked periodically for safety and comfort.
8. After the patient is in restraints, the clinician begins treatment, using verbal intervention.
9. Even in restraints, a majority of patients still take antipsychotic medication in concentrated form.
10. After the patient is under control, one restraint at a time should be removed at five-minute intervals until the patient has only two restraints on. Both of the remaining restraints should be removed at the same time, because it is inadvisable to keep a patient in only one restraint.
11. Always thoroughly document the reason for the restraints, the course of treatment, and the patient's response to treatment while in restraints.

Table data from W R Dubin, K J Weiss: Emergency psychiatry. In *Psychiatry,* vol 2, R Michaels, J O Cavenar, H K H Brodie, A M Cooper, S B Guze, L L Judd, G L Klerman, A J Skolnit, editors, p 9. Lippincott, Philadelphia, 1987. Used with permission.

form available—for example, thioridazine (Mellaril)—use the most similar available drug, such as chlorpromazine.

Benzodiazepines and barbiturates are alternatives to antipsychotics. Since most of the drugs are equally effective, the choice is often based on what is the most rapidly and conveniently available in parenteral form. Commonly used drugs include lorazepam (Ativan) 1 to 2 mg IM or by mouth and amobarbital (Amytal) 250 mg IM or by mouth. Benzodiazepines are also used with patients taking antipsychotics as a short-term augmentation of the antipsychotic to avoid escalating the dose of the antipsychotic simply to provide behavioral control.

Cross-References:

Agitation, homicidal and assaultive behavior, hospitalization, seclusion.

122 / Schizoaffective Disorder

Schizoaffective disorder has been understood in various ways. (1) It may be a type of either schizophrenia or a mood disorder. (2) It may be a combination of both schizophrenia and a mood disorder. (3) It may be completely distinct from either of those disorders. (4) Perhaps most likely, it may comprise a heterogeneous group of disorders that include all three possibilities.

Schizoaffective disorder is less common than either schizophrenia or mood disorders. Emergency presentations resemble hybrids of the disorders. Manic energy, irritability, and a reduced need for sleep may coexist with bizarre ideation or behavior and constricted or inappropriate affects.

CLINICAL FEATURES AND DIAGNOSIS

The clinical signs and symptoms of schizoaffective disorder include all the signs and symptoms of schizophrenia, mania, and depression. The schizophrenic and mood disorder symptoms can present together or in an alternating fashion. The diagnosis may be appropriate when psychotic symptoms have persisted without prominent mood symptoms for at least two weeks but the duration of all symptoms is less than that required for the diagnosis of schizophrenia.

The course can vary from one of exacerbations and remissions to a steadily deteriorating course. Patients with schizoaffective disorder, bipolar type, have a prognosis similar to those with bipolar disorder; those with schizoaffective disorder, depressive type, are prognostically similar to schizophrenia patients. Regardless of type, the same factors that suggest a poor prognosis in schizophrenia are also ominous in schizoaffective disorder. Poor premorbid functioning; an insidious onset; the lack of a precipitant; the predominance of psychotic symptoms, particularly negative and deficit symptoms; an early onset; an unremitting course; and a family history of schizophrenia indicate a poor outcome.

INTERVIEWING AND PSYCHOTHERAPEUTIC GUIDELINES

In interviewing all patients with a history of psychotic symptoms, elicit a history of affective symptoms as well, as they have important treatment implications. However, flight of ideas, distractibility, impulsivity, and intrusiveness can compromise the examination. The schizoaffective disorder patient may be more bizarre or paranoid than the typical mood disorder patient and, consequently, more difficult to interview.

The best approach is a firm, insistent style. Inform the patient explicitly of the structure of the setting, and be prepared to remind the patient of that structure at intervals.

Reduce stimulation as much as possible. Manic patients are sociable and may respond well to the structure provided by the staff and the psychiatrist, but may do much less well in less structured situations.

Patients are likely to be unrealistic about their abilities and prospects, minimizing the consequences of inappropriate behavior and exaggerating their chances of success. The patient's family probably knows best what the patient can tolerate outside the hospital and should be consulted.

Despite seeming to be euphoric, schizoaffective disorder patients are often suicidal. Suicidal ideas may be present even when the patient's mood appears to be elated. Furthermore, the patient's mood is often unstable, and a depressive affect may quickly descend on the patient, carrying with it pessimistic or nihilistic thoughts with attendant suicidal ideation. The risk of the patient's acting on suicidal thoughts in a vulnerable moment if the means are available is significant and must be explored.

EVALUATION AND MANAGEMENT

1. Firm structure is the mainstay of the treatment of schizoaffective patients with manic symptoms. They may require confinement to their rooms and visitor restrictions to reduce stimulation. That limitation offers opportunities to reinforce the patients' appropriate behavior by gradually removing restrictions. Agitation may require locked or unlocked seclusion or restraints.

2. Suicidal ideation should be monitored at frequent intervals. Supervision is adjusted according to the patients' compliance with the prescribed structure and the intensity of their suicidal ideation, if present.

3. Evaluate the patients for concomitant medical problems and substance abuse.

DRUG TREATMENT

If the patient has active psychotic symptoms, the initial treatment of schizoaffective disorder is similar to the treatment of schizophrenia. Antipsychotics alone may be sufficient to terminate both the psychotic symptoms and the manic symptoms.

The treatment of psychosis or agitation can be initiated with agents such as haloperidol (Haldol), fluphenazine (Prolixin), and thiothixene (Navane), all given at 2 to 5 mg by mouth or intramuscularly (IM). Benzodiazepines, such as lorazepam (Ativan) 1 to 2 mg by mouth or IM and clonazepam (Klonopin) 0.5 to 1 mg by mouth, may also be useful for short-term control. Schizoaffective disorder patients may also need treatment with lithium carbonate (Eskalith), anticonvulsants, or antidepressants. Those agents are usually initiated as part of an ongoing outpatient treatment plan or during inpatient care.

Cross-References:

Depression, mania, schizophrenia.

---

123 / Schizophrenia

Schizophrenia is a chronic, relapsing, remitting psychotic disorder with protean manifestations. The premorbid adjustment, the symptoms, and the course are all variable; in fact, schizophrenia is probably a heterogeneous group of disorders. Although the incidence is only 1 per 1,000 persons in the United States, schizophrenia is overrepresented in the emergency room because of the severity of its symptoms, the inability of patients to care for themselves, their lack of insight, and their gradual social deterioration and disaffiliation. Common emergency room and office presentations include distressing hallucinations (which may be loud and distracting, derogatory, or threatening), bizarre behavior, incoherence, agitation, and neglect.

CLINICAL FEATURES AND DIAGNOSIS

No symptom found in schizophrenia in pathognomonic for the disorder. What distinguishes schizophrenia is the course: at least six months of continuous signs of the disturbance, failure to return to the previous level of functioning, and continuing vulnerability to stress. Table B.123–1 lists the diagnostic criteria for schizophrenia.

Patients in the schizophrenic spectrum are driven to seek help for various reasons at various points in the course of the illness. Initially, in cases with a sudden onset, patients are frightened by the confusion of their thought processes; their bizarre, alien thoughts; novel perceptual disturbances; and either a welter of emotions or a deadening of emotional responses. Patients may explicitly wonder if they are losing their minds. Cases with a gradual or insidious onset may present because of school failure, social withdrawal, or bizarre behavior.

As the illness progresses and the psychosocial consequences mount, secondary depression may result in suicidal ideation. Such patients are at high risk not as a result of the psychosis itself but as a result of their understandable demoralization.

Most patients reach a plateau, become knowledgeable about their illness, and do not require hospitalization for exacerbations if good outpatient care is available. However, a disruption in their support system, such as the departure of their therapist or the death of a parent, may result in severe relapses.

Some patients, despite the best of care, follow a downhill course, become totally and permanently disabled, and require custodial care to maintain the basic aspects of nutrition and hygiene. A minority lose insight into the fact of their illness or the psychological nature of their illness and may wander from hospital to hospital, seeking treatment for bizarre somatic complaints. A few patients shun all human contact, are lost to their families, and eke out an existence by eating refuse as they gradually deteriorate physically. They may ultimately be brought to the emergency room by the authorities because of the threat of exposure in winter or obvious medical illness, such as cellulitis of the extremities.

Deterioration in schizophrenia is accelerated by substance abuse. Chemical dependence affects as many as half the schizophrenic patients in some settings and has both direct and indirect deleterious effects.

INTERVIEWING AND PSYCHOTHERAPEUTIC GUIDELINES

Begin by talking with patients about their premorbid conditions, rather than their florid symptoms, to put the patients at ease and to establish a benchmark by which current functioning is measured.

Table B.123-1
Diagnostic Criteria for Schizophrenia

A. Presence of characteristic psychotic symptoms in the active phase: either (1), (2), or (3) for at least one week (unless the symptoms are successfully treated):
  (1) two of the following:
     (*a*) delusions
     (*b*) prominent hallucinations (throughout the day for several days or several times a week for several weeks, each hallucinatory experience not being limited to a few brief moments)
     (*c*) incoherence or marked loosening of associations
     (*d*) catatonic behavior
     (*e*) flat or grossly inappropriate affect
  (2) bizarre delusions involving a phenomenon that the person's culture would regard as totally implausible (e.g., thought broadcasting, being controlled by a dead person)
  (3) prominent hallucinations [as defined in (1)(*b*) above] of a voice with content having no apparent relation to depression or elation, or a voice keeping up a running commentary on the person's behavior or thoughts, or two or more voices conversing with each other

B. During the course of the disturbance, functioning in such areas as work, social relations, and self-care is markedly below the highest level achieved before onset of the disturbance (or, when the onset is in childhood or adolescence, failure to achieve expected level of social development).

C. Schizoaffective disorder and mood disorder with psychotic features have been ruled out, i.e., if a major depressive or manic syndrome has ever been present during an active phase of the disturbance, the total duration of all episodes of a mood syndrome has been brief relative to the total duration of the active and residual phases of the disturbance.

D. Continuous signs of the disturbance for at least six months. The six-month period must include an active phase (of at least one week, or less if symptoms have been successfully treated) during which there were psychotic symptoms characteristic of schizophrenia (symptoms in A), with or without a prodromal or residual phase, as defined below.

Prodromal phase: A clear deterioration in functioning before the active phase of the disturbance that is not due to a disturbance in mood or to a psychoactive substance use disorder and that involves at least two of the symptoms listed below.

Residual phase: Following the active phase of the disturbance, persistence of at least two of the symptoms noted below, these not being due to a disturbance in mood or to a psychoactive substance use disorder.

Prodromal or residual symptoms:
  (1) marked social isolation or withdrawal
  (2) marked impairment in role functioning as wage-earner, student, or homemaker
  (3) markedly peculiar behavior (e.g., collecting garbage, talking to self in public, hoarding food)
  (4) marked impairment in personal hygiene and grooming
  (5) blunted or inappropriate affect
  (6) digressive, vague, overelaborate, or circumstantial speech, or poverty of speech, or poverty of content of speech
  (7) odd beliefs or magical thinking, influencing behavior and inconsistent with cultural norms (e.g., superstitiousness, belief in clairvoyance, telepathy, "sixth sense," "others can feel my feelings," overvalued ideas, ideas of reference)
  (8) unusual perceptual experiences (e.g., recurrent illusions, sensing the presence of a force or person not actually present)
  (9) marked lack of initiative, interests, or energy

Examples: Six months of prodromal symptoms with one week of symptoms from A; no prodromal symptoms with six months of symptoms from A; no prodromal symptoms with one week of symptoms from A and six months of residual symptoms.

E. It cannot be established that an organic factor initiated and maintained the disturbance.

F. If there is a history of autistic disorder, the additional diagnosis of schizophrenia is made only if prominent delusions or hallucinations are also present.

Table B.123-1—*continued*

Classification of course. The course of the disturbance is coded in the fifth digit:

1-Subchronic. The time from the beginning of the disturbance, when the person first began to show signs of the disturbance (including prodromal, active, and residual phases) more or less continuously, is less than two years but at least six months.

2-Chronic. Same as above, but more than two years.

3-Subchronic with acute exacerbation. Reemergence of prominent psychotic symptoms in a person with a subchronic course who has been in the residual phase of the disturbance.

4-Chronic with acute exacerbation. Reemergence of prominent psychotic symptoms in a person with a chronic course who has been in the residual phase of the disturbance.

5-In remission. When a person with a history of schizophrenia is free of all signs of the disturbance (whether or not on medication), "in remission" should be coded. Differentiating schizophrenia in remission from no mental disorder requires consideration of overall level of functioning, length of time since the last episode of disturbance, total duration of the disturbance, and whether prophylactic treatment is being given.

0-Unspecified.

Specify late onset if the disturbance (including the prodromal phase) develops after age 45.

Table from DSM-III-R, *Diagnostic and Statistical Manual of Mental Disorders,* ed 3, revised. Copyright American Psychiatric Association, Washington, 1987. Used with permission.

The next step in a chronological approach to the patient's history is to establish the earliest manifestation that suggested a prodrome, followed by the active-phase symptoms. Thought disorders, lack of motivation, paranoid thinking, and poor insight may all contribute to a difficulty eliciting an adequate history. Collateral contacts may be more revealing than the patient.

Inquire in detail about unusual experiences of any kind. If the patient cannot describe any, ask about specific experiences, beginning with such prepsychotic experiences as déjà vu, numbness, derealization, and depersonalization—matters that are not immediately identified with being psychotic. Florid hallucination may then be broached as the logical next step. If the patient protests the line of questioning, defuse the issue by stating that these are routine medical questions. If necessary, abandon the history of the patient's psychotic symptoms, and shift to questions of mood and cognition, which may be less threatening.

Ask about suicidal ideation; 10 percent of schizophrenic patients die by suicide, usually early in the course of the disorder.

Cognitive examination is also important, as numerous medical conditions may present with signs of schizophrenia, at least early in their course, but do not usually involve cognitive impairment.

EVALUATION AND MANAGEMENT

1. Because of the need for a thorough medical evaluation and the demonstrated efficacy of the psychoeducational aspects of hospitalization, all schizophrenic patients should probably be admitted to the hospital if possible during their first presentation. The hospital provides a supportive environment and exposure to others with similar conditions receiving sim-

ilar treatment. Many questions can be answered quickly by peers and staff members.

2. However, if the patient is strongly opposed to hospitalization, the adverse effects of forcible treatment on any future relationship must be weighed against the risks of outpatient treatment or no treatment. Supervision by the patient's family may make outpatient treatment viable, but it also complicates treatment and may increase the stresses on the patient. No family should be relied on for constant observation. Conditions warranting that degree of concern require hospitalization.

3. Hospital admission late in the course of the illness may be prompted by severe distress related to loud, continuous, derogatory, or threatening voices. Simple, repetitive commands are not typical and probably indicate malingering. In such cases, ascertain from other sources the nonillness variables that are motivating the patient.

4. Paranoia may keep the patient from sleeping and may result in dangerous defensive behavior. Patients sometimes say that they would rather kill themselves than be captured by others. Activity at both extremes, severe apathy and agitation, may necessitate hospital admission.

5. Threatening patients are often chronically ill, do not benefit from treatment, and can be released only after the obligation to protect others is satisfied and if the patients are not a danger to themselves or others. Somatic delusions may result in self-mutilation, autoamputation, or enucleation.

6. Unpredictability is the rule, and a high level of vigilance is indicated. In the hospital, use contracts, periodic checks, and constant observation. However, suicidal ideation in schizophrenic patients is usually a result of depression, rather than psychosis, and in most respects is similar to the suicidal ideation of other people with real losses, failures, and hopelessness about the future.

DRUG TREATMENT

Antipsychotic drugs ameliorate and reduce the signs and symptoms of schizophrenia. Consider low potency antipsychotic drugs (chlopromazine [Thorazine]) if the patient is hyperactive or agitated. Consider high potency antipsychotic drugs (trifluoperazine [Stelazine]) if the patient is withdrawn or lethargic. Clozapine (Clozaril) is used in resistant cases.

In general, both high and low potency drugs are equally effective, but one may work better than another in an individual case.

Start with 25 mg by mouth or intramuscularly (IM) of chlorpromazine and raise the dosage to 300 to 1,800 mg daily for acute attacks. Titrate the dosage upward until the therapeutic effect is achieved. Haloperidol (Haldol) may be used for rapid tranquilization (1 to 10 mg by mouth or IM over 30 to 60 minutes); its daily dosage may go as high as 100 mg. Long-acting depot fluphenazine (Prolixin, Permitil) concentrate/decanoate (25 mg IM) can be effective for 14 to 21 days and is helpful in increasing compliance.

Cross-References:

Brief reactive psychosis, catatonic schizophrenia, chronic schizophrenia in acute exacerbation, delusional disorder, depression, hallucinations, hospitalization, malingering, neologisms, schizoaffective disorder, self-mutilation, suicide, violence.

124 / School Phobia and School Refusal

School phobia is a form of separation anxiety in which children are afraid of school. They may refuse to go to school or endure school with great difficulty because of the overwhelming anxiety that occurs when they are faced with the separation from parental figures that results from attending school.

School refusal may occur for a variety of reasons and under some circumstances may provoke a crisis. Anxiety may contribute to the refusal and may be related to separation from a parent or important caretaker, as in separation anxiety disorder, or anxiety about meeting future expectations, as in overanxious disorder.

CLINICAL FEATURES AND DIAGNOSIS

Anxiety in children often does not appear in a pure form. Overanxious children may also suffer from separation anxiety disorder, avoidant disorder, depression, panic disorder, learning disabilities, and functional enuresis. Each of those problems may contribute to school phobia and refusal in different ways. The overanxious child is persistently concerned about future events and competence in a variety of areas, including athletic, academic, and social performance. Psychophysiological complaints are common in both separation anxiety disorder and overanxious disorder. Children may present with multiple somatic complaints given as the reason for absenteeism. Somatic symptoms secondary to school phobia generally disappear during vacations, holidays, and weekends. True medical illness may result in school refusal. Other causes include family dynamics (such as a dependent parent or caretaker who covertly encourages school refusal), realistic fear caused by victimization at school, and truancy. Children with school phobia have great difficulty in leaving for school; truant children leave readily, claiming to go to school. Truancy is often accompanied by other behavioral problems (for example, fighting and rule breaking). Children with separation anxiety disorder fear that something will happen to them or to their parents or caretakers while they are in school. Depression reduces energy and motivation and results in clinging behavior and school phobia in children.

INTERVIEWING AND PSYCHOTHERAPEUTIC GUIDELINES

The overanxious child may attempt to hide behind the parent and converses with great difficulty. The depressed child may also cling to the parent but may be more easily engaged than the overanxious child. A child with physical complaints should be given a thorough physical examination. The parent provides most of the history. Observe and assess the family dynamics to determine whether the parents are putting the child in a double bind as a result of their own dependence needs. Are the parents encouraging the school phobia?

Explain to both that a return to school is extremely important. The child can be told that he or she need not attend class but that being in the school building itself is part of the therapy. Find out if there is any area of the school (for example, principal's office, gym teacher's office) where the student feels comfortable.

EVALUATION AND MANAGEMENT

1. Perform a thorough medical evaluation to rule out organic illness as the cause of the school refusal. Demonstrating a lack of organic disease helps the clinician in confronting the child and the family with the psychological origin of the symptoms.

2. Perform a full psychiatric evaluation to rule out other psychiatric disorders, such as depression and psychosis, that can cause severe absenteeism.

3. Obtain a history of the child's experience at school. Is the child being teased or bullied? The child's fears may be realistic and amenable to manipulation of the school environment.

4. If school phobia is diagnosed, give the family an explanation of the fear and instructions regarding the implementation of a structured, consistent treatment plan designed to get the child back into school as quickly as possible. It is imperative that the child return to school. The school can be enlisted to aid in the process, which should be carried out with an outpatient therapist. Strategies include having an adult take the child to school and sit in on classes for steadily decreasing amounts of time. A caretaker can telephone the child once daily at school. Any plan needs to address contributing family dynamics. Family therapy or individual psychotherapy for the parents may be needed.

DRUG TREATMENT

Imipramine (Tofranil) can be considered if other treatment modalities are unsuccessful. The medication should be implemented as part of an ongoing therapeutic relationship and should not be initiated in the emergency room.

Cross-References:

Phobia, separation anxiety.

125 / Seclusion

Seclusion is the isolation of a patient in an environment of low stimulation. Seclusion may or may not include locking the door of the room.

CLINICAL FEATURES AND DIAGNOSIS

The indications for seclusion are similar to those for restraints but are less severe. The indications include potential assault, self-injurious behavior, and disorganization to the point of risking self-harm. Seclusion, quiet time, or time out is often an effective alternative to physical restraints and injection with a tranquilizing medication. Many agitated patients, if removed from a stimulating environment that may be provocative, are able to regain behavioral control of themselves. The isolation provides an opportunity for self-reflection in a low-stimulation environment.

Seclusion rooms must be as safe as possible. Remove any potentially dangerous objects from both the patient and the room, and keep the patient under observation.

INTERVIEWING AND PSYCHOTHERAPEUTIC GUIDELINES

In restraint, limits are externally imposed on patients; in contrast, the objective of seclusion is to give patients the opportunity to regain their composure themselves.

Before secluding a patient, describe directly and as specifically as possible the behavior that may lead to seclusion, providing the patient an opportunity to stop the behavior and avoid being secluded. Present yourself to the patient as an ally who is helping prevent seclusion, but indicate that, if the behavior continues, seclusion is inevitable.

If the dangerous behavior does continue, give repeated fair warnings that seclusion may be necessary. Tell the patient that seclusion will be required for a limited time until the behavior has ceased.

Be firm, set clear limits, and prevent escalation of the dangerous behavior. If appropriate, offer medication that may improve the patient's behavioral control and avoid the need for seclusion or restraints.

EVALUATION AND MANAGEMENT

1. Identify the behaviors that may lead to seclusion or restraints.
2. Inform the patient clearly that the behaviors must stop; otherwise, seclusion will be necessary.
3. Have enough staff members available to enforce seclusion if it is needed.
4. If the dangerous or disruptive behavior continues, insist that the patient go into the quiet room, possibly with the door open or unlocked. If

necessary, the patient may be physically forced into the seclusion room, and the door may be locked.

5. Remove any items from the patient that could be used to injure self or others (for example, sharp objects).

6. Check the patient at least every 15 minutes, and give the patient regular and predictable opportunities to show behavioral control and to obtain release from seclusion. Encourage the patient to comply.

7. If agitation or violence persist while the patient is in seclusion (for example, head banging, punching walls, kicking the door), physical restraints or chemical restraint with an injection of tranquilizing medication may be necessary.

8. Clearly document and justify the use of seclusion in the medical record.

DRUG TREATMENT

Seclusion may or may not be used in conjunction with pharmacological agents. If drugs are used, check the patient frequently (at least every 15 minutes) for adverse drug effects.

Cross-References:

Agitation, homicidal and assaultive behavior, hospitalization, restraints.

---

126 / Self-Mutilation

Self-mutilation—most commonly by cutting oneself with a sharp object, such as a knife—may be manipulative or may reflect a genuine intent to do self-harm.

CLINICAL FEATURES AND DIAGNOSIS

In severe cases, patients cut off their own ears, genitals, or other body parts. Burning oneself with cigarettes and inserting objects under the skin are other methods. Head banging, nail biting, and hair pulling are variants sometimes seen in children.

Usually, the problem is long-term, but it can occur impulsively in psychotic patients. The intent is typically not suicide, although self-injurious patients are also prone to suicide attempts, and self-mutilation may precede a suicide attempt. Self-mutilation is more common in females than in males and is more common in patients in their 20s than in older patients.

The common sites of self-injury include the wrists, the arms, and the thighs. The breasts, the face, and the abdomen are less typical sites.

Many patients who cut themselves claim that the experience is painless. The reasons for self-cutting include anger at self or others, tension, a wish to die, and the need to feel pain in order to feel alive. Self-mutilating behavior is also effective in gaining attention. The behavior may be used to manipulate and elicit specific responses.

Patients who are malingering may injure themselves in attempts to obtain either psychiatric or medical-surgical treatment. Patients with factitious disorders may injure themselves to create evidence supporting their need to maintain the sick role.

The most common diagnosis among self-mutilating patients is severe personality disorder, often borderline or antisocial personality disorder. Substance abuse and dependence are commonly associated features.

Self-mutilation in a child who is a victim of child abuse may be an act of aggression toward the abuser that has been directed instead toward the self.

Psychotic patients may injure themselves. The self-mutilating behavior in psychotic patients is sometimes bizarre and may be based on a somatic delusion (for example, that a part of the body is contaminated). In psychotic patients, the self-mutilating act may be unpredictable and impulsive. Patients who are psychotic because of phencyclidine (PCP) intoxication may injure themselves with total disregard for the pain, since the drug causes analgesia, as well as psychosis.

Other types of self-mutilating behavior with typical onset during childhood include head banging and nail biting. Scratching and hair pulling are less common. All may occur as relatively circumscribed stereotypy and habit disorders or in the course of pervasive disorders, such as schizophrenia, mental retardation, autistic disorder, other pervasive developmental disorders, and organic disorders. Lesch-Nyhan syndrome is an X-linked recessive developmental disorder associated with metabolic derangements that can lead to persistent self-mutilating behavior that may require ongoing physical restraint.

INTERVIEWING AND PSYCHOTHERAPEUTIC GUIDELINES

Suspect self-mutilation if other explanations do not easily account for the patient's injuries. Try to determine early in the evaluation whether the patient is psychotic. Explore the possible secondary gain that the self-mutilation provides the patient. If the patient is a child, look for a possible history of child abuse.

Distinguish patients who admit to self-mutilating behavior from patients who are mutilating themselves but deny it. Although the distinction does not always lead to specific interventions, the admitted self-mutilator can be addressed directly, but the denying self-mutilator may be unpredictable and should be treated cautiously.

Consider self-mutilating patients highly dangerous. Maintain clear and firm control of the situation, and clearly inform the patient that continued self-injurious behavior will not be tolerated.

Try to determine whether the self-mutilating behavior is under voluntary control and thus likely to respond to a nonsomatic intervention. Self-mutilating behavior in patients with psychotic disorders, organic disorders, autistic disorder, and other pervasive developmental disorders is less under voluntary control than is self-mutilating behavior in patients with personality disorders.

EVALUATION AND MANAGEMENT

1. Prevent continued self-mutilation with physical restraints if necessary.

2. Perform a complete evaluation, including a medical and psychiatric history, a complete mental status examination, a history of drug and alcohol use, and a physical examination. Examine the patient's body for scars from previous self-mutilating acts.

3. If the patient is a child, look carefully for evidence of possible child abuse.

4. Try to assess the purpose of the self-mutilating behavior: Was it a suicide attempt, or is it due to psychosis? Does it reflect aggression toward another, or is it an act to manipulate the environment and elicit a response from others?

5. Make a definitive psychiatric diagnosis. Self-destructive behavior is a sign of many different diagnoses.

6. If the patient is clearly not psychotic and if the behavior is intended to elicit some specific response from others, use crisis-intervention techniques to reduce the patient's motivation to manipulate others in that way.

7. If the self-mutilation is a suicide gesture, be conservative, and respond to all acts of self-injury as potentially life-threatening. Any other response may deliver a message that the patient must escalate the dangerousness of the self-destructive acts to elicit a definitive intervention.

8. If the patient is psychotic, hospitalization is necessary.

9. Hospitalize nonpsychotic patients if the self-mutilating behavior is likely to continue.

10. During psychiatric hospitalization, maintain one-to-one constant observation to prevent further self-mutilating behavior.

11. Drug treatment and physical restraints are interventions of last resort.

DRUG TREATMENT

The specific drug treatment depends on the definitive diagnosis, rather than on just the self-mutilating behavior.

A sufficient dose of an antipsychotic will eliminate all purposeful behavior, including self-mutilation. But, if the only target symptom is the self-mutilating behavior, tranquilization with antipsychotics, benzodiazepines, or barbiturates is not appropriate for purposes other than providing immediate behavioral control.

The drug treatment plan should focus on long-term management, since self-mutilating behaviors are usually chronic. Drug choice should be based on a definitive diagnosis and a specific treatment of that disorder.

Antipsychotics are indicated if the patient is chronically psychotic. Anticonvulsants such as carbamazepine (Tegretol) may be useful in some organic disorders and in impulse control disorders. β-Blockers—for example, propranolol (Inderal)—are also helpful in reducing violence.

Cross-References:

Agitation, borderline personality disorder, chronic schizophrenia in acute exacerbation, delirium, delusional disorder, hallucinations, homicidal and assaultive behavior, hospitalization, intoxication, malingering, schizophrenia, suicide.

---

127 / Separation Anxiety

Separation anxiety is a type of phobic anxiety that occurs in children during separation or while anticipating separation from a parent or important caretaker. The child's reaction may approach terror or panic. Violence against the person enforcing the separation is possible. School refusal may precipitate a psychiatric emergency. The age at onset is preschool through adolescence. Cases beginning up to 12 years of age are common, but new cases in the teen years are rare.

CLINICAL FEATURES AND DIAGNOSIS

The diagnostic criteria for separation anxiety disorder are listed in Table B.127-1. Morbid fears, preoccupations, and ruminations are characteristic of the disorder. Children become fearful that someone close to them will be hurt or that something terrible will happen to them while they are away from important figures. Fears of getting lost and of being kidnapped and never reunited with their parents are common.

INTERVIEWING AND PSYCHOTHERAPEUTIC GUIDELINES

Parents provide most of the history. The parents and the children should be interviewed separately, if possible, and the children's reactions to efforts to separate them from the parents for the interview should be noted. If children are present during the parents' interviews, the children may accuse the parents of not loving them and may make it difficult for the parents to express their concerns. The children may argue the facts and minimize the problems, fearing that consultation has been sought to curtail their relationships with the parents. However, insisting on separation during early contacts may be both impractical and damaging to the nascent therapeutic relationship.

EVALUATION AND MANAGEMENT

1. Develop a comprehensive treatment plan, particularly in the case of school refusal. Planning should involve the child, the parents, the child's peers, and the school. Encourage the child to attend school, but, if a return to a full school day is overwhelming, arrange a program for the child to gradually increase the time at school.

Table B.127–1
Diagnostic Criteria for Separation Anxiety Disorder

A. Excessive anxiety concerning separation from those to whom the child is attached, as evidenced by at least three of the following:
  (1) unrealistic and persistent worry about possible harm befalling major attachment figures or fear that they will leave and not return
  (2) unrealistic and persistent worry that an untoward calamitous event will separate the child from a major attachment figure (e.g., the child will be lost, kidnapped, killed, or the victim of an accident)
  (3) persistent reluctance or refusal to go to school in order to stay with major attachment figures or at home
  (4) persistent reluctance or refusal to go to sleep without being near a major attachment figure or to go to sleep away from home
  (5) persistent avoidance of being alone, including "clinging to" and "shadowing" major attachment figures
  (6) repeated nightmares involving the theme of separation
  (7) complains of physical symptoms (e.g., headaches, stomachaches, nausea, or vomiting, on many school days or on other occasions when anticipating separation from major attachment figures)
  (8) recurrent signs or complaints of excessive distress in anticipation of separation from home or major attachment figures (e.g., temper tantrums or crying, pleading with parents not to leave)
  (9) recurrent signs of complaints of excessive distress when separated from home or major attachment figures (e.g., wants to return home, needs to call parents when they are absent or when child is away from home)

B. Duration of disturbance of at least two weeks

C. Onset before the age of 18

D. Occurrence not exclusively during the course of a pervasive developmental disorder, schizophrenia, or any other psychotic disorder

Table from DSM-III-R, *Diagnostic and Statistical Manual of Mental Disorders,* ed 3, revised. Copyright American Psychiatric Association, Washington, 1987. Used with permission.

2. Provide psychotherapy directed at increasing the child's autonomy by exploring the unconscious fears underlying the symptoms. Family therapy helps the parents be consistent and supportive and prepares the child for important changes in life.

3. Occasionally, the child and the family are enmeshed to a degree that frustrates any outpatient intervention. Such cases may require hospitalization to interrupt the operation of the family system and to allow for the development of new behavior.

DRUG TREATMENT

Tricyclic and tetracyclic antidepressants effectively reduce panic symptoms. Start imipramine (Tofranil) at a dosage of 25 mg daily and increase it in 25-mg increments up to a total of 150 to 200 mg a day. (Electrocardiographic [ECG] monitoring is needed.) If the child shows no response at that dosage, determine the plasma levels of imipramine and its active metabolite desmethylimipramine. The medication should be initiated by a child psychiatrist as part of an ongoing treatment plan and therapeutic relationship. In most cases, the imipramine should not be started in the emergency room. Diphenhydramine (Benadryl) in dosages of 10 to 25 mg by mouth at bedtime can be used for associated insomnia.

Cross-Reference:
School phobia and school refusal.

128 / Serotonin Syndrome

Serotonin syndrome is a potentially fatal toxic reaction that occurs when serotonergic psychotropic agents, clomipramine (Anafranil), or tryptophan and monoamine oxidase inhibitors (MAOIs) are coadministered.

CLINICAL FEATURES AND DIAGNOSIS

The diagnosis of serotonin syndrome is based on a history of the ingestion of the offending drug combinations and the production of the characteristic signs and symptoms, including hyperthermia, diaphoresis, excitement, rigidity, hyperreflexia, hypotension, headache, tremor, confusion, coma, and death. The syndrome has occurred in patients taking the combination of serotonergic agents and MAOIs or the combination of clomipramine or tryptophan and MAOIs.

The risk of the reaction's occurring in combination with MAOIs is thought to be related to the non-MAOIs' degree of serotonergicity. Therefore, clomipramine and tryptophan are at high risk of causing the syndrome in combination with MAOIs. Serotonin-specific reuptake inhibitors also cause serotonin syndrome in combination with MAOIs.

Reactions can occur even if MAOIs are started several weeks after discontinuing serotonergic agents.

Patients have recovered spontaneously on discontinuation of the psychotropics involved; however, serious medical complications—including disseminated intravascular coagulation, rhabdomyolysis, and death—have occurred.

Tyramine reactions and neuroleptic malignant syndrome (in patients taking antipsychotics) should be considered in the differential diagnosis. A history of antipsychotic drug intake and no history of serotonergic drug intake should indicate neuroleptic malignant syndrome, rather than serotonin syndrome.

INTERVIEWING AND PSYCHOTHERAPEUTIC GUIDELINES

The patients are in medical distress and require prompt medical referral and treatment. Therefore, keep the interview brief and medically oriented. Obtain a history of the patient's ingestion of the agents that can produce the syndrome. Reassure the patient that recovery is likely within days to weeks.

EVALUATION AND MANAGEMENT

1. Obtain the patient's vital signs.
2. Perform a full medical workup, and obtain a medical consultation.
3. Discontinue the offending agents.
4. Give the patient supportive and symptomatic medical care.

DRUG TREATMENT

No specific drug treatment is indicated, as the medical complications dictate management. Avoid offending drug combinations. Intravenous dantrolene (Dantrium) or oral cyproheptadine (Periactin) may be useful in treating serotonin syndrome secondary to the combination of MAOIs and serotonergic agents.

Cross-References:

Hypertensive crisis, neuroleptic malignant syndrome.

---

129 / Sexual Emergencies

Disorders of sexual function may bring patients to your office or to the emergency room. Impotence may occur for the first time in a previously well-functioning person and create overwhelming anxiety. Homosexual panic may happen unexpectedly with dire consequences. Other sexual disorders may so upset the patient's psychological equilibrium that the person involved feels compelled to seek immediate help. In addition, sexual behavior may infringe on the rights or the privacy of others to such an extent that persons are brought to the emergency room against their will for evaluation and management.

Some disorders present first to the medical emergency room, others to the psychiatric emergency room. In almost all cases, however, the physician finds signs and symptoms of mental illness of varying severity that have to be addressed. Some epileptic states, such as temporal lobe disorders, have been associated with sexual aberrations.

DIAGNOSIS AND CLINICAL FEATURES

Algolagnia

Algolagnia encompasses any form of sexual behavior associated with the giving or the receiving of pain.

In *sadism,* pain is inflicted on one person by another; in *masochism,* pain is received by the person or is self-inflicted. Unusual wounds—such as human bites, trunk lacerations (from whip lashings), bleeding of the nipples (in both sexes), and holes in the labia of women or in the prepuce of men (into which metal rings are inserted)—are presumptive signs of sadomasochistic activities.

Analingus

Analingus involves the stimulation of the anus of one person by the mouth, the tongue, or the lips of another.

Foreign objects (for example, bottles and light bulbs) may be inserted into the anus. If they cannot be expelled, emergency evacuation is required.

Anal Intercourse

Anal intercourse occurs most often in homosexual men, but it is also practiced by some heterosexual pairs. The woman may penetrate the man with a dildo that she either wears with a harness or inserts manually. Anal tears, fissures, and hemorrhoids may be sequelae of such activities.

Aphrodisiacs

Aphrodisiacs are substances purported to excite sexual desire. Stimulants, sedatives, hallucinogens, and opioids may be used in an attempt to enhance sexual pleasure. Signs of intoxication or withdrawal from the substance may occur. Some substances (for example, capsaicin) may be rubbed on the genitalia and cause burns. Cantharis (Spanish fly) is toxic and causes hepatorenal damage.

Autoerotic Asphyxiation

Autoerotic asphyxiation involves masturbating while hanging oneself by the neck to heighten the erotic sensations and the intensity of the orgasm through mild hypoxia. Although the persons intend to release themselves from the noose after orgasm, an estimated 500 to 1,000 persons a year accidentally kill themselves by hanging. Most of those who indulge in the practice are male; transvestism is often associated with the habit, and the majority of deaths occur among adolescents. The patient, if found alive, may be brought to the psychiatric emergency room as an attempted suicide; but the clinician should be alert to the possibility of autoerotic asphyxiation, which is usually associated with severe mental disorders, such as schizophrenia and major mood disorders.

Autoeroticism

Autoeroticism involves sexual arousal of oneself without the participation of another person (masturbation). At times, objects are used to enhance the experience. The objects include dildos inserted into the vagina, catheters or other objects inserted into the male or female urethra, and mechanical vibrators (with or without electrical sources), all of which can cause physical damage to the genitalia. Compulsive masturbation may produce penile or vaginal wounds and excoriations.

Bestiality

Bestiality is a sexual deviation in which a person engages in sexual relations with an animal. Both males and females may allow dogs or cats to lick their genitalia, which may cause urethritis, cystitis, or vaginitis. In rural areas, copulation with farm animals can produce vaginal infections and wounds in females and penile abrasions and infections in males.

Castration

Castration is mutilation of the penis or the testicles. Self-castration is carried out by severely ill psychotic persons and by transsexuals who have been denied male-to-female genital surgery and who hope to have a surgical procedure on an emergency basis.

Coprolalia

Coprolalia is the compulsive use of vulgar or obscene words. It is most often found in men who approach women in public places with lewd and graphic invitations to engage in sex acts of various kinds. Patients with Tourette's disorder may have coprolalia as an associated manifestation.

Coprophilia

In coprophilia, sexual pleasure is associated with feces. Men or women may eat feces (coprophagia) or play with feces (their own or their partners' feces). Local infections of the mouth or the eyes and systemic infections (for example, hepatitis and parasitic infestation) may result.

Diaphragm

A diaphragm is a dome-shaped contraceptive device, usually made of rubber, that obstructs the cervical os. On occasion, a woman is unable to remove her diaphragm, and she arrives at the medical emergency room or doctor's office with that complaint. Tampons may also unknowingly remain in the vagina for long periods, with resulting infections.

Dildo

A dildo is an artificial penis made of rubber, silicone, or latex that is used by both men and women. It may cause physical tears of the vaginal or anal areas or produce chronic anal dilation and encopresis. Chronic anal dilation is most often found in homosexual men who repeatedly experience anal penetration.

Exhibitionism

Exhibitionism is a sexual disorder characterized by a compulsive need to expose one's body, particularly the genitals. It almost always occurs in men, who may be apprehended and brought to the emergency room for evaluation.

Frottage

Frottage is a sexual disorder in which men touch or rub their bodies against the breasts or buttocks of women in crowded places, such as subways. The perpetrator may be brought to the emergency room.

Koro

Koro is an acute anxiety reaction characterized by the patient's fear that his penis is shrinking and may disappear into his abdomen, in which case he will die. It is most common in Asians and is a psychiatric emergency because it may result in suicide.

Priapism

Priapism is a persistent penile erection accompanied by severe pain. It may occur as a side effect of some psychotropic drugs, such as trazodone (Desyrel). It is a true medical emergency that requires the removal of blood from the engorged penile cavernosa by mechanical or surgical drainage. Without timely intervention, thrombosis and gangrene may develop.

Scopophilia

Also known as voyeurism, scopophilia is characterized by the compulsive desire to view sex organs or sex acts. Persons with the disorder are often apprehended as peeping Toms and brought for psychiatric evaluation.

Urolagnia

Urolagnia is a sexual disorder characterized by getting sexual pleasure from drinking urine or being urinated on. Skin, eye, or mouth infections may result.

INTERVIEWING AND PSYCHOTHERAPEUTIC GUIDELINES

If questions about sex are indicated, inquire in language that is familiar to the patient. Questions should be as specific as possible. A professional manner helps elicit truthful responses with a minimum of patient embarrassment and shame. Asking about sex practices is especially important to determine whether or not the patient is at risk for human immunodeficiency virus (HIV) infection and other sexually transmitted diseases.

EVALUATION AND MANAGEMENT

1. Treatment is geared first to the presenting complaint; physical injuries require immediate medical attention.

2. No specific therapy for the underlying sexual disorder is given on an emergency basis; however, diagnose the disorder, and recommend a treatment plan.

3. Most persons with sexually deviant behavior experience severe guilt and shame, and you can motivate such patients for psychiatric treatment. In addition, you have the opportunity to provide reliable information to patients about sex, possibly for the first time.

4. Referral to a sex therapy clinic (one that is associated with a medical school is best) can be made for the definitive treatment of a wide range of sexual disorders.

DRUG TREATMENT

There is no drug treatment for these disorders. When anxiety is a major component, antianxiety agents may be of help. If there is an underlying psychosis, antipsychotic agents may be useful. Impulsive behavior may respond to serotonergic agents.

Cross-References:

Homosexual panic, impotence, rape and sexual abuse.

---

130 / Starvation

Starvation involves a series of physiological changes that the body undergoes in the course of reduced food intake. Psychiatric disturbances may lead to inanition, but starvation also produces secondary psychiatric symptoms, including intense preoccupation with food, food hoarding and stealing, binge eating, food dreams, sleep disturbance, loss of sexual interest, reduced concentration, decreased alertness, diminished ambition, and social withdrawal. Depression and a mild organic mental syndrome may result. Physical changes include a loss of fat, reduced muscle mass, reduced thyroid metabolism, cold intolerance, and difficulty in maintaining the core body temperature. Cardiac muscle condition and conduction are affected by cardiac muscle loss, atrial and ventricular premature contractions, ventricular tachycardia, and sudden death. The gastrointestinal effects are bloating, constipation, and abdominal pain. Menstrual irregularities are common, and amenorrhea ultimately develops in the course of starvation. Lanugo, edema, leukopenia, and osteoporosis are frequently found.

CLINICAL FEATURES AND DIAGNOSIS

Starvation may be deliberately self-induced for cultural reasons, as in hunger strikes, or may result from true anorexia, anorexia nervosa, or schizophrenic apathy. True anorexia is the loss of appetite and may occur in depression, grief, and anxiety disorders. The appetite is not affected in anorexia nervosa. Instead, patients with anorexia nervosa have a marked preoccupation with food, cook elaborate meals, eat surreptitiously, and binge eat. In addition, they suffer from a disturbance of body image, with the persistent belief that they are fat, despite all evidence to the contrary.

The elderly are vulnerable to starvation because of preexisting physical debilitation, dementia, social isolation, and poverty.

Schizophrenic persons among the homeless mentally ill may suffer starvation as a result of complete self-neglect. Hematological changes are common in those people partly because of nutritional reasons and partly because of lice infestation. They often deny any evidence of illness or social deterioration. Most will eat if meals are provided, but they do not have the motivation to obtain food. Some are too apathetic or paranoid to take meals that are offered to them.

INTERVIEWING AND PSYCHOTHERAPEUTIC GUIDELINES

Patients with social reasons to starve themselves and those with true anorexia are usually able to provide a reliable history. Patients with anorexia nervosa, however, are resistant. Schizophrenic patients may also be resistant, but the examiner need not focus directly on appetite and weight loss but can question patients indirectly and concretely. How do the patients support themselves? If they have money, how much do they spend on food? What do they like to eat? Some homeless mentally ill maintain an adequate, if unsanitary, diet by regular visits to the refuse cans of restaurants or by other scavenging. If that is the case, the patients should be able to describe the activity in some detail.

EVALUATION AND MANAGEMENT

1. Any patient with significant weight loss or decreased appetite should be evaluated medically to rule out any underlying physical illness (for example, malignancy). Starvation without complicating mental illness responds to feeding and vitamin supplementation.

2. Starving patients may require admission to the hospital to ensure an adequate intake of food. Involuntary hospitalization in such circumstances is controversial in some jurisdictions, as inanition may not be viewed as an imminent danger. However, most physicians agree that involuntary hospitalization is warranted in extreme cases. Once hospitalized, most patients respond to coaxing to eat.

3. In anorexia nervosa, a 20 percent reduction from the patient's ideal weight or significant electrolyte disturbances, particularly hypokalemia, suggest the need for hospital admission. The threat of hospitalization can be used to set limits on further starvation as long as binging and vomiting do

not derange the patient's electrolytes. Patients with anorexia nervosa do not respond to simple reasoning and advice.

4. Occasionally, electroconvulsive therapy (ECT) may be indicated for severe depression with inanition.

5. In severe cases, a nasogastric tube can be used.

DRUG TREATMENT

Anorexia in the case of depressed patients and apathy in the case of schizophrenic patients respond to treatment of the underlying condition.

Cross-Reference:

Anorexia nervosa.

---

131 / Suicide

Suicide is intentional self-inflicted death. Suicidal ideation and attempted suicide are among the most common emergency presentations. Common themes in suicide include a crisis that causes intense suffering and feelings of hopelessness and helplessness, conflicts between survival and unbearable stress, a narrowing of the patient's perceived options, and the wish to escape. Suicidal ideation occurs in vulnerable persons in response to many kinds of stressors at any age and may be present for long periods without resulting in an attempt.

CLINICAL FEATURES AND DIAGNOSIS

Identifying suicidal patients is a crucial but difficult task. Studies reveal that male sex, white race, advancing age, and social isolation increase the risk of completed suicide. Patients with family histories of suicide attempts or completions are at increased risk, as are patients with histories of chronic pain, recent surgery, or chronic physical illness. Also at increased risk are patients who are unemployed, live alone, put their affairs in order, or have an anniversary of a loss.

Eighty percent of patients who commit suicide have a mood disorder and 25 percent are alcohol dependent. Suicide is the cause of death for 15 percent of people in those two groups. The risk for alcoholic persons is particularly high in the six months after a major loss. Schizophrenia is a less common disorder and, therefore, accounts for a lower number of suicides, but 10 percent of persons with schizophrenia die by suicide.

The best hope for suicide prevention lies in the early detection and treatment of those contributory psychiatric disorders.

The role of prior suicide attempts in suicide risk assessment is complex. The majority of completed suicide victims have made no prior attempts; they are successful the first time. Although anyone who has made a prior suicide attempt has a demonstrated capacity for self-destructive behavior, only 10 percent of persons who attempt suicide are successful within 10 years.

A substantial number of deliberately self-aggressive persons cut or burn themselves in a clearly nonlethal manner with no intention of killing themselves. A variety of motives may be present, including deliberate manipulation and unconscious rage at significant others. Diagnostically, the patients may meet the criteria for antisocial or borderline personality disorder, or the behavior may coexist with other bizarre ideation and behavior in schizophrenia.

Especially disturbing and medicolegally challenging are parasuicides, who repeatedly and, to some extent, predictably engage in near-lethal behavior while denying suicidal ideation. The most common variant is the patient who takes repetitive, unintentional drug overdoses. Such patients appear to have personality disturbances without major psychiatric symptoms. They often demand their release from the hospital as soon as they recover from the acute intoxication, sometimes sooner, and it is difficult to justify treating them coercively. However, it is wise to detain such persons involuntarily if the frequency of their parasuicidal behavior escalates.

INTERVIEWING AND PSYCHOTHERAPEUTIC GUIDELINES

There is no truth to the myth that talking about suicide in a clinical setting induces it. Patients may spontaneously describe suicidal ideation. If they do not, question them directly.

Start by asking if the patients have ever felt like giving up or have felt that they would be better off dead. That approach carries little stigma and can be endorsed by most people.

Then talk about exactly what thoughts the patients have had and document the thoughts. Once the subject has been broached, use words like "killing" and "dying," rather than "hurting," since some patients are confused about the point of the question and most do not want to hurt themselves, even if they do want to kill themselves.

Ask the following questions: How frequent are your suicidal thoughts? Has your preoccupation with suicidal ideas increased? Have you simply had morbid thoughts, or have you thought about exactly how you might kill yourself? Have you thought casually or seriously about killing yourself? Have you considered any particular method?

Take into consideration the patients' age and sophistication and how well the patients' stated intentions match their methods. A woman of normal intelligence who insists that she wants to die and would take six to eight aspirin tablets to do so provokes less concern than does a child who makes the same statement.

Are the chosen means of committing suicide available to the patients? Have they taken any active steps, such as accumulating pills and settling their affairs? How pessimistic are they? Can they imagine any way in which things might improve?

That last question assists with both assessment and treatment, as patients may suggest some avenues of escape from their dilemma. If they do not, are they hopeless about the future? If so, are their fears realistic or delusional? A young man who is hopeless because his wife has left him is at less risk than a man who is convinced without foundation that he is dying of cancer and that everyone is withholding the truth.

Obtain a history from significant others if the patient is uncooperative.

EVALUATION AND MANAGEMENT

1. When evaluating suicidal patients, do not leave them alone; remove any potentially dangerous objects from the room.

2. When evaluating a patient who has just made a suicide attempt, assess whether the attempt was planned or impulsive and determine the lethality, the patient's chance of discovery (for example, was the patient alone, and did the patient notify anyone?), the patient's reactions to being saved (is the patient disappointed or relieved?), and whether the factors that led to the attempt have changed.

3. Management depends to a large degree on diagnosis. Patients with severe depression may be treated as an outpatient if their families can supervise them closely and if treatment can be initiated rapidly. Otherwise, hospitalization may be necessary.

4. The suicidal ideation of alcoholic patients generally remits with abstinence in a few days. No specific treatment is required in most cases. If depression persists after the physiological signs of alcohol withdrawal have resolved, a high suspicion of major depression is warranted. All suicidal patients who are intoxicated by alcohol or drugs must be reassessed when they are sober.

5. Suicidal ideas in schizophrenic patients must be taken seriously, as they tend to use violent and sometimes bizarre methods of high lethality.

6. Patients with personality disorders benefit mostly from empathic confrontation and assistance with resuming a rational, responsible approach to the problem that precipitated the crisis and to which they have usually contributed. The involvement of family or friends and environmental manipulation may be helpful in resolving the crisis that led to the attempted suicide.

7. Long-term hospitalization is recommended for the conditions that contribute to self-mutilation, but brief hospitalization does not usually affect such habitual behavior. Parasuicides may also benefit from long-term rehabilitation, and a brief period of stabilization may be necessary from time to time, but no short-term treatment can be expected to significantly alter their course.

DRUG TREATMENT

A patient in crisis because of a death or other event with a limited time course may function better after receiving mild sedation as needed, particularly if sleep has been disturbed. Benzodiazepines are the drugs of choice, and a typical regimen is lorazepam (Ativan) 1 mg one to three times a day for two weeks. The patient's irritability may be increased by the regular use of a benzodiazepine, and irritability is a risk factor for suicide, so benzodiazepines should be used with caution in hostile patients. Only small quantities of the medication should be provided, and the patient should be followed up within days.

Antidepressants are the definitive treatment for many patients who present with suicidal ideas, but it is not typical to begin antidepressants in the emergency room. If prescribed, however, a definite follow-up appointment should be made, preferably on the following day.

Cross-References:
Alcohol withdrawal, depression, hospitalization, self-mutilation.

---

132 / Sundowner Syndrome

Sundowner syndrome is seen in the elderly, usually at night. It is characterized by drowsiness, confusion, disorientation, transient psychotic symptoms, ataxia, and falling as a result of being overly sedated with medications. It is also called sundowning.

CLINICAL FEATURES AND DIAGNOSIS

Sundowner syndrome is a variant of delirium and may present dramatically with delusions and hallucinations. Depression, anxiety, and irritability can be the presenting symptoms. Some patients are demanding and uncooperative and attempt to leave the hospital against medical advice. Sundowner syndrome may be secondary to the sensory deprivation that occurs when elderly, cognitively impaired patients are placed in a new environment, such as a hospital.

INTERVIEWING AND PSYCHOTHERAPEUTIC GUIDELINES

The key to interviewing any disorganized patient, whatever the cause, is to gently but firmly impose a high degree of structure. The first questions may be abstract, but, as soon as the patient fails to respond appropriately, substitute concrete questions. Rambling, pointless responses may be interrupted after a brief unstructured speech sample has been obtained.

Ask the patient about delusions, hallucinations, and suicidal and aggressive ideas, even if the answers are fragmentary and inconsistent.

Document cognitive deficits by the use of the Mini-Mental State Examination.

The patients' irritability and poor responses should not provoke the physician to discontinue an examination in frustration.

EVALUATION AND MANAGEMENT

1. Management focuses on establishing and treating the underlying condition.

2. Restraints may be necessary. A waist or camisole restraint may suffice to prevent wandering. Two-point or three-point restraints (legs together constituting one point) may be necessary if the patient is agitated or aggressive. Patients attempting to leave should be restrained and held for the consultant. Emergency treatment should proceed while awaiting the consultation.

3. Parenteral medication may be preferable to the prolonged use of restraints and may be administered under the emergency exception to the doctrine of informed consent. In fact, patients with sundowner syndrome are incapable of informed consent, and the physician who allows such patients to leave or fails to render appropriate treatment because of their refusal may be liable for any damages that result.

4. The use of clocks, calendars, radios, and televisions and the presence of family or friends at the bedside may be useful in treating sundowner syndrome secondary to sensory deprivation.

DRUG TREATMENT

For agitation, lorazepam (Ativan) may be given in 1 to 2 mg doses by mouth or intramuscularly (IM). Low-dose antipsychotics—for example, haloperidol (Haldol) 0.5 mg—at bedtime may be of use in treating sundowner syndrome in elderly demented patients. However, if the syndrome is the result of medication excess, use only supportive or restraining methods.

Cross-References:

Anticholinergic intoxication, confusion, delirium, dementia, disorientation, hallucinations, restraints.

---

133 / Syncope (Fainting)

Syncope is the brief loss of consciousness, usually not lasting longer than 15 seconds, caused by decreased perfusion, generally in the carotid arteries and occasionally in the vertebral-basilar system. True syncope has a wide array of causes, and the transient loss of consciousness has many other nonvascular causes. The most common causes are vasovagal dysfunction, orthostatic hypotension, cardiac arrhythmia, and, much less often, vertebral-basilar artery insufficiency. The most commonly associated psychiatric disorder is blood-injury phobia, in which fainting is common on exposure to a phobic stimulus because of a vasovagal mechanism. However, many psychotropic medications have orthostatic hypotension as a side effect.

CLINICAL FEATURES AND DIAGNOSIS

Begin the assessment of syncope with a medication history, and continue with the patient's postural vital signs, auscultation of the heart and the neck, a thorough neurological examination, and an electrocardiogram (Table B.133-1). Do not ascribe alterations in the patient's mental state to a psychiatric condition until you have thoroughly considered possible medical causes, some of which are life-threatening or disabling.

The psychiatric causes of syncope have historically included hysteria and, recently, anxiety disorders. Fainting was at one time a culturally accepted response to stress among women and was described as hysterical. It is still the kind of dramatic attention-seeking behavior that, although now not common, suggests the diagnosis of histrionic personality disorder.

Exposure to blood, the threat of injury, or the news of illness can provoke a vasovagal episode, resulting in syncope. That type of phobic response is unusual. More commonly, simple phobia results in autonomic arousal, resembling panic. If the patient can avoid phobic stimuli, the condition results in little distress. Occasionally, blood-injury phobia causes delayed medical attention. Because of avoidance, few phobics are seen in clinical settings, but they are common in the community. Although most simple phobias are fears of animals and have their onset in childhood, blood-injury phobias typically begin in adolescence. Unlike panic disorder, the phobia may be causatively related. Patients are invariably aware that their fears are excessive or unreasonable.

INTERVIEWING AND PSYCHOTHERAPEUTIC GUIDELINES

The loss of consciousness for any reason is a frightening experience and should be taken seriously, regardless of the patient's personality type. Patients with blood-injury phobia may be aware of the antecedents of the phobia, since the stimulus that provoked the original episode remains in the patient's memory and is not associated with significant intrapsychic conflict.

In the patient who appears to be genuinely unconcerned, that unconcern may be *la belle indifférence* and may point to a conversion disorder.

The symptom is not deliberately produced, as in factitious disorder, and the cause of the patients' distress is outside their awareness. The particular manifestations of hysterical symptoms may be determined by prior exposure to others with similar behaviors. Indirect questioning about the context of the episode and the history of both the family and the patient is helpful. A supportive approach may uncover evidence of a strong affect associated with conflicting reactions to a recent real or imagined event involving significant others.

EVALUATION AND MANAGEMENT

1. If organic causes have been eliminated, no specific management is required for psychogenic syncope.

Table B.133–1
Clinical Approach to Syncope

Evaluation and Assessment	Clinical Syndrome	Second-Order Evaluation
History		
Provocation		
Upright position	Postural hypotension	
Recumbent position	Hysteria, hyperventilation, hypoglycemia, arrhythmia	
Exercise	Aortic stenosis, IHSS,[1] arrhythmia	
Emotional stress	Vasodepressor, hyperventilation	
Food intake	Fasting or reactive hypoglycemia	Blood sugar
Drugs and toxin exposure	Iatrogenic or abuse	
Duration		
Prolonged	Aortic stenosis, IHSS	
Seconds	Hypoglycemia, hysteria, cerebrovascular disease, arrhythmia	
Premonitory symptoms		
None	Arrhythmia, postural hypotension	
Palpitations	Arrhythmia	
Vagal	Vasodepressor	
Dyspnea, light-headedness, numbness	Hyperventilation	
Neurological symptoms	Cerebrovascular disease	EEG, CT, MRI, lumbar puncture
Physical examination		
Orthostatic hypotension		
Tachycardia	Volume loss	Tests for volume loss, adrenal insufficiency
Normal heart rate	Autonomic postural hypotension	Tests for integrity of autonomic and voluntary nervous systems (tabes, diabetes, β-blockers, or other drug-related cause)
Carotid pulse, cardiac murmur	Left ventricular outflow obstruction, localized vascular disease	Echocardiogram, ECG, carotid duplex, catheterization
Carotid sinus massage	Carotid sinus hypersensitivity	
Voluntary hyperventilation	Hyperventilation	
Electrocardiogram		
Heart block, bilateral bundle branch block		
Sinus bradycardia, block, arrest	Bradycardia	Prolonged monitoring, resting or ambulatory; stress test, pacing and His bundle electrophysiologic studies
Supraventricular tachycardia, WPW[2]	Tachycardia	
PVCs[3] or ventricular tachycardia	Tachycardia	

Adapted from R J Noble: The patient with syncope. JAMA *237*: 1375, 1977. Used with permission.
Table from L Goldfrank, N A Lewin, M A Howland, R S Weisman: Diets. In *Goldfrank's Toxicologic Emergencies*, L Goldfrank, N E Flomenbaum, N A Lewin, R S Weisman, M A Howland, editors, p 297. Appleton Lange, Norwalk, Conn, 1990.
[1]IHSS = ideopathic hypertrophic subaortic stenosis
[2]WPW = Wolff-Parkinson-White syndrome
[3]PVCs = premature ventricular contractions

2. Blood-injury phobias do not respond to simple reassurance, since the patients are already aware that their fears are unrealistic.

3. If the patient is unable to avoid the stimulus on a regular basis, a variety of behavioral techniques have been developed involving systematic exposure to the phobic stimulus.

DRUG TREATMENT

If orthostatic hypotension is the result of adrenergic side effects of medication, the dosage may require adjustment. Encourage oral hydration. Some patients respond to fludrocortisone (Florinef) 0.025 to 0.05 mg twice a day. High-potency antipsychotics may be used instead of low-potency drugs. If the patient must remain on a particular drug because of poor responses to other drugs, as happens with monoamine oxidase inhibitors, use pressor drugs.

If a phobic patient must be regularly exposed to a phobic situation, a β-blocker, such as atenolol (Tenormin) 50 to 100 mg as needed, may be sufficient.

Benzodiazepines may be useful for a short time if the patient is overwhelmed, but regular use must be weighed against the risks of benzodiazepine dependence.

Cross-References:

Panic disorder; phobia; urinary retention, psychogenic.

---

134 / Tardive Dyskinesia

Tardive dyskinesia is a movement disorder caused by antipsychotics. It occurs late in the course of treatment, rarely fewer than six months after the start of treatment. The syndrome consists of abnormal, involuntary, irregular, choreoathetoid movements of the tongue, head, trunk, and limbs.

CLINICAL FEATURES AND DIAGNOSIS

The severity of the movements ranges from minimal—often not noticeable by untrained people, including the patient—to grossly incapacitating. Perioral movements are generally the earliest and most common signs and include darting, twisting, and protruding movements of the tongue; chewing and lateral jaw movements; lip puckering; and facial grimacing. Finger movements and hand clenching are also common. Even relatively minor movements of the upper extremities may interfere with coordination and result in disability. Torticollis, retrocollis, trunk twisting, and pelvic thrusting may be incapacitating when they are frequent.

The movements are exacerbated by stress and disappear during sleep. Elderly patients, particularly women, are especially vulnerable, as are patients with mood disorders and brain damage.

The risk increases with the length of antipsychotic treatment. However, the course of tardive dyskinesia is variable. It may remain stable on the same antipsychotic dosage or progress; if antipsychotics are discontinued, the movements may diminish or disappear completely, particularly in mild cases detected in the early stages.

The diagnosis is made by administering the Abnormal Involuntary Movement Scale (AIMS) (Table B.134-1). Consider a number of other diagnoses, including perioral (rabbit) syndrome, bruxism, senile chorea, edentulous dyskinesia, Meige's disease, Parkinson's disease, Huntington's chorea, Wilson's disease, Sydenham's chorea, Tourette's disorder, and dystonia musculorum deformans. Abnormal movements sometimes emerge when the antipsychotic dosage is reduced. The relation of withdrawal emergent dyskinesias to tardive dyskinesia is unclear, but the withdrawal dyskinesias are generally regarded as early tardive dyskinesia masked by high dosages but uncovered by dosage reduction. Tardive movements can be suppressed, at least temporarily, by increasing the antipsychotic dosage. Antiparkinsonian agents may worsen tardive dyskinesia.

INTERVIEWING AND PSYCHOTHERAPEUTIC GUIDELINES

Discuss tardive dyskinesia as soon as you have established trust with the patient and it is clear that the patient will be receiving maintenance antipsychotics. It is probably not necessary to broach the subject during the acute phase, since the onset of tardive dyskinesia is delayed. However, an informed-consent dialogue concerning the potentially serious side effect is essential. Conducted at the appropriate time, the dialogue shows your concern for the patient's welfare, and it fosters responsible behavior by the patient.

EVALUATION AND MANAGEMENT

1. Refer the patient for a neurological consultation; laboratory evaluation, including ceruloplasmin; and either a computed tomography (CT) scan or magnetic resonance imaging (MRI) to rule out other movement disorders.

2. Currently, no treatment for tardive dyskinesia is widely recommended. The condition can be permanent. Approaches to the problem can be divided into prevention, early diagnosis, and management.

3. Prevention is achieved by using antipsychotic medications only when they are clearly indicated and in the lowest effective dosage.

4. Early diagnosis is made possible by regular examinations, preferably with the AIMS. Repeat examinations at 6-to-12-month intervals are recommended.

5. Once abnormal movements are detected, a neurological consultation is in order, and regular ratings are imperative.

Table B.134–1
Abnormal Involuntary Movement Scale (AIMS)
Examination Procedure

Patient Identification	Date

Rated by	

Either before or after completing the examination procedure, observe the patient unobtrusively at rest (e.g., in waiting room).

The chair to be used in this examination should be a hard, firm one without arms.

After observing the patient, rate him or her on a scale of 0 (none), 1 (minimal), 2 (mild), 3 (moderate) and 4 (severe) according to the severity of symptoms.

Ask the patient whether there is anything in his or her mouth (i.e., gum, candy, etc.) and, if so, to remove it.

Ask the patient about the *current* condition of his or her teeth. Ask patient if he or she wears dentures. Do teeth or dentures bother patient *now.*

Ask patient whether he or she notices any movement in mouth, face, hands or feet. If yes, ask patient to describe and indicate to what extent they *currently* bother patient or interfere with his or her activities.

0	1	2	3	4	Have patient sit in chair with hands on knees, legs slightly apart, and feet flat on floor. (Look at entire body for movements while in this position.)

0	1	2	3	4	Ask patient to sit with hands hanging unsupported. If male, between legs, if female and wearing a dress, hanging over knees. (Observe hands and other body areas.)

0	1	2	3	4	Ask patient to open mouth. (Observe tongue at rest within mouth.) Do this twice.

0	1	2	3	4	Ask patient to protrude tongue. (Observe abnormalities of tongue movement.) Do this twice.

0	1	2	3	4	Ask the patient to tap thumb, with each finger, as rapidly as possible for 10 to 15 seconds; separately with right hand, then with left hand. (Observe facial and leg movements.)

0	1	2	3	4	Flex and extend patient's left and right arms. (One at a time.)

0	1	2	3	4	Ask patient to stand up. (Observe in profile. Observe all body areas again, hips included.)

0	1	2	3	4	*Ask patient to extend both arms outstretched in front with palms down. (Observe trunk, legs, and mouth.)

0	1	2	3	4	*Have patient walk a few paces, turn and walk back to chair. (Observe hands and gait.) Do this twice.

*Activated movements.

DRUG TREATMENT

If possible, reduce or discontinue the antipsychotics. Anticholinergic drugs do not benefit tardive dyskinesia and may aggravate it. Clozapine (Clozaril) offers an alternative agent that may be considered, although the risk of fatal agranulocytosis probably outweighs the impairment of mild involuntary movements.

The decision to discontinue or decrease the dosage of an antipsychotic should not be made in the emergency room, as it requires a risk-benefit analysis in the context of an ongoing treatment plan. If tardive dyskinesia is diagnosed in the emergency room, notify the patient's treating physician.

Cross-References:

Akathisia; akinesia; dyskinesia; dystonia, acute; perioral (rabbit) tremor; tic; tremor.

---

135 / Temporal Lobe Epilepsy

A *seizure* is a transient, paroxysmal pathophysiological disturbance of cerebral function that is caused by the spontaneous excessive discharge of cortical neurons. Complex partial seizures are those that begin locally and spread and that result in disturbances of consciousness. *Temporal lobe epilepsy* is a complex partial seizure with a focus in the temporal lobe that is likely to present with behavior problems resulting in diagnostic confusion. A patient may be brought to the emergency room or your office with a history of sudden, irrational, agitated, and possibly violent behavior. On examination, the patient appears to be sleepy and confused, with no memory for the events in question.

CLINICAL FEATURES AND DIAGNOSIS

The diagnosis is made on the basis of the patient's history and is supported by electroencephalography (EEG). The history may be divided into preictal, ictal, postictal, and interictal symptoms.

Preictal events, auras, may or may not occur or may occur irregularly. They include autonomic sensations (for example, stomach fullness, hunger, nausea, and blushing), cognitive events (for example, déjà vu, déjà jamais, hallucinations, and forced thinking), affective states (for example, fear, depression, and elation), and automatisms (for example, lip smacking and chewing).

The ictal event is characterized by a three-to-five-minute loss of consciousness and by disorganized, disinhibited behavior. Violence is rare; since the patient is unconscious, any aggressive behavior is random, undirected, and disorganized. Patients may experience dissociative phenomena, including changes in personality, characteristics, handedness, and speech. Prolonged dissociation secondary to complex partial status epilepticus may resemble catatonia.

After the seizure, the patient may experience a variable period of postictal confusion and, possibly, bizarre or agitated behavior. The postictal confusion passes, but amnesia for the ictal period remains, and the patient's memory is cloudy for events in the preictal and postictal periods.

INTERVIEWING AND PSYCHOTHERAPEUTIC GUIDELINES

Cognitive assessment is crucial, as delirium is associated with high mortality. Any recurrent abrupt and spontaneous onset and remission of a psychiatric disturbance should increase the suspicion of epilepsy. Obtaining the patient's history from the family is usually critical because of the patient's amnesia during the ictal period. A patient who does appear to be conscious and responsive during a seizure and who remembers events during the seizure is probably experiencing pseudoseizures or attempting to produce factitious symptoms.

EVALUATION AND MANAGEMENT

1. The mainstay of management during the ictal event is restraint to prevent injury. Episodes are generally brief, and patients are usually in the postictal period by the time they reach the emergency room or your office.

2. The patients' sensoria may be clouded, and their activities should be restricted until normal cognition is restored. At that point, if no family member has been reached, the patient is usually able to clarify the situation. No further short-term care is necessary unless seizures recur or psychosis is present.

3. If psychosis is present, evaluation and treatment proceed as for other psychoses, except for the medication used.

DRUG TREATMENT

Temporal lobe epilepsy responds to phenytoin (Dilantin) and carbamazepine (Tegretol). Determine the anticonvulsant level for any suspected seizure patient, and adjust the dosage accordingly. A negligible phenytoin level suggests noncompliance and necessitates loading the patient with phenytoin 1,000 mg orally divided into two doses separated by about four hours. The usual maintenance dosage is then 300 mg once daily. Carbamazepine must be titrated with close monitoring of the granulocyte count because of the idiosyncratic occurrence of agranulocytosis. The initial dosage is 200 mg twice daily, increased in 200 mg increments after plasma-level monitoring.

Recurrent seizures (status epilepticus) is treated with parenteral diazepam (Valium) and, if necessary, a general anesthetic.

Temporal lobe epilepsy is not responsive to antipsychotics.

Cross-References:

Anticonvulsant intoxication, blackouts, confusion, delirium, disorientation, epilepsy, fugue state, violence.

---

136 / Terminal Illness

Terminal illness is not simply a biological event leading to death; it involves a complex psychological process of adaptation that varies among individual patients and cultures. Reactions to having a terminal illness may be measured or extreme. Common reactions to a serious, potentially fatal diagnosis include numbness, frank disbelief, and diffuse anger. Healthy responses, reflecting some degree of acceptance, include sadness and fear. The most worrisome initial manifestation is the lack of an emotional response.

CLINICAL FEATURES AND DIAGNOSIS

In general, people die as they have lived. Frank psychopathology in reaction to having a terminal illness is relatively rare. Most adults have developed the psychic apparatus necessary to cope with the stress of dying.

Cognitive equilibrium is maintained by subdividing the process of dying into components, putting things into a favorable perspective, and temporarily minimizing the consequences. Denial is used constructively in that phase. Catastrophic fantasies may be reassessed and better intermediate situations discovered by seeking information, adopting a concrete problem-solving approach, and finding meaningful, realistic alternative short-term goals.

Affective equilibrium is maintained by suppressing the emotions, ventilating, seeking the support of others, and, eventually, accepting reality. The natural consequence of the process is bereavement. Insomnia, appetite disturbances, anxiety, and a depressed mood are common at some points in the process.

Although psychiatric symptoms are present, a psychiatric diagnosis is not reached unless the patient shows both distress and impairments in function. Assess the patient for suicidal ideation, and conduct a thorough evaluation.

INTERVIEWING AND PSYCHOTHERAPEUTIC GUIDELINES

Show respect for the patient's mind and spirit, and care for the patient's body. Try to allow the patient to be the executive decision maker. Educating the patient facilitates the decision-making process. Most decisions can be anticipated and options presented in advance, while the patient is in the best frame of mind.

At some point, try to involve the patient's family, and provide them with emotional and physical support.

Avoid making the patient's important decisions. Emergency treatment may be withheld if patients have given advance directives to have physicians make all the treatment decisions. A number of states now provide a process by which patients may document their treatment wishes and may designate an alternate decision maker.

EVALUATION AND MANAGEMENT

1. Provide patients with accurate and appropriate data.
2. Allow patients to ventilate their fears. Reassure them that they will not be abandoned.
3. Ascertain patients' priorities and defer to the patients' definitions of quality of life.

4. Help patients maintain hope.

5. At some point, make the transition from a primary objective of curing to caring. Palliation may be more appropriate than aggressive treatment.

6. Avoid overly zealous treatment, especially if the treatment conflicts with patients' or the family's wishes.

7. As death nears and with it the specter of failure, avoid the tendency of health care providers to withdraw.

DRUG TREATMENT

The terminally ill must always be kept free from disabling pain; the liberal use of narcotic preparations is encouraged. The phase of coping with a catastrophic condition is one of the few clear indications for the use of sedatives. Family members, particularly spouses, may also be severely affected, and, given the importance of family members in supporting the patient, hypnotics may be appropriate. Dependence liability is low in that population. The short-acting benzodiazepines are probably best. Lorazepam (Ativan) 0.5 to 1 mg by mouth one to three times a day and at bedtime, alprazolam (Xanax) 0.5 to 1 mg by mouth two times a day and at bedtime, or oxazepam (Serax) 10 to 30 mg by mouth two times a day and at bedtime in the early days or weeks can minimize the fear of loss of control while the patient and the family regroup.

Cross-References:

Anxiety, grief and bereavement.

---

137 / Thyrotoxicosis

Thyrotoxicosis results from the sustained elevation of plasma levels of free thyroid hormone. The resulting psychological state is best described as tense dysphoria. Common causes of thyrotoxicosis include Graves' disease, toxic multinodular goiter, thyroiditis, and exogenous iodide.

CLINICAL FEATURES AND DIAGNOSIS

Patients with hyperthyroidism report heat intolerance, excessive sweating, weight loss despite hyperphagia, increased bowel movements, palpitations, fine tremor, and hyperkinesis. Insomnia, irritability, episodic anxiety, affective lability, and rapid tangential speech are typical. Despite motor restlessness and hyperkinesis, energy levels are usually subjectively depressed. Thyrotoxicosis may eventuate in psychosis or delirium.

Muscle wasting is common, particularly the muscles of the limb girdles. Deep tendon reflexes are hyperactive. Tachycardia, paroxysmal arrhythmias, and cardiomegaly occur with increased contractility, increased cardiac output, and increased pulse pressure mediated by catecholamines. Tachycardia is maintained even during sleep. The skin is moist and velvety smooth, with vasodilation. The hair is fine and thin. Patients with Graves' disease may have pretibial myxedema and vitiligo. Ocular signs include fixed stare, lid lag, infrequent blinking, widened palpebral fissures, and exophthalmos. However, goiter, tachycardia, and exophthalmos may not be present in all cases. Laboratory evaluation reveals undetectable thyroid-stimulating hormone (TSH), blunted thyrotropin-releasing hormone (TRH), and elevated serum T_4, T_3, and free thyroxin index.

Both hyperthyroid and hypothyroid patients can appear depressed, especially hypothyroid patients. Hyperthyroidism may also present as mania or anxiety. Apathetic hyperthyroidism, which occurs predominately in the elderly, is indistinguishable from major depression with melancholia. It may present as dementia.

INTERVIEWING AND PSYCHOTHERAPEUTIC GUIDELINES

Interview techniques depend on the clinical status of the patient. Apathetic depressed patients need gentle encouragement when you ask specific questions that are not too taxing. Patients with organic disorders may need frequent reorientation and repetition of questions and information. Anxious patients need reassurance, support, and a calm environment. Manic and psychotic patients need redirection, limit setting, and a nonstimulating environment.

EVALUATION AND MANAGEMENT

1. Consider the diagnosis of hyperthyroidism in all patients with psychotic, mood, anxiety, and organic disorders.

2. Order thyroid function tests (for example, TSH, T_4, T_3) as part of the routine evaluation of such patients.

3. Psychopathology secondary to thyrotoxicosis may remit with the reduction of circulating hormone levels.

DRUG TREATMENT

β-Blockers—for example, propranolol (Inderal) 10 to 40 mg by mouth four times a day—reduce arrhythmias, tremor, and many behavioral symptoms but not muscle wasting. Lithium (Eskalith) has also been used. Agitated patients can be sedated with oxazepam (Serax) 10 to 30 mg by mouth, estazolam (ProSom) 0.5 to 1 mg by mouth, lorazepam (Ativan) 1 to 2 mg by mouth or intramuscularly (IM), or alprazolam (Xanax) 0.25 to 0.5 mg by mouth. Long-term therapy involves the use of propylthiouracil to block synthesis; it inhibits the deiodination of all iodothyronines. Radioactive iodine is effective but may result in permanent hypothyroidism that requires replacement therapy.

Cross-References:

Anxiety, delirium, tremor.

138 / Tic

Tics are rapid, brief involuntary movements, vocalizations, or sensations. When they begin suddenly in school, the child may be brought to the emergency room or your office.

CLINICAL FEATURES AND DIAGNOSIS

Tics may be single or multiple, simple or complex, transient or long-term. Tourette's disorder is marked by the combination of motor and vocal tics. The onset is in childhood. Tics are usually not disabling in and of themselves, but they are significant if they are noticeable to other people and elicit comment or curiosity. Occasionally, particular tics are disruptive or result in orthopedic or dermatological complications.

Tic disorders as a group are (1) involuntary; (2) rapid, brief, sudden, and ejaculatory; (3) recurrent, repetitive, and stereotypical; (4) non-rhythmic, occurring at irregular intervals; (5) purposeless, inappropriate, and an end in themselves; and (6) irresistible but able to be suppressed for varying periods.

Simple motor tics, such as eye and head movements, are the most common initial symptoms. Complex motor tics include hitting oneself, jumping, touching oneself or others, and echopraxia (repeating the movements of others). Simple vocal tics are inarticulate noises, such as throat clearing, grunts, coughs, barks, high-pitched noises, and word accentuation. Complex vocal tics range from single words to sentences. Coprolalia (involuntary use of socially unacceptable expressions) is dramatic but not typical, occurring in about 20 percent of tic patients. Sensory tics are recurrent feelings of heaviness, emptiness, tickling, cold, heat, or other sensations in the skin, the bones, the muscles, or the joints.

Tics may be suppressed for only brief periods. The symptoms change in type and severity over time. Psychosocial factors are probably not significant in the development of tic disorders.

Tics are distinguished from compulsions in that tics are involuntary and compulsions have a volitional component, although the urge to enact the compulsive behavior may be experienced as overwhelming. Simple motor tics lack the premovement electrical potential found in voluntary movements.

Family history studies suggest a link among simple tics, Tourette's disorder, and obsessive-compulsive disorder, but the only established comorbid condition is attention-deficit hyperactivity disorder. A history of tremor and other involuntary movements should be obtained.

INTERVIEWING AND PSYCHOTHERAPEUTIC GUIDELINES

Remember that tic patients are not psychotic or retarded. Be careful not to patronize them or laugh at them. Empathize with the difficulties they encounter as a result of their condition.

EVALUATION AND MANAGEMENT

1. Perform a complete psychiatric evaluation, with attention in the differential diagnosis to such conditions as schizophrenia with bizarre movements, medication-induced abnormal movements, and comorbid conditions (for example, attention-deficit hyperactivity disorder).

2. Obtain a neurological consultation. Rule out Tourette's disorder.

3. Evaluate the patient for depressive symptoms, including suicidal ideation and immature behavior, which occasionally necessitate hospitalization.

4. Refer the patient to a support group for help with social stigmatization and other problems.

DRUG TREATMENT

The mainstay of treatment for tics has been high-potency antipsychotics. Haloperidol (Haldol) decreases 70 to 90 percent of tics in 80 percent of patients. Pimozide (Orap) and clonazepam (Klonopin) have been effective in some cases. Treatment is initiated with 0.25 mg of haloperidol at bedtime; the dosage is increased 0.25 mg at weekly intervals. Serotonergic agents have been reported to be of use.

Cross-References:
Obsessions and compulsions, tremor.

---

139 / Toluene and Other Inhalant Intoxication and Withdrawal

Toluene or methylbenzene is a volatile solvent readily available in glue, paint, and shoe polish. Glue is placed in a bag, and the fumes are inhaled, sometimes by placing the head in the bag as well. The practice is known as sniffing, bagging, and huffing. The inhaled substances are rapidly absorbed, and the effects are virtually immediate. A drunken presentation is most common.

Another commonly available, highly toxic inhalant is trichloroethane, which is present in liquid paper correction fluid. In fact, hydrocarbons occur in numerous products in varying combinations and concentrations (Table B.139–1).

Table B.139–1
Composition of Abused Hydrocarbon Solvents

Inhalant	Chemical Constituents
Acrylic paint	Toluene
Aerosols	Fluorocarbons, nitrous oxide
Dyes	Acetone, methylene chloride
Gasoline	Hydrocarbons, tetraethyl lead
Glues and adhesives	Toluene, benzene, xylene, acetone, naphtha, *n*-hexane, trichloroethylene, tetrachloroethylene, trichloroethane, carbon tetrachloride
Lighter fuel	Butane
Nail polish remover	Acetone, amyl acetate
Paints, varnishes, and lacquers	Trichloroethylene, methylene chloride, toluene
Polystyrene cements	Acetone, toluene, trichloroethylene, hexane
Rubber cement	Benzene, hexane, trichloroethylene
Shoe polish	Chlorinated hydrocarbons, toluene
Spot remover	Trichloroethane, trichloroethylene, carbon tetrachloride
Typewriter correction fluid	Trichloroethane, trichloroethylene, perchloroethylene

Table from L R Goldfrank, A G Kulberg, E A Bresnitz: Occupational and environmental toxins. In *Goldfrank's Toxicologic Emergencies,* L Goldfrank, N E Flomenbaum, N A Lewin, R S Weisman, M A Howland, editors, p 764. Appleton Lange, Norwalk, Conn, 1990.
Adapted from J A Vale, T J Meredith: Solvent abuse. In *Clinical Management of Poisoning and Overdose,* L Haddad, J Winchester, editors, p 801. Saunders, Philadelphia, 1982, and D G Wyse: Deliberate inhalation of volatile hydrocarbons: A review. Can Med Assoc J *108*: 71, 1973. Used with permission.

CLINICAL FEATURES AND DIAGNOSIS

Inhalant intoxication is diagnosed according to the criteria in Table B.139–2. The symptoms begin within five minutes of intake and resolve in one to two hours.

Inhalants are generally not drugs of choice but are used by young persons when other drugs are not readily available or affordable. Inhalant abuse is usually a social activity undertaken in groups. The relatively few solitary sniffers are often heavy users who are psychologically disturbed. Schizoid features are common in those users. Some tolerance and dependence may develop with chronic use.

The physical signs include swollen, red eyes; blurred vision; tremor; ataxia; hyporeflexia; diplopia; residue on the face, the hands, and the clothes; irritation of the nose, the lungs, and the throat; a rash around the nose and the mouth; and breath odors.

The sequelae are serious and involve multiple systems. Inhalant abuse is associated with hepatic, pulmonary, muscular, cardiac, immunological, renal, and neurological damage. Static encephalopathy results from both the hydrocarbons and the lead present in some paints. Cerebellar damage can result from long-term use. Occasional deaths by asphyxiation have occurred when the user becomes confused and fails to uncover the nose and the mouth.

Because of the serious acute and chronic effects of hydrocarbon inhalants, they are considered separately from the volatile nitrates, which follow the same route of administration but are different in their effects and treatment.

Withdrawal after long-term heavy use may produce such symptoms as delusions, agitation, disorientation, tachycardia, tremulousness, seizures,

Table B.139–2
Diagnostic Criteria for Inhalant Intoxication

A. Recent use of an inhalant

B. Maladaptive behavioral changes (e.g., belligerence, assaultiveness, apathy, impaired judgment, impaired social or occupational functioning)

C. At least two of the following signs:
(1) dizziness
(2) nystagmus
(3) incoordination
(4) slurred speech
(5) unsteady gait
(6) lethargy
(7) depressed reflexes
(8) psychomotor retardation
(9) tremor
(10) generalized muscle weakness
(11) blurred vision or diplopia
(12) stupor or coma
(13) euphoria

D. Not due to any physical or other mental disorder

Table from DSM-III-R, *Diagnostic and Statistical Manual of Mental Disorders,* ed 3, revised. Copyright American Psychiatric Association, Washington, 1987. Used with permission.

and hallucinations. Symptoms of withdrawal begin within hours to days after the discontinuation of toluene use.

INTERVIEWING AND PSYCHOTHERAPEUTIC GUIDELINES

Look for subtle cognitive deficits in substance abusers who are not currently intoxicated. Preexisting organic conditions are common in patients who are heavy users, and the relative contributions of the premorbid condition and the heavy use may be difficult to establish without detailed testing.

If organicity is present, speak in simple terms, repeating yourself as needed. Give simple explanations of the procedures while providing support and reassurance.

EVALUATION AND MANAGEMENT

1. As with other intoxications, restraints may be necessary to prevent injury to the patient or others. Neurological sequelae are not progressive once the offending agent is removed.

2. A thorough medical evaluation—including a complete blood count, blood urea nitrogen, liver function tests, creatinine and toxicology screen—should be performed because of possible organ system damage and multiple substance abuse.

3. Abstinence is the only treatment. No services are specifically devoted to those who abuse inhalants. Inhalant abusers most often use multiple substances and qualify for placement according to the drug abused.

DRUG TREATMENT

As with other forms of intoxication, antipsychotics have no advantage and may aggravate organic presentations of inhalant abuse. Agitation may be safely managed with lorazepam (Ativan) 1 to 2 mg parenterally, repeated as necessary at 30-minute intervals until the patient is calm. Withdrawal can also be treated with lorazepam 1 to 2 mg by mouth, intramuscularly (IM), or intravenously (IV) repeated every 30 minutes as needed until the patient is calm.

Cross-References:

Intoxication, phencyclidine or similarly acting arylcyclohexylamine intoxication, psychotropic drug withdrawal, volatile nitrates.

---

140 / Tremor

Tremor is an involuntary oscillating movement of parts of the body (for example, the limbs or the head) that results from alternating contractions of opposing muscle groups.

CLINICAL FEATURES AND DIAGNOSIS

Fine tremors that occur at rest are typical of anxiety, fatigue, and toxic and metabolic disorders. Coarse tremors are seen in Parkinson's disease and cerebellar disease. Tremors may also be classified by the phase of movement. A static tremor is present when the limb is at complete rest, as in Parkinson's disease. An action tremor may be of the postural type, present while sustaining any posture and throughout movement, or the intention type, absent while sustaining any posture and during early movement but worsening when a target is approached.

The differential diagnosis of tremor is wide and includes a physiological variety, benign essential or familial tremor, and senile tremor. Other causes include anxiety, hyperthyroidism, caffeine, hallucinogens, stimulants, cocaine, opioid withdrawal, alcohol withdrawal, benzodiazepine withdrawal, and numerous psychotropic medications. Sedatives and alcohol may be used for anxiety and essential tremor, so those conditions may suddenly appear to be much worse during abstinence. Occasionally, a persistent movement disorder may be attributable to hallucinogen abuse in the distant past.

Lithium (Eskalith) can produce a 7-to-16-per-second action tremor that is similar in appearance to essential tremor. Wilson's disease typically first manifests with tremor before progressing to athetoid movements. Cerebellar lesions caused by tumors, vascular and degenerative diseases, and multiple sclerosis result in intention tremors.

INTERVIEWING AND PSYCHOTHERAPEUTIC GUIDELINES

Conduct a medically oriented interview, paying close attention to the patient's medication history. Reassure the patient that treatment is often effective.

EVALUATION AND MANAGEMENT

1. Management begins with a thorough medical and psychiatric workup to resolve the differential diagnostic issues.
2. A neurological consultation may be needed.

DRUG TREATMENT

Drug treatment of tremor depends on the cause. Tremor caused by benzodiazepine withdrawal may require no specific treatment if the benzodiazepine was used in therapeutic dosages for weeks to months. If the drug was used in very high dosages for months or sometimes in therapeutic amounts for a period of years, seizures may result when it is withdrawn, and detoxification may be indicated. Drugs with a long half-life are less likely to be associated with an abstinence syndrome than drugs with a short half-life.

Tremor alone caused by alcohol withdrawal does not require alcohol detoxification, but a rapid pulse and other signs of withdrawal suggest an increased level of concern. Prophylactic thiamine and folate are always appropriate treatments.

Pseudoparkinsonism caused by antipsychotics is easily managed, if severe, with benztropine (Cogentin) 1 to 2 mg intramuscularly (IM). Oral administration of benztropine is almost as rapid as IM administration. Maintenance treatment with 1 to 6 mg a day in divided doses should then be continued. An alternative is diphenhydramine (Benadryl) 50 mg, which has the advantage of sedation.

Historically, sedatives have been used to treat tremor, but they have been replaced by the more effective, less abusable β-blockers, which may be used either intermittently for performance anxiety or continuously for essential tremor. Atenolol (Tenormin) 50 mg orally is often sufficient for episodic anxiety; atenolol 50 mg twice daily may be given if necessary. Lithium-induced tremor can be treated with β-blockers or with a reduction of the lithium dosage.

Cross-References:

Akathesia, alcohol withdrawal, anxiety, parkinsonism, phobia.

141 / Urinary Retention, Psychogenic

Psychogenic urinary retention is the transient inability to urinate because of emotional conflicts. Urinary retention may occur in schizophrenia, depression, and social phobia (shy bladder). Numerous psychotropic medications also cause urinary dysfunction, primarily as a result of their anticholinergic properties and particularly in overdoses. Psychogenic urinary retention may be accompanied by indifference, but urinary retention caused by toxicity is painful and requires urgent treatment.

CLINICAL FEATURES AND DIAGNOSIS

Psychogenic urinary retention is usually diagnosed by the process of exclusion after a variety of urodynamic studies. The emotional conflicts central to the diagnosis may be conscious or unconscious. If the conflicts are conscious, unfortunate experiences during socialization as a child may condition anxiety, fear of exposure, and shame on urination under certain circumstances—for example, in public places. The anxiety may grow and include a broad range of conditions. Avoidance becomes habitual. In those cases the patients are generally aware of the pattern of events that led to the difficulty in urinating.

If the patient's conflicts are unconscious, urinary retention is classified as a conversion disorder, formerly referred to as hysteria. The symptom is modeled on the patient's prior experience of others with urinary retention or the patient's own chance experience of difficulty in urinating. The disorder is precipitated by some internal threat outside the patient's conscious awareness and arises during extreme psychosocial stress. Conflicts about dependence, self-determination, and sexuality are common. Histrionic and dependent personality disorders contribute to the patient's vulnerability to conversion symptoms.

The onset is usually in adulthood, and women are affected more than men. Intermediate cases with varying degrees of conscious and unconscious motivation and insight also occur.

INTERVIEWING AND PSYCHOTHERAPEUTIC GUIDELINES

Patients with conscious anxiety readily describe the antecedents of their symptoms, and a straightforward history is sufficient for diagnosis. However, patients with unconscious conflicts and an established secondary gain do not respond well to the suggestion that the problem is psychogenic. Since the symptom serves a protective function and is a source of gratification, such patients resist uncovering the issues. Therefore, a subtle approach is suggested. Question the patients thoroughly about their histories, but do not directly focus on their toilet training or other emotionally charged issues.

Devote particular attention to the stressful events that surrounded the onset of the urinary problems, but do not suggest a causative role.

Ascertain the patients' exposure and modeling by enquiring about family members with similar problems. That approach spares patients the threat of sudden confrontation with the source of their conflicts and allows the examiner to identify the problem without triggering increased defensiveness.

EVALUATION AND MANAGEMENT

1. The management of urinary retention includes intermittent catheterization. Most patients then resume spontaneous urination, although recurrences are common.

2. Urinary retention caused by schizophrenia or depression requires treatment of the primary condition.

3. By the time of the psychiatric consultation, self-catheterization may be established. Self-catheterization carries with it an attendant risk of infections, and it perpetuates the patient's emotional problems and maladaptive behavior. However, because of the importance of the symptom to the patient, unconscious resistance may interfere with evaluation and treatment. Hospitalization may be necessary to ensure valid assessment and treatment compliance.

4. Successful treatment ultimately depends on resolving the underlying conflicts about dependence and on altering the patterns of reinforcement with behavior therapy. Problems with voiding tend to persist, and recurrences of urinary retention are common.

DRUG TREATMENT

Short-acting benzodiazepines may be useful for anxiety-based retention. Alprazolam (Xanax) 0.5 to 1 mg by mouth, oxazepam (Serax) 10 to 30 mg by mouth, estazolam (ProSom) 0.5 to 1 mg by mouth, or lorazepam (Ativan) 1 to 2 mg by mouth may induce urination within one hour. Anticholinergic-induced urinary retention may be treated with bethanechol (Urecholine) 2.5 to 5 mg subcutaneously.

Cross-Reference:
Phobia.

---

142 / Violence

Violence is physical aggression inflicted by one person on another. When it is directed toward oneself, it is referred to as self-mutilation or suicidal behavior. Violence can be due to a wide range of psychiatric disorders, but it may also occur in normal people who cannot cope with life stresses in less severe ways. Violence and threats of violence are frequently encountered in psychiatric emergency settings and are frequent causes of psychiatric consultations. The physician and the staff members must know how to rapidly initiate a procedure for the prevention of escalating violence. The procedure may involve behavioral, pharmacological, and psychosocial interventions.

CLINICAL FEATURES AND DIAGNOSIS

The psychiatric conditions most commonly associated with violence include such psychotic disorders as schizophrenia and mania (particularly if the patient is paranoid or is experiencing command hallucinations), intoxication with alcohol and drugs, withdrawal from alcohol and sedative-hypnotics, catatonic excitement, agitated depression, personality disorders that are characterized by rage and poor impulse control (for example, borderline and antisocial personality disorders), and organic disorders (especially those with frontal and temporal lobe involvement). See Table B.142–1 for diagnoses associated with violent behavior.

Other risk factors for violence include a statement of intent, a specific plan, the availability of the means of violence, male sex, young age (15 to 24 years), low socioeconomic status, poor social support system, past history of violence, other antisocial acts, poor impulse control, history of suicide attempts, and recent stressors. A history of violence is the best predictor of violence. Additional important factors include a history of childhood victimization; childhood history of the triad of bed-wetting, fire setting, and cruelty to animals; criminal record; military or police service; reckless driving; and family history of violence.

The first goal with the potentially violent patient is the prevention of immediate violence. The next objective is to make a diagnosis that will lead to a treatment plan, including measures to minimize the likelihood of subsequent violence.

INTERVIEWING AND PSYCHOTHERAPEUTIC GUIDELINES

Be supportive and nonthreatening to potentially violent patients. However, be firm, and present clear limits that can be enforced with physical restraint if necessary. Set limits by offering choices (for example, medication or restraints), instead of provocative directives ("Take this medicine now"). Tell the patients directly that violence is not acceptable. Reassure the patients that they are safe. Convey an attitude of calm and control. Offer the patients medication to help them relax.

EVALUATION AND MANAGEMENT

1. *Protect yourself.* Assume that violence is always a possibility, and never allow yourself to be surprised by a sudden violent act. Never interview an armed patient. The patient should always surrender the weapon to a security guard. Know as much as possible about the patient before the

Table B.142–1
Diagnoses Associated with Violent Behavior

A. Psychotic disorders
   1. Schizophrenia (especially paranoid or catatonic)
   2. Mania
   3. Paranoid disorders
   4. Postpartum psychosis

B. Organic mental disorders
   1. Delirium
   2. Drug intoxication or withdrawal

C. Personality disorders
   1. Antisocial
   2. Paranoid and others with transient psychosis

D. Situational problems
   1. Domestic quarrels (spouse abuse)
   2. Child abuse
   3. Homosexual panic

E. Brain disorders
   1. Seizure disorders
   2. Structural defects (trauma, encephalitis)
   3. Mental retardation and minimal brain dysfunction

F. Dissociative states

Table from N Hanke: *Handbook of Emergency Psychiatry,* p 109. Collamore Press, Lexington, Mass, 1984. Used with permission.

interview. Never interview a potentially violent patient alone or in an office with the door closed. Consider removing neckties, necklaces, and other articles of clothing or jewelry you are wearing that the patient can grab or pull. Stay within sight of other staff members. Leave physical restraint to the staff members who are trained for that. Do not give the patient access to areas where weapons may be available (for example, a crash cart or a treatment room). Do not sit close to a paranoid patient, who may feel that you are threatening. Keep yourself at least an arm's length away from any potentially violent patient. Do not challenge or confront a psychotic patient. Be alert to the signs of impending violence. Always leave yourself a route of rapid escape in case the patient attacks you. Never turn your back on the patient.

2. The signs of impending violence include recent violent acts against people or property, clenched teeth and fists, verbal threats (menacing), weapons or objects potentially usable as weapons (for example, a fork, an ice pick, an ashtray), psychomotor agitation (considered by many to be an important indicator), alcohol or drug intoxication, paranoid delusions, and command hallucinations.

3. Be sure that sufficient staff members are on hand to safely restrain the patient. Call for staff assistance before the patient's agitation has escalated. Often, a show of force through the presence of several able-bodied staff members is sufficient to prevent a violent act.

4. Physical restraint should be performed only by those who are trained to do so. For patients with suspected phencyclidine (PCP) intoxication, physical restraints (especially limb restraints) should be avoided, since self-injuries may occur. Usually, a benzodiazepine or an antipsychotic is given

immediately after physical restraints are applied to provide a chemical restraint, but the drug choice depends on the diagnosis. Provide a nonstimulating environment.

5. Make a definitive diagnostic evaluation, including the patient's vital signs, physical examination, and psychiatric history. Evaluate the patient's suicide risk, and create a treatment plan that provides for the management of potential subsequent violence. Elevated vital signs may suggest withdrawal from alcohol or sedative-hypnotics.

6. Explore possible psychosocial interventions to reduce the risk of violence. If violence is related to a specific situation or person, try to separate the patient from that situation or person. Try family interventions and other manipulations of the environment. Would the patient still be potentially violent while living with other relatives?

7. Hospitalization may be necessary to detain the patient and to prevent violence. Constant observation may be necessary, even on a locked inpatient psychiatric ward.

8. If psychiatric treatment is not appropriate, you may involve the police and the legal system.

9. Intended victims must be warned if there is a continued possibility of danger (for example, if the patient is not hospitalized).

DRUG TREATMENT

Drug treatment depends on the specific diagnosis. Benzodiazepines and antipsychotics are used most often for tranquilization. Fluphenazine (Prolixin), thiothixene (Navane), trifluoperazine (Stelazine), or haloperidol (Haldol), all given at 5 mg by mouth or intramuscularly (IM) or lorazepam (Ativan) 2 mg by mouth or IM may be tried initially. If the patient is already taking an antipsychotic, give more of the same drug. If the patient's agitation has not decreased in 20 to 30 minutes, repeat the dose. Avoid antipsychotics in patients at risk for seizures. Benzodiazepines may be ineffective in patients who are tolerant; benzodiazepines may cause disinhibition, which can potentially worsen the violence. For patients with epilepsy, first try an anticonvulsant—for example, carbamazepine (Tegretol)—and then a benzodiazepine. Chronically violent patients with organic disorders sometimes respond to β-blockers, such as propranolol (Inderal).

Cross-References:

Agitation, homicidal and assaultive behavior, intermittent explosive disorder, phencyclidine or similarly acting arylcyclohexylamine intoxication, rape and sexual abuse, restraints, seclusion, self-mutilation, suicide.

143 / Vitamin B$_{12}$ Deficiency

Neurological symptoms and personality change or confusion combined with anemia may suggest *vitamin B$_{12}$ deficiency*. Although megaloblastic anemia is typical in vitamin B$_{12}$ deficiency, mental symptoms may precede the development of anemia. The psychiatric symptoms include irritability, psychomotor agitation or retardation, depression, neurovegetative disturbances, delirium, dementia, and schizophrenialike symptoms. The neurological complaints include paresthesias, weakness, poor coordination, and an unsteady gait.

CLINICAL FEATURES AND DIAGNOSIS

Patients with vitamin B$_{12}$ deficiency are typically in middle to late life with malabsorption secondary to pernicious anemia. Strict vegetarians are also at risk and may have a folate intake inadequate to prevent anemia. Gastrectomy and bacterial and parasitic competition account for some cases.

The onset is insidious. Anemia develops gradually and hence is tolerated, but it may result in pallor, mild splenomegaly, and jaundice. The patient may have a low-grade fever. B$_{12}$ deficiency is one of several deficiencies that cause glossitis. The loss of fine motor skills is related to the loss of vibratory sensation and two-point discrimination. Patchy central nervous system (CNS) degeneration ultimately results.

Psychiatrically, the condition is classified as an organic mental syndrome, whether its major psychiatric manifestation is affective, cognitive, or perceptual. The diagnosis is critical, as the condition is one of the few treatable types of dementia, and it is gradually progressive if untreated. A routine complete blood count (CBC) may reveal the classic megaloblastic anemia. A low B$_{12}$ level confirms the diagnosis.

INTERVIEWING AND PSYCHOTHERAPEUTIC GUIDELINES

Detailed neurological and cognitive examinations are essential. For the cognitive examination use a structured instrument, such as the Mini-Mental State Examination. Reassure the patient that they will improve with treatment.

EVALUATION AND MANAGEMENT

1. Parenteral vitamin B$_{12}$ rapidly corrects many manifestations of vitamin B$_{12}$ deficiency, including fever, anemia, and glossitis.
2. Establish the underlying cause.
3. A transfusion is generally not required.

4. Neurological deficits do not respond well to vitamin B_{12} replacement, and advanced cases may be left with persistent neurological or psychiatric sequelae and require rehabilitation.

DRUG TREATMENT

Vitamin B_{12} 100 μg daily should be administered parenterally for 10 to 14 days and then given monthly. Any excess vitamin B_{12} is excreted in the urine. If sedation is necessary, lorazepam (Ativan) 1 to 2 mg by mouth or oxazepam (Serax) 10 to 30 mg by mouth may be given safely at frequent intervals in the short term.

Cross-References:

Dementia, Korsakoff's syndrome, Wernicke's encephalopathy.

144 / Volatile Nitrates

The *volatile nitrates,* principally amyl nitrite and isobutyl nitrite or rush, are liquid inhalants that are used as aphrodisiacs and stimulants. The desired effects are anal smooth muscle dilation, delayed ejaculation, and euphoria. Approximately half of all volatile nitrate abusers find the experience unpleasant because of the resulting throbbing headache, nausea, and lightheadness or syncope. The effect is brief, so patients do not present with acute nitrate intoxication. However, nitrates are often used with other substances and in the setting of other high-risk behaviors. Methemoglobinemia may occur in vulnerable persons. There is no associated abstinence syndrome.

Although the route of administration is similar to that of hydrocarbon inhalants, the toxicity of hydrocarbon inhalants is much greater than that of volatile nitrates.

CLINICAL FEATURES AND DIAGNOSIS

The signs and symptoms of nitrate abuse are related to smooth muscle relaxation and include intense peripheral vasodilation, flushing, hypotension, and reflex tachycardia. Subjectively, the effect is experienced as warmth, a rapid pulse, throbbing headache, and dizziness. Cerebral vasodilation results in a pulsatile headache. Nitrates are also irritants and may cause tracheobronchitis. Crusty skin lesions may be noted around the nose and the lips. Long-term users have a yellowish facial tint. Nitrates are flammable liquids, and burns may result. Foreign bodies may be lodged in the rectum.

In patients with defective heme-reducing systems, methemoglobinemia is a potentially fatal consequence of exposure to nitrates. Patients with methemoglobinemia present with cyanosis and respiratory distress that is unresponsive to oxygen therapy. The arterial blood appears to be chocolate brown, although the partial pressure of oxygen (pO_2) remains normal. Transient ST segment and T wave changes may be present on the electrocardiogram (ECG).

INTERVIEWING AND PSYCHOTHERAPEUTIC GUIDELINES

Nitrate abuse has declined as a result of its association with acquired immune deficiency syndrome (AIDS) during early investigations and as a result of its criminalization in some jurisdictions. Nitrate abusers are at risk for other substance abuse; the patient's drug of choice may be marijuana, alcohol, stimulants, or (least likely) hallucinogens. Obtain a thorough substance-abuse history from the patient. Sexual activity involving nitrate abuse should prompt a thorough sexual history.

EVALUATION AND MANAGEMENT

1. In most patients, the symptoms pass quickly after cessation of nitrate use, and no specific treatment is indicated.

2. Direct your efforts at drug counseling, taking advantage of any current adverse consequences to promote efforts to enroll the patient in rehabilitation.

3. Human immunodeficiency virus (HIV) testing and AIDS education may be indicated.

DRUG TREATMENT

Mild methemoglobinemia resolves within 24 to 72 hours with conservative management. If angina or an altered mental state occurs or if methemoglobinemia exceeds 30 percent, methylene blue 1 to 2 mg per kilogram of body weight as a 1 percent solution may be administered intravenously (IV) over five minutes.

Cross-References:

Nitrous oxide intoxication, toluene and other inhalant intoxication and withdrawal.

---

145 / Wernicke's Encephalopathy

Wernicke's encephalopathy is characterized by ophthalmoplegia, weakness, a staggering gait, and confusion in the long-term alcoholic person. The diagnosis is critical, since the acute encephalopathy is treatable with thiamine and usually resolves in a matter of days; if untreated, the condition progresses to Korsakoff's syndrome. Other signs of thiamine deficiency may also be present, such as cardiovascular disease.

CLINICAL FEATURES AND DIAGNOSIS

The hallmark of Wernicke's encephalopathy is confusion, so a reliable history is difficult to obtain. In addition, the patient may not be currently drinking, making the association with alcohol difficult to establish. The confusion is marked by apathy, slowed responses, and disorientation, despite gross awareness, lack of drowsiness, and superficially appropriate behavior.

The patient's apathy may impress the casual examiner as a lack of effort. A thorough examination, however, reveals that the patient cannot retain new information, despite repeated efforts.

The ocular symptoms are related to sixth cranial nerve palsy and include internal strabismus, dysconjugate gaze, and nystagmus. A staggering gait is present even in the absence of acute intoxication.

INTERVIEWING AND PSYCHOTHERAPEUTIC GUIDELINES

The patient's apathetic demeanor and superficial cooperation may foster an unfortunate lack of concern or even antipathy in the physician. A disposition made too rapidly because of bias will frustrate an accurate diagnosis, with catastrophic results. A structured approach to the diagnosis of organic mental syndromes is always suggested. An appropriate and reliable screening tool is the Mini-Mental State Examination. Do not ignore disturbances of consciousness, as they are associated with a high rate of serious occult medical illness and subsequent mortality.

EVALUATION AND MANAGEMENT

1. A neurological examination is necessary to establish the diagnosis.

2. The onset may be sudden or gradual, and it is unrelated to the presence of alcohol, so the patient may present in any stage of intoxication or withdrawal.

3. A thiamine level may confirm the diagnosis, but treatment should proceed without awaiting the results.

4. The short-term treatment is the correction of the nutritional deficiency. Early Wernicke's encephalopathy is largely reversible with timely treatment. The remainder of the patient's care is directed at alcohol detoxification and rehabilitation. Admission to a medical service is usually indicated.

5. Observe the patient closely to prevent self-harm secondary to the confused state.

DRUG TREATMENT

Alcohol-dependent patients should be given thiamine 100 mg parenterally and subsequently placed on daily supplements of thiamine 100 mg, folic acid 1 mg, and multivitamins. Elevated vital signs, tremor, and vomiting are consistent with concurrent alcohol withdrawal and can be treated with diazepam (Valium) 5 mg intravenously (IV) or lorazepam (Ativan) 2 mg intramuscularly (IM) or IV repeated at 30-minute intervals until the withdrawal symptoms are controlled. The total benzodiazepine dose during the first 24 hours may then be tapered by 20 percent a day.

Cross-References:

Alcohol hallucinosis, alcohol idiosyncratic intoxication, alcohol intoxication, alcohol overdose, alcohol seizures, alcohol withdrawal, alcohol withdrawal delirium, amnesia, confusion, Korsakoff's syndrome.

Specific Poisons: Symptoms and Treatment

Poison	Symptoms	Treatment
Acetaminophen	Early: Often asymptomatic; mild nausea, vomiting, diaphoresis, pallor; beginning signs of hepatotoxicity; oliguria Later (at 24–48 h): Nausea & protracted vomiting, right upper quadrant pain, jaundice, coagulation defects, hypoglycemia, encephalopathy, hepatic failure; renal failure, myocardiopathy may occur	Emesis; gastric lavage and/or charcoal. Monitor plasma drug levels for prognosis: if > 160–200 μg/mL at 4 h, hepatic damage may occur; if > 300 μg/mL at 4 h, hepatic damage is almost certain. If given before 18 h, oral acetylcysteine (Mucomyst) 140 mg/kg to start and 70 mg/kg q 4 h for 4 to 18 doses has been effective in preventing significant hepatotoxicity
Acetanilid Aniline (indelible) inks Aniline oils Chloroaniline Phenacetin (acetophenetidin)	Cyanosis due to formation of methemoglobin & sulfhemoglobin, dyspnea, weakness, vertigo, anginal pain, rashes & urticaria, vomiting, delirium, depression, respiratory & circulatory failure	(1) Inhalation: Give O_2; support respiration. Blood transfusion. For severe cyanosis, methylene blue 1–2 mg/kg IV (2) Skin: Remove clothing & wash area with copious soap & water; then as in (1) (3) Ingestion: Give ipecac emetic; if this fails, gastric lavage and/or charcoal; then as in (1)
Acetic acid: see Acids & alkalis		
Acetone Ketones Model airplane glues, cements Nail polish remover	Inhalation: Bronchial irritation, pulmonary congestion & edema, decreased respirations, dyspnea, drunkenness, stupor, ketosis Ingestion: As above except direct pulmonary effect	Remove from source; evacuate stomach except for small amounts; support respiration; give O_2 & fluids; correct metabolic acidosis
Acetonitrile Cosmetic nail adhesive	Converted to cyanide, with usual symptoms & signs	Manage as for cyanide
Acetophenetidin: see Acetanilid		
Acetylene gas: see Carbon monoxide		

Poison	Symptoms	Treatment
Acids & alkalis 　Acids 　　Acetic 　　Hydrochloric 　　Nitric 　　Phosphoric	Corrosive burns from inhalation, skin contact, eye contact, & ingestion; local pain. In general, alkali is more damaging to the GI tract	Skin or eye: Flush with water for 15 min Ingestion: Dilute with water or milk; *do not stimulate vomiting;* consider gastric lavage if large amounts of alkali granules have been consumed
Sulfuric (some drain or toilet bowl cleaners, some dishwasher detergents) 　Alkalis 　　Ammonia water (ammonium hydroxide) 　　Potassium hydroxide (potash) 　　Sodium hydroxide (caustic soda, lye) 　　Carbonates of the above 　　Detergent powders 　　Some drain or toilet bowl cleaners; some dishwasher detergents	Drooling & stridor are suggestive of damage Note: Even in the absence of mouth lesions, strong alkalis (pH > 10.5–11.0) can burn the esophagus; esophagoscopy is advised	Hospitalize; give opiates for pain; treat shock if present; endoscopy is recommended; tracheostomy may be needed; for verified esophageal burns, give antibiotics & dexamethasone 1 mg/m^2 BSA q 6 h or equivalent for 2–3 wk

Airplane glues, cements (model-building): see Acetone; Benzene; Petroleum distillates

Alcohol, ethyl (ethanol) 　Brandy, whiskey, & other liquors	Emotional lability, impaired coordination, flushing, nausea & vomiting, stupor to coma, respiratory depression	Emesis; gastric lavage; support respiration; IV glucose to prevent hypoglycemia, dialysis if blood levels > 300–350 mg/dL; generous fluid administration as serum alcohol increases serum osmolarity
Alcohol, isopropyl 　Rubbing alcohol	Dizziness, incoordination, stupor to coma, gastroenteritis, hypotension; *no* retinal injury	Emesis; gastric lavage; IV glucose; correct dehydration & electrolyte changes; dialysis
Alcohol, methyl (methanol, wood alcohol) 　Antifreeze 　Paint solvent 　Solid canned fuel 　Varnish	Very toxic: 60–250 mL (2–8 oz) fatal in adults; 8–10 mL (2 tsp) in children. Latency period 12–18 h; headache, weakness, leg cramps, vertigo, convulsions, dimness of vision, decreased respiration	Combat acidosis with IV sodium bicarbonate; give 10% ethanol/ 5% dextrose solution IV; initially, a loading dose of 0.7 gm/kg of ethanol to impede methanol metabolism is infused over 1 h followed by 0.1–0.2 gm/kg/h to maintain a blood ethanol level of 100 mg/dL; investigate use of 4-methylpyrazole (currently pending FDA approval); *hemodialysis*

Aldrin: see DDT

Alkalis: see Acids & alkalis

Poison	Symptoms	Treatment
Aminophylline Caffeine Theophylline	Wakefulness, restlessness, anorexia, vomiting, dehydration, convulsions; with hypersensitivity, immediate vasomotor collapse may occur. Adults are more susceptible than children	If ingested, use emetic or charcoal (avoid emesis if seizures are imminent). Stop medication; obtain theophylline blood level; phenobarbital or diazepam for convulsions; give parenteral fluids; maintain BP; if serum level > 50–100 mg/dL, consider dialysis; consider using a β-blocker, eg propranolol, if patient is nonasthmatic

Amitriptyline: see Tricyclic antidepressants

Ammonia gas	Irritation of eyes & respiratory tract; cough, choking; abdominal pain	Flush eyes with tap water for 15 min. *No gastric lavage or emetic.* If severe, positive pressure O_2 to manage pulmonary edema; support respiration

Ammonia water: see Acids & alkalis

Ammoniated mercury: see Mercury

Ammonium carbonate: see Acids & alkalis

Ammonium fluoride: see Fluorides

Ammonium hydroxide: see Acids & alkalis

Amobarbital: see Barbiturates

Amphetamines Amphetamine sulfate, phosphate Dextroamphetamine Methamphetamine Phenmetrazine	Increased activity, exhilaration, talkativeness, insomnia, irritability, exaggerated reflexes, anorexia, dry mouth, arrhythmia, anginal chest pain, heart block, psychoticlike states and inability to concentrate or sit still	Emesis, lavage, or charcoal may be effective long after ingestion because of recycling via gastric mucosa Sedate with chlorpromazine 0.5–1 mg/kg IM or orally q 30 min as needed; reduce external stimuli; hypothermia; combat cerebral edema; hemodialysis. Use of β-blockers may be helpful in nonasthmatics

Amyl nitrite: see Nitrites

Aniline: see Acetanilid

Ant poison: see DDT (chlordane); Thallium salts

Antidepressants: see Tricyclic antidepressants

Antifreeze: see Alcohol, methyl; Ethylene glycol

Antihistamines	Excitation or depression, drowsiness, nervousness, disorientation, hallucinations, tachycardia, arrhythmias, hyperpyrexia, delirium, convulsions	Ipecac emesis (avoid emesis if seizures are imminent), gastric lavage, charcoal; support respiration/BP; control seizures with diazepam; physostigmine 0.5–2 mg (adults), 0.02 mg/kg (children) IM or IV (slowly) only after all else fails. (Caution: *Seizures* [see Physostigmine])

Antimony: see Arsenic & antimony

Antineoplastic agents Methotrexate Mercaptopurine Vincristine	Effects on hematopoietic system, nausea, vomiting	Emesis > lavage; supportive care; "leucovorin rescue"; observe for postacute problems (beyond 24–48 h)

Poison	Symptoms	Treatment

Arsenic & antimony
  Antimony compounds
    Stibophen
    Tartar emetic
  Arsenic
    Donovan's solution
    Fowler's solution
    Herbicides
    Paris green
    Pesticides
	Throat constriction, dysphagia; burning GI pain; vomiting, diarrhea; dehydration; pulmonary edema; renal failure; liver failure	Emesis; gastric lavage, then a demulcent; chelation with penicillamine; BAL if patient cannot take oral medication; hydration; treat shock, pain; sorbitol or saline cathartic (sodium sulfate 15–30 gm in water)

Arsine gas	Acute hemolytic anemia	Transfusions; diuresis
Atropine: see Belladonna		
Automobile exhaust: see Carbon monoxide		

Barbiturates
  Amobarbital
  Meprobamate
  Pentobarbital
  Phenobarbital
  Secobarbital
	Headache, confusion, ptosis, excitement, delirium, loss of corneal reflex, respiratory failure, coma	Empty stomach up to 24 h after ingestion. If immediately after, use ipecac emetic; if sedated, use lavage and charcoal with cuffed endotracheal tube. Good nursing care; support respiration, give O_2; correct any dehydration. Rarely dialysis, especially for long-acting barbiturates where alkalinization hastens excretion

Barium compounds
  (soluble)
  Barium acetate
    carbonate
    chloride
    hydroxide
    nitrate
    sulfide
  Depilatories
  Fireworks
  Rodenticides
	Vomiting, abdominal pain, diarrhea, tremors, convulsions, hypertension, cardiac arrest	To precipitate barium in stomach, give 60 gm sodium or magnesium sulfate orally. Then emesis or gastric lavage. Control convulsions with diazepam; atropine s.c., IM, or IV 0.5–1 mg (adults), 0.01 mg/kg (children) for colic; sublingual nitroglycerin 1/100–1/50 for hypertension; O_2 for dyspnea & cyanosis; quinidine 100–300 mg (adults), 6 mg/kg (children) to prevent ventricular fibrillation; correct hypokalemia

Belladonna
  Atropine
  Hyoscyamine
  Hyoscyamus
  Scopolamine (Hyoscine)
  Stramonium
	Dry skin & mucous membranes; pupils dilated; flushing, hyperpyrexia; tachycardia, restlessness; coma; respiratory failure; convulsions	Emesis or charcoal; support respiration. May need to catheterize bladder. Physostigmine 0.5–2 mg (adults), 0.02 mg/kg (children) IM or IV (slowly) may reverse peripheral and central effects, but use only for severe problems. (Caution: *Seizures* [see Physostigmine])

Benzene
  Benzol
  Hydrocarbons
  Model airplane glue
  Toluene
  Toluol
  Xylene
	Dizziness, weakness, headache, euphoria, nausea, vomiting, ventricular arrhythmia, paralysis, convulsions; with chronic poisoning, aplastic anemia, leukemia	If sizable ingestion (> 0.5–1 mL/kg), emesis or cautious gastric lavage. Give O_2; support respiration; monitor ECG—ventricular fibrillation can occur early. Control seizures with diazepam. Blood transfusion for severe anemia. *Do not give epinephrine*

γ-Benzene hexachloride
  BHC
  Hexachlorocyclohexane
  Lindane
	Irritability, CNS excitation, muscle spasms, atonia, clonic & tonic convulsions, respiratory failure, pulmonary edema	Emesis immediately after ingestion; gastric lavage; diazepam for convulsions. Avoid all oils—they promote absorption. Charcoal hemoperfusion prn

Benzin, benzine: see Petroleum distillates		

Poison	Symptoms	Treatment
Benzodiazepines Dalmane Librium Valium	Sedation to coma, particularly if accompanied by alcohol	Emesis; lavage; supportive care; suicidal precautions
Benzol: see Benzene		
BHC: see γ-Benzene hexachloride		
Bichloride of mercury: see Mercury		
Bichromates: see Chromic acid		
Bishydroxycoumarin: see Warfarin		
Bismuth compounds	Poorly absorbed. Ulcerative stomatitis, anorexia, headache, rash, renal tubular damage	Ipecac emesis; gastric lavage; respiratory support; BAL
Bitter almond oil: see Cyanides		
Bitter almond oil, artificial: see Nitrobenzene		
Bleach, chlorine: see Hypochlorites		
β-Blockers	Hypotension, bradycardia, seizures, cardiac arrhythmias	Monitor closely, evacuate stomach. If symptomatic, initiate glucagon 3–5 mg IV or in saline; consider cardiac pacing
Borates Boric acid	Nausea, vomiting, diarrhea, hemorrhagic gastroenteritis, weakness, lethargy, CNS depression, convulsion, "boiled lobster" skin rash, shock	Ipecac emesis; gastric lavage; remove from skin; prevent or treat electrolyte changes & shock; control convulsions. Rarely, dialysis for severe poisoning
Boric acid: see Borates		
Brandy: see Alcohol, ethyl		
Bromates: see Chlorates		
Bromides	Nausea, vomiting, rash (may be acneiform), slurred speech, ataxia, confusion, psychotic behavior, coma, paralysis	Ipecac emesis, gastric lavage for acute ingestion; stop use as medication; promote mild diuresis by hydration & sodium chloride IV; ethacrynic acid is specifically useful. Hemodialysis only if severe
Bromine: see Chlorine		
Bulan: see DDT		
Cadmium Solder	Severe gastric cramps, vomiting, diarrhea; dry throat, cough, dyspnea; headache; shock, coma; brown urine, renal failure ("ouch-ouch disease")	Ipecac emesis; gastric lavage with milk or albumin; respiratory support; hydration; intermittent positive pressure breathing (IPPB) for pulmonary edema. Give edetate calcium disodium, *not BAL*
Caffeine: see Aminophylline		
Calomel: see Mercury		
Camphor Camphorated oils	Camphor odor on breath, headache, confusion, delirium, hallucinations, convulsions, coma	Ipecac emesis (avoid emesis if seizures are imminent), charcoal, or gastric lavage. Prevent & treat convulsions with diazepam; support respiration. Lipid dialysis is still being explored

Poison	Symptoms	Treatment
Canned fuel, solid: see Alcohol, methyl		
Cantharides Cantharidin Spanish fly	Skin and mucous membranes irritated, vesicles; nausea, vomiting, bloody diarrhea; burning pain in back and urethra; respiratory depression; convulsions, coma; abortion, menorrhagia	Avoid all oils; ipecac emesis; support respiration; treat convulsions; maintain fluid balance; no specific antidote
Carbamates	Usually less intense than those for organophosphates	See management of organophosphates, except for pralidoxime (2-PAM)
Carbolic acid: see Phenols		
Carbon bisulfide: see Carbon disulfide		
Carbon dioxide	Dyspnea, weakness, tinnitus, palpitations	Respiratory support; O_2
Carbon disulfide Carbon bisulfide	Garlic-breath odor irritability, weakness, manic depression, narcosis, delirium, mydriasis, blindness, parkinsonism, convulsions, coma, paralysis, respiratory failure	Wash skin; emesis; gastric lavage; O_2; diazepam sedation; support respiration & circulation
Carbon monoxide Acetylene gas Automobile exhaust Carbonyl iron Coal gas Furnace gas Illuminating gas Marsh gas	Toxicity varies with length of exposure, concentration inhaled, respiratory & circulatory rates. Symptoms vary with % carboxyhemoglobin in blood. Headache, vertigo, dyspnea, confusion, dilated pupils, convulsions, coma	100% O_2 by mask; respiratory support if needed; obtain carboxyhemoglobin level immediately. *Avoid all stimulants.* Hyperbaric O_2 appears to be effective if carboxyhemoglobin is > approx. 25%; primary value may be at level of cytochrome
Carbon tetrachloride Cleaning fluids (nonflammable)	Nausea, vomiting, abdominal pain, headache, confusion, visual disturbances, CNS depression, ventricular fibrillation, renal injury, hepatic injury	Wash from skin; emesis or gastric lavage; give O_2; support respiration; monitor renal & hepatic function & treat appropriately. *Avoid alcohol, epinephrine, ephedrine*
Carbonates (ammonium, potassium, sodium): see Acids & alkalis		
Caustic soda: see Acids & alkalis		
Chloral hydrate Chloral amide	Drowsiness, confusion, shock, coma; respiratory depression; renal injury, hepatic injury	Ipecac emesis; gastric lavage; respiratory support; look for concomitant ingestions
Chlorates Bromates Nitrates Permanent wave neutralizers	Vomiting, nausea, diarrhea, cyanosis (methemoglobin), toxic nephritis, shock, convulsions, CNS depression, coma, jaundice	Ipecac emesis; gastric lavage; transfusion for severe cyanosis; *do not use methylene blue for chlorates or bromates.* Treat shock; O_2; consider dialysis for complex cases
Chlordane: see DDT		
Chlorinated lime: see Chlorine		

Poison	Symptoms	Treatment

Chlorine (see also Hypochlorites)
    Bromine
    Chlorinated lime
    Chlorine water
    Tear gas
	Inhalation: Severe respiratory & ocular irritation, glottal spasm, cough, choking, vomiting; pulmonary edema; cyanosis
	Ingestion: Irritation, corrosion of mouth & GI tract, possible ulceration or perforation; abdominal pain, tachycardia, prostration, circulatory collapse
		Inhalation: O_2; respiratory support; watch for & treat pulmonary edema
		Ingestion: Ipecac emesis; gastric lavage; treat shock

Chloroaniline; see Acetanilid		

Chloroform
    Ether
    Nitrous oxide
    Trichloromethane
	Drowsiness, coma; with nitrous oxide, delirium	Inhalation: Respiratory, cardiac, and circulatory support
		Ingestion: Ipecac emesis; gastric lavage; observe for renal and hepatic damage

Chlorophenothane: see DDT		
Chlorothion: see Organophosphates		
Chlorpromazine: see Phenothiazine		
Chromates: see Chromic acid		

Chromic acid
    Bichromates
    Chromates
    Chromium trioxide
	Corrosive due to oxidation. Ulcer and perforated nasal septum; severe gastroenteritis; shock, vertigo, coma; nephritis	Milk or water to dilute; BAL (or penicillamine) for severe symptoms; fluids & electrolytes, with caution, to support renal function

Chromium trioxide: see Chromic acid		
Cimetidine; ranitidine	Slight dryness & drowsiness; can alter metabolism of concomitant drugs	No specific antidotal treatment available: maintain a focus on metabolism of other drugs
Clonidine	Sedation; periodic apnea; hypotension	Emesis; lavage; supportive care; tolazoline IV & dopamine drip; naloxone 5 μg/kg up to 2–20 mg, repeated as necessary
Coal gas: see Carbon monoxide		
Cobaltous chloride: see Nitrogen oxides		
Cocaine	Stimulation, then depression; nausea & vomiting; loss of self-control, anxiety, hallucinations; sweating; respiratory difficulty progression to failure; cyanosis; circulatory failure; convulsions	Emetic early; charcoal or gastric lavage; if needed, IV propranolol, with extreme caution, for arrhythmias, diazepam for excitation; O_2 respiratory & circulatory support. Observe for myocardial or pulmonary disorder (usually occurs prior to emergency room arrival)
Codeine: see Narcotics		

Copper salts
    Cupric sulfate, acetate,
        subacetate
    Cuprous chloride, oxide
    Zinc salts
	Vomiting, burning sensation, metallic taste, diarrhea, pain, shock, jaundice, anuria, convulsions	Emesis; gastric lavage; penicillamine or BAL; electrolyte & fluid balance; respiratory support; monitor GI tract; treat shock, control convulsions; monitor for hepatic & renal failure

Corrosive sublimate: see Mercury		

Poison	Symptoms	Treatment
Creosote; cresols: see Phenols		

Cyanides
  Bitter almond oil
  Hydrocyanic acid
  Nitroprusside
  Potassium cyanide
  Prussic acid
  Sodium cyanide
  Wild cherry syrup
	Tachycardia, headache, drowsiness, hypotension, coma, convulsions, death; venous blood bright red; *very rapidly lethal* (1–15 min)	*Speed essential.* Remove from source if inhaled; immediate emesis or lavage, amyl nitrite inhalation, 0.2 mL (1 ampule) 30 sec of each min, 100% O$_2$, support respiration; 10 mL 3% sodium nitrite 2.5–5 mL/min IV (in child: 10 mg/kg) then 25–50 mL 25% sodium thiosulfate at 2.5–5 mL/min IV; repeat the above if symptoms recur. Use Lilly cyanide kit

DDD: see DDT		

DDT (chlorophenothane)
  Aldrin
  Bulan
  Chlordane
  Chlorinated organic
    insecticides
  DDD
  Dieldrin
  Dilan
  Endrin
  Heptachlor
  Methoxychlor
  Prolan
  Toxaphene
	Vomiting (early or delayed); paresthesias, malaise; coarse tremors, convulsions; pulmonary edema, ventricular fibrillation, respiratory failure	Emesis; gastric lavage if not convulsing, or charcoal; diazepam or phenobarbital to prevent & control tremors & convulsions; avoid epinephrine & sudden stimuli; parenteral fluids; monitor for renal & hepatic failure

Deodorizers, household: see Naphthalene; Paradichlorobenzene		
Depilatories: see Barium compounds		
Desipramine: see Tricyclic antidepressants		
Detergent powders: see Acids & alkalis		
Dextroamphetamine: see Amphetamines		
Diazinon: see Organophosphates		
Dicumarol: see Warfarin		
Dieldrin: see DDT		
Diethylene glycol: see Ethylene glycol		
Dilan: see DDT		
Dinitrobenzene: see Nitrobenzene		

Dinitro-o-cresol
  Herbicides
  Pesticides
	Fatigue, thirst, flushing; nausea, vomiting, abdominal pain; hyperpyrexia, tachycardia, loss of consciousness; dyspnea, respiratory arrest. Also absorbed through skin	Emesis; gastric lavage; fluid therapy; O$_2$; anticipate renal & hepatic toxicity; no specific antidote. Rinse skin with detergents

Diphenoxylate with atropine	Lethargy, nystagmus, pinpoint pupils, tachycardia, coma, respiratory depression (Note: toxicity may be delayed up to 12 h)	Ipecac emesis, gastric lavage; activated charcoal; naloxone; admit all children for observation if ingestion is verified
Dipterex: see Organophosphates		
Dishwasher detergents: see Acids & alkalis		
Diuretics, mercurial: see Mercury		

Poison	Symptoms	Treatment
Doxepin: see Tricyclic antidepressants		
Drain cleaners: see Acids & alkalis		
Endrin: see DDT		
Ergot derivatives	Thirst, diarrhea, vomiting, lightheadedness, burning feet; convulsions, hypotension, coma, abortion; gangrene of feet; cataract	Ipecac emesis; gastric lavage; benzodiazepine or short-acting barbiturate for convulsions; papaverine 60 mg IV, 1–2 mg/kg IV for children
Eserine: see Physostigmine		
Ethanol: see Alcohol, ethyl		
Ether: see Chloroform		
Ethyl alcohol: see Alcohol, ethyl		
Ethyl biscoumacetate: see Warfarin		
Ethylene glycol Diethylene glycol Permanent antifreeze	Eye contact: iridocyclitis Ingestion: Inebriation but no alcohol odor on breath; nausea, vomiting; carpopedal spasm, lumbar pain; oxalate crystalluria; oliguria progressing to anuria & acute renal failure; respiratory distress, convulsions, coma	Flush eyes Ingestion: Emesis; gastric lavage, support respiration, correct electrolyte imbalance (anion gap); give ethanol (see Alcohol, methyl); hemodialysis
Explosives: see Barium compounds (fireworks); Nitrogen oxides		
Ferric salts: see Iron		
Ferrous gluconate, ferrous sulfate: see Iron		
Fireworks: see Barium compounds		
Fluorides Ammonium fluoride Hydrofluoric acid Rat poisons Roach poisons Sodium fluoride Soluble fluorides generally	Inhalation: Intense eye, nasal irritation; headache; dyspnea, sense of suffocation, glottal edema, pulmonary edema, bronchitis, pneumonia; mediastinal & subcutaneous emphysema from bleb rupture Skin & mucosa: Superficial or deep burns Ingestion: Salty or soapy taste; in large doses; tremors, convulsions, CNS depression; shock; renal failure	Inhalation: O_2, respiratory support: prednisone for chemical pneumonitis (adults 30–80 mg/day in divided doses); manage pulmonary edema Skin: Copious flushing with cold water; debride white tissue; inject 10% calcium gluconate locally or intra-arterially & apply magnesium oxide paste Ingestion: Ipecac emesis; gastric lavage—leave aluminum hydroxide gel, calcium, or magnesium hydroxide or chloride in stomach; IV glucose & saline; 10% calcium gluconate, 10 mL IV (1 mL/kg in child); monitor for cardiac irritability; treat shock & dehydration

Poison	Symptoms	Treatment
Formaldehyde Formalin (Note: May contain methyl alcohol)	Inhalation: Irritation of eyes, nose, respiratory tract; laryngeal spasm & edema; dysphagia; bronchitis, pneumonia Skin: Irritation, coagulation necrosis; dermatitis, hypersensitivity Ingestion: Oral & gastric pain, nausea, vomiting, hematemesis, shock, hematuria, anuria, coma, respiratory failure	Inhalation: Flush eyes with saline: O_2; support respiration Skin: Wash copiously with soap & water Ingestion: Give water or milk to dilute; treat shock; correct acidosis with sodium bicarbonate; support respiration; observe for perforations

Fowler's solution: see Arsenic & antimony

Fuel, canned; see Alcohol, methyl

Fuel oil: see Petroleum distillates

Furnace gas: see Carbon monoxide

Gamma benzene hexachloride: see γ-Benzene hexachloride

Gas
  Acetylene, automobile exhaust, coal, furnace, illuminating, marsh: see Carbon monoxide
  Ammonia: see Ammonia gas
  Nerve: see Organophosphates
  Sewer, volatile hydrides: see Hydrogen sulfide
  Tear: see Chlorine

Gasoline: see Petroleum distillates

Glues, model airplane: see Acetone; Benzene; Petroleum distillates

Glutethimide	Drowsiness, areflexia, mydriasis, hypotension, respiratory depression, coma	Ipecac emesis; gastric lavage, activated charcoal; support respiration, maintain fluid & electrolyte balance; hemodialysis may help; treat shock

Guaiacol: see Phenols

Halogenated hydrocarbons: see DDT

H_2 blockers	Minor GI problems; may alter the concentration level of other drugs	Nonspecific supportive measures

Heptachlor: see DDT

Herbicides: see Arsenic & antimony; Dinitro-o-cresol

Heroin: see Narcotics

HETP (hexaethyl tetraphosphate): see Organophosphates

Hexachlorocyclohexane: see γ-Benzene hexachloride

Hormones—single acute oral overdose—no toxicity

Hydrides, volatile: see Hydrogen sulfide

Hydrocarbons: see Benzene

Hydrocarbons, halogenated: see DDT

Hydrochloric acid: see Acids & alkalis

Hydrocyanic acid: see Cyanides

Hydrogen chloride, fluoride: see Nitrogen oxides

Poison	Symptoms	Treatment
Hydrogen sulfide Alkali sulfides Phosphine Sewer gas Volatile hydrides	"Gas eye" (subacute keratoconjunctivitis), lacrimation & burning; cough, dyspnea, pulmonary edema; caustic skin burns, erythema, pain; profuse salivation, nausea, vomiting, diarrhea; confusion, vertigo; sudden collapse & unconsciousness	Give O_2, support respiration; amyl nitrite & sodium nitrite as for cyanide (*no thiosulfate*)

Hyoscine, hyoscyamine, hyoscyamus: see Belladonna

Hypochlorites Bleach, chlorine Javelle water	Usually mild pain & inflammation of oral & GI mucosa; cough, dyspnea, vomiting; skin vesicles	Usual 6% household preparations require little except milk dilution; treat shock; esophagoscopy only if concentrated forms have been ingested

Illuminating gas: see Carbon monoxide

Imipramine: see Tricyclic antidepressants

Indelible markers: see Acetanilid—usually no problem

Ink, aniline; see Acetanilid—usually no problem

Insecticides: see DDT; Organophosphates; Paradichlorobenzene; Pyrethrum

Iodine	Burning pain in mouth & esophagus; mucous membranes stained brown; laryngeal edema; vomiting, abdominal pain, diarrhea; shock, nephritis, circulatory collapse	Give milk, starch, or flour orally; gastric lavage; fluid & electrolytes; treat shock; tracheostomy for laryngeal edema
Iodoform Triiodomethane	Dermatitis; vomiting; cerebral depression, excitation; coma; respiratory difficulty	Skin: Wash with sodium bicarbonate or alcohol Ingestion: Emetic or gastric lavage; respiratory support

Iron
Carbonyl iron: see
  Carbon monoxide
Ferric salts
Ferrous salts
  Ferrous gluconate
  Ferrous sulfate
Vitamins with iron (Note: Children's chewables with iron are remarkably safe)
	Vomiting, upper abdominal pain, pallor, cyanosis, diarrhea, drowsiness, shock; concern if > 40–70 mg/kg of elemental iron ingested	Ipecac emesis, gastric lavage; if serum iron > 400–500 mg/dL at 3–6 h, give deferoxamine 1 gm IV (maximal rate of 15 mg/kg/h) or 1–2 gm IM q 3–12 h (urine turns red within 2 h; if no color change, no further dose is needed); for shock, give deferoxamine 1 gm IV (maximal rate 15 mg/kg/h); exchange transfusion

Isoniazid (INH)	CNS stimulation, seizures, obtundation, coma	Emesis; lavage; diazepam sedation; pyridoxine (mg for mg INH ingested) up to 200 mg slowly IV for seizures, repeat prn; $NaHCO_3$ for acidosis

Isopropyl alcohol: see Alcohol, isopropyl

Javelle water: see Hypochlorites

Kerosene: see Petroleum distillates

Ketones: see Acetone

Poison	Symptoms	Treatment
Lead Lead salts Solder Some paints & painted surfaces	Acute inhalation: Insomnia, headache, ataxia, mania, convulsions Acute ingestion: Thirst, burning abdominal pain, vomiting, diarrhea, CNS symptoms as above	Combine treatment with BAL and CaEDTA; D-penicillamine (PCA) also used
Lead, tetraethyl	Vapor inhalation, skin absorption, ingestion: CNS symptoms—insomnia, restlessness, ataxia, delusions, mania, convulsions	Supportive treatment; eg, diazepam, chlorpromazine, fluid & electrolytes; eliminate the source
Lime, chlorinated: see Chlorine		
Lindane: see γ-Benzene hexachloride		
Liquor: see Alcohol, ethyl		
Lithium salts	Nausea, vomiting, diarrhea, tremors, drowsiness, renal failure, diabetes insipidus	Acute: Emesis; diazepam—consider dialysis Chronic: Reduce dose; supportive therapy
Lye: see Acids & alkalis		
Lysergic acid diethylamide (LSD)	Confusion, hallucinations, hyperexcitability—coma. Flashbacks	Supportive therapy; diazepam; chlorpromazine (50–100 mg IM in adults)
Malathion: see Organophosphates		
Marsh gas: see Carbon monoxide		
Meperidine: see Narcotics		
Meprobamate: see Barbiturates		
Mercurial diuretics: see Mercury		
Mercuric chloride: see Mercury		
Mercury All mercury compounds Ammoniated mercury Bichloride of mercury Calomel Corrosive sublimate Diuretics Mercuric chloride Mercury vapor Merthiolate	Acute: Severe gastroenteritis, burning mouth pain, salivation, abdominal pain, vomiting; colitis, nephrosis, anuria, uremia. Skin burns from alkyl & phenyl mercurials Chronic: Gingivitis, mental disturbance, neurologic deficits Mercury vapor: severe pneumonitis	Gastric lavage, activated charcoal; give penicillamine (or BAL). Chelation therapy; maintain fluid & electrolyte balance; hemodialysis for renal failure; observe for GI perforation Skin: Scrub with soap & water Lungs: Supportive care
Merthiolate: see Mercury—usually no problem		
Metaldehyde	Nausea, vomiting, retching, abdominal pain, muscular rigidity, hyperventilation, convulsions, coma	Emesis, if not spontaneous; supportive therapy; diazepam
Methadone: see Narcotics		
Methamphetamine: see Amphetamines		
Methanol: see Alcohol, methyl		
Methoxychlor: see DDT		
Methyl alcohol: see Alcohol, methyl		

Poison	Symptoms	Treatment
Mineral spirits: see Petroleum distillates		
Model airplane glues, solvents: see Acetone; Benzene; Petroleum distillates		
Morphine: see Narcotics		
Moth balls, crystals, repellent: see Naphthalene; Paradichlorobenzene		
Nail polish remover: see Acetone		
Naphtha: see Petroleum distillates		

Naphthalene (see also Paradichlorobenzene)
  Deodorizer cakes
  Moth balls, crystals, repellent cakes
	Contact: dermatitis, corneal ulceration
	Inhalation: Headache, confusion, vomiting, dyspnea
	Ingestion: Abdominal cramps, nausea, vomiting; headache, confusion; dysuria; intravascular hemolysis; convulsions. Hemolytic anemia in persons with G6PD deficiency
		Contact: Remove clothing if formerly stored with naphthalene moth balls; flush skin and eyes
		Ingestion: Ipecac emesis, gastric lavage; blood transfusion for severe hemolysis; alkalize urine for hemoglobinuria; control convulsions

Naphthols: see Phenols		

Narcotics
  Alphaprodine
  Codeine
  Heroin
  Meperidine
  Methadone
  Morphine
  Opium
  Propoxyphene
	Pinpoint pupils, drowsiness, shallow respirations, spasticity, respiratory failure	Do not give emetics. Gastric lavage, charcoal, respiratory support. Naloxone 5 μg/kg IV to awaken & improve respiration; if patient does not respond, give 2–20 mg naloxone (dosage may need to be repeated as often as 10–20 times); fluids IV to support circulation

Neostigmine: see Physostigmine		
Nerve gas agents: see Organophosphates		
Nicotine: see Tobacco		
Nitrates: see Chlorates		
Nitric acid: see Acids & alkalis		

Nitrites
  Amyl nitrite
  Butyl nitrite
  Nitroglycerin
  Potassium nitrite
  Sodium nitrite
	Methemoglobinemia, cyanosis, anoxia, GI disturbance, vomiting, headache, dizziness, hypotension, respiratory failure, coma	Ipecac emesis, gastric lavage; O$_2$; for methemoglobinemia, 1% methylene blue 1–2 mg/kg slowly IV; when > 40% methemoglobin, transfusion with whole blood

Nitrobenzene
  Artificial bitter almond oil
  Dinitrobenzene
	Bitter almond odor (suggests cyanides), drowsiness, headache, vomiting, ataxia, nystagmus, brown urine, convulsive movements, delirium, cyanosis, coma, respiratory arrest	See Acetanilid

Poison	Symptoms	Treatment
Nitrogen oxides (see also Chlorine, Hydrogen sulfide, and Sulfur dioxide)		

Air contaminants that form atmospheric oxidants; liberated from missile fuels, explosives, agricultural wastes
  Cobaltous chloride
  Fluorine
  Hydrogen chloride
  Hydrogen fluoride
	Delayed onset of symptoms with nitrogen oxides unless heavy concentration; other irritant gases give warnings—local burning in eye, nasal, pharyngeal mucous membranes. Fatigue, cough, dyspnea, pulmonary edema; later, bronchitis, pneumonia	Bed rest; O_2 as soon as symptoms develop; for excessive pulmonary foam: suction, postural drainage, tracheostomy; to prevent pulmonary fibrosis: prednisone 30–80 mg/day (adults) and dexamethasone 1 mg/m² BSA (children) have been used

Nitroglycerine: see Nitrites		
Nitrous oxide: see Chloroform		
Nortriptyline: see Tricyclic antidepressants		

Oils
  Aniline: see Acetanilid
  Fuel, lubricating: see Petroleum distillates		

OMPA (octamethyl pyrophosphoramide): see Organophosphates		
Opiates: see Narcotics		

Organophosphates
  Chlorothion
  Demeton
  Diazinon
  Dipterex (trichlorfon)
  HETP (hexaethyl tetraphosphate)
  Malathion
  Nerve gas agents
  OMPA (octamethyl pyrophosphoramide)
  Parathion
  Systox
  TEPP (tetraethyl pyrophosphate)
	Nausea, vomiting, abdominal cramping, excessive salivation; increased pulmonary secretion, headache, rhinorrhea, blurred vision, miosis; slurred speech, mental confusion; breathing difficulty, frothing at mouth, coma. Absorbed through skin, via inhalation, or orally	Remove clothing, flush & wash skin. Empty stomach; atropine: adults 2 mg, children 0.01 mg/kg IV or IM q 15–60 min, if no signs of atropine toxicity, repeat as needed; pralidoxime chloride (PAM): adults 1–2 gm, children 20–40 mg/kg, IV over 15–30 min, repeat in 1 h if needed; O_2; support respiration; correct dehydration. *Do not use morphine or aminophylline.* Attendant should avoid self-contamination

Oxalates: see Oxalic acid		

Oxalic acid
  Ethylene glycol
  Oxalates
	Burning pain in throat, vomiting, intensive pain; hypotension, tetany, shock; glottal & renal damage; oxaluria	Give milk or calcium lactate; careful gastric lavage if at all; 10% calcium gluconate 10–20 mL IV; pain control, saline IV for shock; demulcents by mouth; watch for glottal edema & stricture

Paint solvents: see Mineral spirits (under Petroleum distillates): Turpentine		
Paints: see Lead		

Paradichlorobenzene
  Insecticide
  Moth repellent
  Toilet bowl deodorant
	Abdominal pain, nausea, vomiting, diarrhea, seizures, tetany	Ipecac emesis, gastric lavage; fluid replacement; diazepam for seizure control

Paraldehyde	Paraldehyde odor on breath, incoherent, pupils contracted, respirations depressed, coma	Ingestion: Ipecac emesis, gastric lavage; support respiration, O_2
Paraquat	Immediate: GI pain and vomiting; within 24 h: respiratory failure	Emesis, fuller's earth plus Na_2SO_4; limit O_2; call poison center or manufacturer
Parathion: see Organophosphates		
Paris green: see Arsenic & antimony		

Poison	Symptoms	Treatment
Pentobarbital: see Barbiturates		
Permanent wave neutralizers (bromates): see Chlorates		
Pesticides: see Arsenic & antimony; Barium compounds; DDT; Dinitro-*o*-cresol; Fluorides; Organophosphates; Paradichlorobenzene; Phosphorus; Pyrethrum; Thallium salts; Warfarin		
Petroleum distillates Asphalt Benzine (benzin) Fuel oil Gasoline Kerosene Lubricating oils Mineral spirits Model airplane glue Naphtha Petroleum ether Tar	Vapor inhalation: Euphoria; burning in chest; headache, nausea, weakness; CNS depression, confusion; dyspnea, tachypnea, rales Ingestion: burning throat & stomach, vomiting, diarrhea; pneumonia, only if aspiration has occurred Aspiration: Early acute pulmonary changes	Since major problems are consequential to aspiration, as opposed to GI absorption, in most instances no gastric evacuation is warranted; gastric lavage only with rapid-onset depression from large amounts ingested; arterial blood gas levels to monitor care; supportive care for pulmonary edema; O_2, respiratory support
Petroleum ether: see Petroleum distillates		
Phenacetin: see Acetanilid		
Phencyclidine (PCP)	"Spaced-out" unconscious; hypertension	Quiet environment; prolonged gastric lavage; propanolol & diazepam
Phenmetrazine: see Amphetamines		
Phenobarbital: see Barbiturates		
Phenols Carbolic acid Creosote Cresols Guaiacol Naphthols	Corrosive. Mucous membrane burns; pallor, weakness, shock; convulsions in children; pulmonary edema; smoky urine; respiratory, cardiac, & circulatory failure	Remove clothing, wash external burns. Lavage with water, activated charcoal. *Do not use alcohol or mineral oil.* Demulcents; pain relief; O_2; support respiration; correct fluid imbalance; watch for esophageal stricture (rare)
Phenothiazine Chlorpromazine Prochlorperazine Promazine Trifluoperazine (etc)	Extrapyramidal tract symptoms (ataxia, muscular & carpopedal spasms, torticollis), usually idiosyncratic; overdose results in dry mouth, drowsiness, coma, hypothermia, respiratory collapse. Leukopenia, jaundice, coagulation defect, skin rashes	Ipecac emesis, charcoal, or gastric lavage; diphenhydramine 2–3 mg/kg IV or IM for extrapyramidal symptoms; diazepam for convulsions; warm patient. Avoid levarterenol & epinephrine; dialysis is of no benefit
Phenylpropanolamine	Nervousness, irritability, *hypertension* plus other sympathomimetic effects	Supportive therapy; diazepam; treat hypertension with phentolamine (Regitine 5 mg) or nitroprussides
Phosphoric acid: see Acids & alkalis		

Poison	Symptoms	Treatment
Phosphorus (yellow or white) Rat poisons Roach powders (Note: Red phosphorus is unabsorbable & nontoxic)	3 Stages of symptoms: 1st—Garlicky taste; garlic odor on breath; local irritation, skin & throat burns, nausea, vomiting, diarrhea 2nd—Symptom-free 8 h to several days 3rd—Nausea, vomiting, diarrhea, liver enlargement, jaundice, hemorrhages, renal damage, convulsions, coma Toxicity enhanced by alcohol, fats, digestible oils	Protect patient & attendant from vomitus, gastric washing, feces. If phosphorus is imbedded in skin, keep patient's body submerged in water. Gastric lavage copiously—some still recommend potassium permanganate (1:5000) or cupric sulfate (250 mg in 250 mL water); mineral oil 100 mL (to prevent absorption) & repeat in 2 h; combat shock; vitamin K_1 IV; transfusion with fresh blood
Physostigmine Eserine Neostigmine (Prostigmin) Pilocarpine Pilocarpus	Dizziness, weakness, vomiting, cramping pain; pupils dilated, then contracted	Atropine sulfate 0.6 to 1 mg (adults), 0.01 mg/kg (children) s.c. or IV with repeat doses prn. (Caution: *Using physostigmine to counter anticholinergics is associated with a 15% seizure rate*)
Pilocarpine, pilocarpus: see Physostigmine		
Potash: see Acids & alkalis		
Potassium bichromate, potassium chromate: see Chromic acid		
Potassium carbonate: see Acids & alkalis		
Potassium cyanide: see Cyanides		
Potassium hydroxide: see Acids & alkalis		
Potassium nitrate: see Chlorates		
Potassium nitrite: see Nitrites		
Potassium permanganate	Brown discoloration & burns of oral mucosa, glottal edema; hypotension; renal involvement	Gastric lavage, demulcents; maintain fluid balance
Prochlorperazine: see Phenothiazine		
Prolan: see DDT		
Promazine: see Phenothiazine		
Propoxyphene: see Narcotics		
Propranolol	Confusion and seizures	Emesis; lavage; supportive care; diazepam sedation; pacemakers and glucagon (0.05 mg/kg stat plus 2–5 mg/h) have been effective
Prostigmin: see Physostigmine		
Protriptyline: see Tricyclic antidepressants		
Prussic acid: see Cyanides		
Pyrethrum Pyrethrin	Allergic response (including anaphylactic reactions, skin sensitivity) in sensitive people. Otherwise low toxicity, unless vehicle is a petroleum distillate (see that entry)	For sizable ingestion, emesis if patient is alert; otherwise, endotracheal tube & gastric lavage; wash skin well

Poison	Symptoms	Treatment
Rat poison: see Barium compounds; Fluorides; Phosphorus; Thallium salts; Warfarin		
Resorcinol (resorcin)	Vomiting, dizziness, tinnitus, chills, tremor, delirium, convulsions, respiratory depression, coma	Emetic or gastric lavage; support respiration
Roach poison: see Fluorides; Phosphorus; Thallium salts		
Rodenticides (rat poison): see Barium compounds; Fluorides; Phosphorus; Thallium salts; Warfarin		
Rubbing alcohol: see Alcohol, isopropyl		
Scopolamine: see Belladonna		
Secobarbital: see Barbiturates		
Sewer gas: see Hydrogen sulfide		

Silver salts
  Silver nitrate
  (Note: Chloride, bromide, iodide, & oxide salts are usually benign)
	Stain on lips (white, brown, then black); gastroenteritis, shock, vertigo, convulsions	Gastric lavage with saline (0.9% sodium chloride) solution; control pain; control convulsions with diazepam

Smog: see Sulfur dioxide		
Soda, caustic: see Acids & alkalis		
Sodium carbonate: see Acids & alkalis		
Sodium cyanide: see Cyanides		
Sodium fluoride: see Fluorides		
Sodium hydroxide: see Acids & alkalis		
Sodium nitrite: see Nitrites		
Solder: see Cadmium; Lead		
Stibophen: see Arsenic & antimony		
Stramonium: see Belladonna		
Strychnine	Restlessness, hyperacuity of hearing, vision, etc; convulsions from minor stimuli, complete muscle relaxation between convulsions, perspiration; respiratory arrest	Isolate & restrict stimulation to prevent convulsions. Activated charcoal orally; control convulsions with IV diazepam, curariform drugs; support respiration; acid diuresis with ammonium chloride or ascorbic acid; gastric lavage *after* convulsions are controlled
Sulfur dioxide Smog	Respiratory tract irritation; sneezing, cough, dyspnea, pulmonary edema	Remove from contaminated area, give O_2; positive pressure breathing, respiratory support
Sulfuric acid: see Acids & alkalis		
Syrup of wild cherry: see Cyanides		
Systox: see Organophosphates		
Tar: see Petroleum distillates		
Tartar emetic: see Arsenic & antimony		
Tear gas: see Chlorine		
TEPP: see Organophosphates		
Tetraethyl lead: see Lead, tetraethyl		

Poison	Symptoms	Treatment
Thallium salts (formerly used in: Ant poison Rat poison Roach poison)	Abdominal pain (colic), vomiting (may be bloody), diarrhea (may be bloody), stomatitis, excessive salivation; tremors, leg pains, paresthesias, polyneuritis, ocular & facial palsy; delirium, convulsions, respiratory failure; loss of hair about 3 wk after poisoning	Ipecac emesis, gastric lavage; treat shock, control convulsions with diazepam; chelation therapy is still experimental. Contact local poison center for latest information.

Theophylline: see Aminophylline

Thyroxine	Most are asymptomatic; rarely, increasing irritability progressing to thyroid storm in 5–7 days	Emesis; observation at home; diazepam; consider antithyroid preparations and propranolol *only* if actual symptoms occur
Tobacco Nicotine	Excitement, confusion, muscular twitching, weakness, abdominal cramps, clonic convulsions, depression, rapid respirations, palpitations, collapse, coma, CNS paralysis, respiratory failure	Ipecac emesis, gastric lavage; activated charcoal; support respiration, O_2; diazepam for convulsions; wash skin well if contaminated

Toilet bowl cleaners, deodorizers; see Acids & alkalis; Paradichlorobenzene

Toluene, toluol; see Benzene

Toxaphene: see DDT

Trichlorfon: see Organophosphates

Trichloromethane: see Chloroform

Tricyclic antidepressants Amitriptyline Desipramine Doxepin Imipramine Nortriptyline Protriptyline	Anticholinergic effects (eg, blurred vision, urinary hesitation); CNS effects (eg, drowsiness, stupor, coma, ataxia, restlessness, agitation, hyperactive reflexes, muscle rigidity, & convulsions); CVS effects (tachycardia & other arrhythmias, bundle branch block, impaired conduction, congestive heart failure). Respiratory depression, hypotension, shock, vomiting, hyperpyrexia, mydriasis, & diaphoresis may also be present	Symptomatic & supportive; emesis (avoid emesis if seizures are imminent), charcoal, gastric lavage; monitor vital signs & ECG; maintain airway & fluid intake. Sodium bicarbonate as a rapid IV injection (0.5–2 mEq/L), repeat periodically to maintain blood pH $>$ 7.45, precludes development of arrhythmias. Diazepam controls most CNS problems; only if symptoms persist should physostigmine salicylate (slowly IV) be used to reverse both CNS and cardiac manifestations of overdosage— adults: 2 mg with repeat of 1–4 mg prn at 20- to 60-min intervals; children: 0.5 mg repeated prn at 5-min intervals to maximum 2 mg

Trifluoperazine: see Phenothiazine

Triiodomethane: see Iodoform

Turpentine Paint solvent Varnish	Turpentine odor; burning oral & abdominal pain, coughing, choking, respiratory failure; nephritis	Emesis (alert patient) if $>$ 1–4 oz; gastric lavage; support respiration; O_2; control pain; monitor renal function

Varnish: see Alcohol, methyl; Turpentine

Poison	Symptoms	Treatment
Verapamil; nifedipine; diltiazem	Nausea, vomiting, mental confusion, bradycardia, hypotension	Emesis; atropine has reversed bradycardia; avoid β-agonists
Vitamins—single acute oral ingestion of isolated or multiple dose form—no toxicity		
Warfarin Bishydroxycoumarin Dicumarol Ethyl biscoumacetate Superwarfarins	Single ingestion not serious, multiple overdoses result in coagulopathy; even with "super" drugs, most are uneventful	For hemorrhagic manifestations, vitamin K_1 till prothrombin time is normal, transfusion with fresh blood if necessary
Wax, floor: see Carbon tetrachloride		
Whiskey: see Alcohol, ethyl		
Wild cherry syrup: see Cyanides		
Wood alcohol: see Alcohol, methyl		
Xylene: see Benzene		
Zinc salts: see Copper salts		

Adapted from *The Merck Manual of Diagnosis and Therapy,* ed 16, R Berkow, editor, p 2686. Merck & Co, Rahway, N J, 1992. Used with permission.

Drugs and Classes of Drugs Used in the Treatment of Major Psychiatric Disorders

Aggression (see Episodic dyscontrol disorder)
Akathisia (see Drug-induced extrapyramidal movement disorders)
Alcohol-related disorders
    β-Adrenergic receptor antagonists
    Benzodiazepines
    Carbamazepine
    Lithium
Anorexia nervosa (see Eating disorders)
Anxiety (also see specific anxiety disorder)
    Antihistamines
    Barbiturates and other similarly acting drugs
    Benzodiazepines
Bipolar disorder
    Benzodiazepines (especially clonazepam)
    Calcium channel inhibitors
    Carbamazepine
    Dopamine receptor antagonists
    Lithium
    L-Tryptophan
    Valproic acid
Bulimia nervosa (see Eating disorders)
Cyclothymia (see Bipolar disorder)
Delusional disorder (see Schizophrenia)
Depressive disorder
    Benzodiazepines (especially alprazolam)
    Bupropion
    Carbamazepine
    Lithium
    Monoamine oxidase inhibitors
    Serotonin-specific reuptake inhibitors
    Sympathomimetics
    Thyroid hormones
    Trazodone
    Tricyclic and tetracyclic antidepressants
    L-Tryptophan
Drug-induced extrapyramidal movement disorders
    β-Adrenergic receptor antagonists
    Amantadine
    Anticholinergics
    Antihistamines
    Benzodiazepines
Dysthymia (see Depressive disorder)
Dystonias (see Drug-induced extrapyramidal movement disorders)
Eating disorders
    Lithium
    Monoamine oxidase inhibitors
    Serotonin-specific reuptake inhibitors
    Tricyclic and tetracyclic antidepressants
Episodic dyscontrol disorder
    β-Adrenergic receptor antagonists
    Buspirone
    Carbamazepine
    Dopamine receptor antagonists
    Lithium
    Valproic acid
Generalized anxiety disorder
    β-Adrenergic receptor antagonists
    Barbiturates and other similarly acting drugs

Benzodiazepines
Buspirone
Serotonin-specific reuptake inhibitors
Tricyclic and tetracyclic antidepressants
Obsessive-compulsive disorder
   Serotonin-specific reuptake inhibitors
   Tricyclic and tetracyclic antidepressants (especially clomipramine)
Opioid-related disorders
   Clonidine
   Methadone
Panic disorder (with and without agoraphobia)
   β-Adrenergic receptor antagonists
   Benzodiazepines (especially alprazolam and clonazepam)
   Monoamine oxidase inhibitors
   Serotonin-specific reuptake inhibitors
   Tricyclic and tetracyclic antidepressants
Parkinsonism (see Drug-induced extrapyramidal movement disorders)
Phobias (see also Panic disorder)
   β-Adrenergic receptor antagonists
   Benzodiazepines
Posttraumatic stress disorder
   Monoamine oxidase inhibitors
   Serotonin-specific reuptake inhibitors
   Tricyclic and tetracyclic antidepressants
Psychosis (see Schizophrenia)
Rabbit syndrome (see Drug-induced extrapyramidal movement disorders)
Schizoaffective disorder (see Depressive disorder, Bipolar disorder, and Schizophrenia)
Schizophrenia
   Benzodiazepines
   Carbamazepine
   Clozapine
   Dopamine receptor antagonists
   Lithium
Sleep disorders
   Antihistamines
   Barbiturates and other similarly acting drugs
   Benzodiazepines
   Chloral hydrate
   Sympathomimetics
   L-Tryptophan
Violence (see Episodic dyscontrol disorder)

References

Abrams R C, Alexopoulos G S: Substance abuse in the elderly: Alcohol and prescription drugs. Hosp Community Psychiatry *38:* 1288, 1987.

Anderson A A, Ghali A Y, Bansil R K: Weapon carrying among patients in a psychiatric emergency room. Hosp Community Psychiatry *40:* 845, 1989.

Barraclough B, Bunch J, Nelson B S: A hundred cases of suicide: Clinical aspects. Br J Psychiatry *125:* 355, 1974.

Bassu K E C, Minden S, Apster R: Geriatric emergencies: Psychiatric or medical. Am J Psychiatry *140:* 539. 1983.

Beck J C, White K A, Gage B: Emergency psychiatric assessment of violence. Am J Psychiatry *148:* 1562, 1991.

Beckett A, Summergrad P, Manschreck T: Symptomatic HIV infection of the CNS in a patient without evidence of immune deficiency. Am J Psychiatry *144:* 1242. 1987.

Bengelsdorf H, Alden D C: A mobile crisis unit in the psychiatric emergency room. Hosp Community Psychiatry *38:* 662, 1987.

Beskow J: Suicide and mental disorders in Swedish men. Acta Psychiatr Scand Suppl *277:* 5, 1979.

Blank C A, Mascitti-Mazur J E: Violence in Philadelphia emergency departments reflects national trends. J Emerg Nurs *17:* 318, 1991.

Boyer W F, Bakalar N H, Lake C R: Anticholingergic prophylaxis of acute haloperidol-induced acute dystonic reactions. J Clin Psychopharmacol *7:* 264, 1987.

Brizer D A: Psychopharmacology and the management of violent patients. Psychiatr Clin North Am *11:* 551, 1988.

Dorpat T, Ripley H: A study of suicide in the Seattle area. Compr Psychiatry *1:* 349, 1960.

Dubin W R: Evaluating and managing the violent patient. Ann Emerg Med *10:* 481, 1981.

Ellison J M, Blum N R, Barsky A J: Frequent repeaters in a psychiatric emergency service. Hosp Community Psychiatry *40:* 958, 1989.

Ellison J M, Hughes D H, White K A: An emergency psychiatry update. Hosp Community Psychiatry *40:* 250, 1989.

Ellison J M, Jacobs D: Emergency psychopharmacology: A review and update. Ann Emerg Med *15:* 962, 1986.

Epstein L G, Shearer L R, Goudsmit L: Neurological and neuropathological features of human immunodeficiency virus in children. Ann Neurol *23:* 19, 1988.

Faulstick M E: Psychiatric aspects of AIDS. Am J Psychiatry *144:* 551, 1987.

Fauman B J: Psychiatric residency training in the consideration of alternatives to hospitalization. Psychiatr Clin North Am *8:* 609, 1985.

Fauman M A, Fauman B J: The differential diagnosis of organic based psychiatric disturbance in the emergency department. JACEP *6:* 315, 1977.

Fisher W H, Geller J L, Altaffer F, Bennett M B: The relationship between community resources and state hospital recidivism. Am J Psychiatry *149:* 385, 1992.

Frommer D A, Kulig K W, Mark J A, Rumack B: Tricyclic antidepressant overdose: A review. JAMA *257:* 521, 1987.

Geller J L: "Anyplace but the state hospital." Hosp Community Psychiatry *42:* 145, 1991.

Johnson M C: Alcohol, street drugs and prescribed psychoactive medications: Seeking clarity in a "witches brew." Consult *1:* 2, 1987.

Marson D C, McGovern M P, Pomp H C: Psychiatric decision making in the emergency room: A research overview. Am J Psychiatry *145:* 918, 1988.

Morgan S L: Families' experiences in psychiatric emergencies. Hosp Community Psychiatry *40:* 1265, 1989.

Murphy G, Wetzel R: The lifetime risk of suicide in alcoholism. Arch Gen Psychiatry *47:* 383, 1990.

Murphy G E: On suicide prediction and prevention. Arch Gen Psychiatry *40:* 343, 1983.

Nicholi A M: The nontherapeutic use of psychoactive drugs. N Engl J Med *108:* 925, 1983.

Olfson M: Psychiatric emergency room dispositions of HMO enrollees. Hosp Community Psychiatry *40:* 639, 1989.

Perry S W, Markowitz J: Psychiatric interventions for AIDS: Spectrum disorders. Hosp Community Psychiatry *37:* 1001, 1986.

Puryear D A, Lovitt R, Miller D A: Characteristics of elderly persons seen in an urban psychiatric emergency room. Hosp Community Psychiatry *42:* 802, 1991.

Robins E, Murphy G, Wilkinson R: Some clinical considerations in the prevention of suicide based on a study of 134 successful suicides. Am J Public Health *49:* 888, 1959.

Roy A: Family history of suicide. Arch Gen Psychiatry *40:* 971, 1983.

Roy A: Risk factors for suicide in psychiatric patients. Arch Gen Psychiatry *39:* 1089, 1982.

Roy A: Self-destructive behavior. Psychiatr Clin North Am *8:* 215, 1985.

Roy A: Suicide in chronic schizophrenia. Br J Psychiatry *141:* 171, 1982.

Roy A, DeJong J, Linnoila M: Cerebrospinal fluid monoamine metabolites and suicidal behavior in depressed patients: A five-year follow-up study. Arch Gen Psychiatry *46:* 609, 1989.

Roy A, Linnoila M: Alcoholism and suicide. Suicide Life Threat Behav *16:* 244, 1986.

Roy A, Segal N, Centerwall B, Robinette D: Suicide in twins. Arch Gen Psychiatry *48:* 29, 1991.

Sanguineti V R, Brooks M O: Factors related to emergency commitment of chronically mentally ill patients who are substance abusers. Hosp Community Psychiatry *43:* 237, 1992.

Saxena K: Glue sniffing and other deliriants. Top Emerg Med *7:* 55, 1985.

Shaffer D: The epidemiology of teen suicide: An examination of risk factors. J Clin Psychiatry *49:* 36, 1988.

Slaby A E: Emergency psychiatry: An update. Hosp Community Psychiatry *32:* 687, 1981.

Slaby A E: Emergency psychiatry in the general hospital: Staffing, training, and leadership issues. Gen Hosp Psychiatry *3:* 306, 1981.

Solomon P, Gordon B: Outpatient compliance of psychiatric emergency room patients by presenting problems. Psychiatr Q *59:* 271, 1988.

Stelzer J, Elliot C A: A continuous-care model of crisis intervention for children and adolescents. Hosp Community Psychiatry *41:* 562, 1990.

Stewart J T, Myers W C, Burket R C, Lyles W B: A review of pharmacotherapy of aggression in children and adolescents. J Am Acad Child Adolesc Psychiatry *29:* 269, 1990.

Szuster R R, Schanbacher B L, McCann S C: Characteristics of psychiatric emergency room patients with alcohol- or drug-induced disorders. Hosp Community Psychiatry *41:* 1342, 1990.

Tancredi L R: Emergency psychiatry and crisis intervention: Some legal and ethical issues. Psychiatr Ann *12:* 799, 1982.

Theinhaus O J, Rowe C, Woellert P, Hillard J R: Geropsychiatric emergency services: Utilization and outcome predictors. Hosp Community Psychiatry *41:* 1301, 1988.

Waller F S: Hospital and room security: The next decade. J Health Prot Manage *7:* 43, 1991.

Waxman H M, Dubin W, Klein M, Weiss K J, Carner E A: Geriatric psychiatry in the emergency department: Evaluation and treatment of geriatric and nongeriatric admissions. J Am Geriatr Soc *32:* 343, 1984.

Weissberg M: Chained in the emergency department: The new asylum for the poor. Hosp Community Psychiatry *42:* 317, 1991.

Index

Note: Page number followed by t indicates table; page number followed by f indicates figure.

for exacerbation of chronic schizophrenia, 157–158
for grandiosity, 210
for group hysteria, 215
for hallucinations, 217
for hallucinogen hallucinosis, 220
in head trauma patients, 225
for homosexual panic, 229
for hyperventilation, 238–239
for hypochondriasis, 241
for illusions, 244
for impending death of psychogenic origin, 246
for insomnia, 257–258
    with dementia, 182
    with depression, 186
    with grief/bereavement, 213
for intermittent explosive disorder, 259–260
for intoxication, 261
intramuscular, 8
for Korsakoff's syndrome, 264
lethal dose of, 129
and leukopenia/agranulocytosis, 265
for mania, 271–272
for mutism, 278
for nutmeg intoxication, 285
for obsessive-compulsive disorder, 286–287
for panic attacks, 88
for panic disorder, 276, 299
pharmacology of, 123t–124t
for phencyclidine intoxication, 307
for phenylpropanolamine toxicity, 308
for phobias, 310
for posttraumatic stress disorder, 317
for psychogenic blindness, 135
for psychogenic urinary retention, 369
for psychotic symptoms associated with depression, 186
for psychotropic drug withdrawal, 320
for rape victim, 323
for restraint, 325–326
safety of, 128
for schizoaffective disorder, 328
for sedation of abused spouse, 74
for self-mutilation, 338
side effects of, 86, 137, 260, 272, 372
for suicide prevention, 349–350
for syncope, 354
for tension headaches, 223
for terminally ill patient, 360
therapeutic index, 128–129
toxicity
    signs of, 220, 307, 383
    treatment of, 383
for violent patient, 372
for Wernicke's encephalopathy, 376–377
withdrawal, 320, 321t
    treatment of, 320
    tremor caused by, 366–367
Benzol, toxicity, symptoms and treatment, 382
Benztropine
    abuse, in schizophrenic patients, 157
    dosage and administration
        for agitation, 86

for akathisia, 90
for akinesia, 91
for antipsychotic-induced pseudoparkinsonism, 367
for antipsychotic side effects, 157
for arrhythmias caused by psychotropic drug withdrawal, 321
for catatonia, 154
for dystonia, 201
    and parkinsonism, 199
for laryngeal dystonia, 201
for parkinsonism, 303, 304t
for perioral (rabbit) tremor, 305
prophylactic use of, for antipsychotic-induced dystonia, 201
Bereavement. *See* Grief/bereavement
Berocca C, dosage and administration, for alcohol withdrawal, 103t
Bestiality, 343
Bethanechol, dosage and administration, for anticholinergic-induced urinary retention, 369
BHC, toxicity, symptoms and treatment, 382
Bichloride of mercury, toxicity, symptoms and treatment, 390
Bichromates, toxicity, symptoms and treatment, 385
Biperidin, 304t
Bipolar disorder
    depression in, 184, 186
    drugs used in treatment of, 401
    lifetime prevalence of, 270
    mania in, 270
    postpartum psychosis in, 313–314
Bishydroxycoumarin, toxicity, symptoms and treatment, 397
Bismuth compounds, toxicity, symptoms and treatment, 383
Bitter almond oil, toxicity, symptoms and treatment, 386, 391
Blackouts, 133–134
    in barbiturate intoxication, 128
    clinical features and diagnosis of, 133
    definition of, 133
    drug treatment for, 133
    evaluation and management of, 133
    interviewing and psychotherapeutic guidelines for, 133
Bleach, chlorine, toxicity, symptoms and treatment, 389
Blindness
    hysterical, 135
    organic conditions causing, 135
    psychogenic, 134–135
        clinical features and diagnosis of, 134
        drug treatment for, 135
        evaluation and management of, 135
        interviewing and psychotherapeutic guidelines for, 134
β-Blocker(s)
    for akathisia, 90, 157, 199
    for amphetamine intoxication, 109
    for anxiety disorders, 125
    for claustrophobia, 159
    for cocaine-induced tachycardia/hypertension, 162